NATURAL HEALTH
SECRETS
FROM AROUND
THE WORLD

NATURAL HEALTH SECRETS FROM AROUND THE WORLD

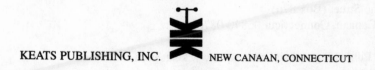

Edited by Glenn W. Geelhoed, M.D.
and Jean Barilla, M.S.

KEATS PUBLISHING, INC.   NEW CANAAN, CONNECTICUT

Natural Health Secrets From Around the World is intended solely for informational and educational purposes, and not as medical advice. Please consult a medical or health professional if you have questions about your health.

NATURAL HEALTH SECRETS FROM AROUND THE WORLD
Copyright © 1995 by Shot Tower Books, Inc.

Keats edition published 1997 by arrangement with Shot Tower Books, Inc.

Library of Congress Cataloging-in-Publication Data

Natural health secrets / edited by Glenn W. Geelhoed and Jean R. Barilla.
     p.   cm.
   Originally published by Shot Tower Books, Inc., 1995.
   Includes bibliographical references and index.
   ISBN 0-87983-805-1
   1. Alternative medicine.   2. Herbs—Therapeutic use.   3. Traditional medicine.
I. Geelhoed, Glenn W., 1942–   . II. Barilla, Jean.
R733.N365   1997
615.5—dc21   97-13973
                                                        CIP

Printed in the United States of America

Keats Publishing, Inc.
27 Pine Street (Box 876)
New Canaan, Connecticut 06840-0876

Keats Publishing website address: www.keats.com

DOCTOR'S FOREWORD

For many of us, the words "folklore" and "folk remedy" bring to mind old wives' tales and superstitions. But even a traditionally trained doctor will admit that these words also represent the accumulated wit and wisdom of millions of people. And although nearly all of the remedies you will read about in this book preceded the discovery of the scientific method, these "natural experiments" have passed a different test. They have helped people in the past and are still helping people now.

Hippocrates' first rule of treatment, *"Primum non nocere,"* remains a good rule in evaluating any known or suspected therapeutic agent; that is, "first of all, do no harm." Certainly, some harm may come from postponing medical attention that might be effective for treatable conditions, or from forgoing curative treatment in favor of homely remedies that provide only symptomatic relief. But given these precautions, there are still many serious conditions for which orthodox medical treatments are ineffective, leaving those affected to cope on their own.

While it is true that folklore may be based partly on superstition and unfounded magical beliefs, some folk remedies have been proven effective in experimental situations — and many times we can give scientific explanations for why they work. For example, the antimalarial quinine was long ago discovered from the cinchona of Jesuit bark; salicylates such as aspirin were found in birch bark; and the vitamin C we now understand and value so highly was already being used unknowingly when James Lynn gave a lime a day to British seamen with scurvy. In such cases, the practice came first, and the scientific proof came later. These remedies for which there is now scientific proof should indicate that there is much more to learn from folk medicine.

To find new ways to deal with old problems, we must keep an open mind. We must get to know our international neighbors better.

We often look upon people in more primitive parts of the world as "backward" because they don't have access to our own sophisticated medical systems. Backward they may be, in fact, since they seem to have not yet developed the myriad of afflictions that plague those populations who have industrialized modern lifestyles — and hospitals filled with heart disease, cancer and stroke patients which are rare in the "developing world." Rather than the fascination we often express for the "exotic" tropical infections these "primitive" world populations exhibit, we might pause to note what is conspicuously absent or rare among them — degenerative diseases that now constitute the major morbidity among first world populations. People who live to their senior years in these "less privileged" environments are often healthier, free of the worry and physical debility of heart attacks, vascular disease, diabetes, functional colon abnormalities, appendicitis, gallstones, varicose veins, hiatal hernias, most cancers and a variety of diseases said to be associated with the inevitable "aging process."

It is axiomatic that disease is most effectively treated at its earliest stages; and the most effective, least expensive medical process is disease prevention. Senior citizens in the developing world, constrained by limited resources, have handled many of their problems with ingenuity and simple coping mechanisms.

The time has come for us to ask why these people do not have the more common degenerative disorders that we have in over-abundance. And to ask, "What can we learn from them in this shared life experience for better health?"

We must remain receptive to the collective wisdom of a wide range of human experience, and combine this wisdom with scientific awareness. After all, even modern medicine itself is a part of that collective human experience. And if we combine it with the distillates of centuries of pre-scientific "research" from around the world, we can bring a full range of intelligence to the management of human health problems, big and small. The bottom line is: People everywhere have secrets, not just to subsist — but to thrive.

— Glenn W. Geelhoed, A.B., B.S., M.D., D.T., M.H., M.A., M.P.H., F.A.C.S.
  Professor of Surgery
  Professor of International Medical Education
  George Washington University, Washington, D.C.

TABLE OF CONTENTS

    Aloe, chamomile, Chinese angelica, cucumber, echinacea, essential oils, honey, ice, lemon, lemon balm, oatmeal, papaya, soapwort, vinegar, vitamin A, vitamin B, water, zinc

    Black currants, coconut, exercise, fo-ti-tieng, ginkgo, ginseng, gotu kola, honey, longevity soup, royal jelly, vitamin B, vitamin C, yerba mate, yogurt

    Bioflavonoids, broth, ephedra, eucalyptus, exercise, fenugreek, ginkgo, honey, horseradish, nettle, vitamin C

    Artichokes, asparagus, chaste berries, chives, chocolate, clams, damiana, dates, fenugreek, honey, hops, jasmine, kino gum, lavender, licorice, magnolia, oysters, peppers, rice bran oil, roses, saw palmetto, sesame seeds, soybeans

    Alfalfa, caffeine, caraway, dandelion, dill, ginger

INTRODUCTION

You are holding in your hands a compendium of natural health secrets from all over the globe — centuries of folk wisdom from just about every culture that has ever existed on this planet. These time-tested secrets have been passed down from generation to generation. And now, in *Natural Health Secrets From Around the World*, we are passing them on to you. In these pages, you will find more than 1,600 proven ways to keep yourself and your family strong and healthy — to soothe the minor aches and pains of daily living, and even prevent serious illness.

In today's high-tech world, it's sometimes hard to imagine that for thousands of years, people couldn't just pop over to the corner drugstore to pick up a bottle of something or other whenever they needed relief. Instead, they used what they had to cure their ills. Willow bark for headaches, ginger for an upset stomach, moldy bread to protect cuts and scrapes against infection are just a few of the countless remedies they found in Mother Nature's pharmacy.

For years, practitioners of modern medicine scoffed at these "primitive" folk treatments. But the tables have turned. Researchers are discovering that folk cures not only work, in many cases they are even better than chemically manufactured commercial drugs. They are at least as effective — and almost always cheaper, gentler and safer.

Scientists are also learning more about the important role nutrition plays in preventing disease. And here, again, they are learning that the old ways are the best ways. That the simple, low-fat, high-fiber foods our ancestors ate were far healthier than the fancy, pre-packaged, overly processed foods most Americans fill their grocery carts (and bellies) with today. That the diets of all the ancient cultures in the world — Orientals, Mediterraneans, Africans, Indians, South Americans — are the main reason these people are far less likely to suffer from killer diseases like cancer and heart disease that plague Western society.

Whether you've been interested in natural health alternatives for just a few months, or for many years, chances are you've had difficulty getting the information you need. Until now. Because *Natural Health Secrets From Around the World* is the most comprehensive book that's ever been published on the subject. This isn't just a quick-fix guide, it's a resource for total health — chock-full of home remedies, ancient secrets, helpful hints, informative illustrations and solid advice.

■ You'll find specific recommendations for over 100 common ailments, complete with instructions on how to make your own healing medications.

■ You'll learn the difference between compresses and poultices, between decoctions and infusions, between tinctures and teas — and how to make them all.

■ You'll find countless beauty secrets — some that date back to Cleopatra — for your hair, your skin, your teeth and your nails — along with instructions for making your own cleansers, shampoos, moisturizers, facials and massage oils.

■ You'll find a section on nutrition — everything you need to know about healthy eating — along with a handy chart that lists all the essential vitamins and minerals, their benefits, and their best food sources.

■ You'll learn about alternative healing methods like yoga, meditation, t'ai chi, shiatsu, akido, aromatherapy and naturopathy.

■ You'll find a section on natural "wonder drugs" — honey, ginger, fish oils, garlic, onions, ginseng, aloe — that are so effective in treating so many different problems that some people actually label them "panaceas" (cure-alls).

■ You'll find a section on relaxation and stress-management techniques — another on natural ways to keep your energy levels at their peak — and yet another on ancient (and modern) secrets of longevity.

■ You'll find numerous exercise suggestions, including specific exercises to relieve arthritis, backache and stress.

■ We've even included a section on natural ways to keep your pets happy, healthy and well fed.

■ We've added a glossary, a section on herbal preparations, and many, many recipes — for everything from love potions to bug repellents to energy shakes. And though you'll find just about every ingredient mentioned in your own garden or kitchen cabinet, we've included pages and pages of listings to help you find any items that might not be available locally.

As you can see, we've done the work for you. Now all you have to do is take advantage of this world of collective wisdom.

ALTERNATIVE HEALING METHODS

Not so long ago, if you had a taste for international cuisine, you were out of luck. Sure, there were a few Chinese-American restaurants and a few Americanized Italian places, but if you were in the mood for some real Thai, Indian or Ethiopian cuisine, you had to search far and wide to find a restaurant — especially if you didn't live in a major urban area.

Until recently, Western medicine has been the same. Your menu of choices for health care was limited to standard, orthodox, mainstream medicine. Only if you looked hard enough, lived in a major metropolitan area and knew the right people could you find alternatives.

Now things are changing dramatically. In 1993, the New England Journal of Medicine, arguably the most respected medical journal in the world, reported that Americans are turning to alternative health treatments in larger and larger numbers. Interest is so high that a new magazine, the *Journal of Alternative and Complimentary Medicine* was recently established to publish work being done in alternative health care. Even the high-tech world of the Internet, also known as the "Information Superhighway," is loaded with information about alternative medicine and has become one of the leading places for distributing alternative therapies.

"ALTERNATIVE MEDICINE" DOESN'T MEAN "QUACKERY"

In the 1800s, hucksters traveled the country in horse-drawn wagons selling "miracle" cures to unsuspecting settlers. Sly operators that they were, these unscrupulous con men would come into a new town, set up their brightly colored wagons in the town square, and work the gathering crowd up into a frenzy using important sounding (but meaningless) scientific jargon, bold banners and promises that what they sold — often just concoctions of alcohol and drugs such as morphine or cocaine — would "cure all yer ills."

Though the Food and Drug Administration put an end to all that quackery in the 1900s, medical con artists still exist. However, just because a medicine or treatment hasn't been approved by the medical establishment, that doesn't mean it's bad. For years, Western medicine dismissed treatments like acupuncture and chiropracty as quackery. Now we know that both may have their places as alternative therapies.

Western medicine often ignores the connection between the mind and body, but most alternative and folk traditions emphasize the importance of that link. Though they may be completely new to you, most of the therapies we'll discuss in this chapter have a long, proven track record (thousands of years and millions of people for some of them!). While we suggest you try those that appeal to you, we want to emphasize that you should not forego curative conventional treatments for serious ailments.

THE ORIENTAL TRADITION

For centuries, some of the most successful and sophisticated alternative healing methods have been found in the East. China, Japan and India have long-standing medical traditions that include acupuncture, the different martial arts, shiatsu massage, yoga and the Ayurveda system of India.

Avoiding Quack Cures

In 1992, the U.S. Federal Trade Commission published a pamphlet called "Health Claims: Separating Fact From Fiction" that contains an excellent checklist for separating quack cures from those that really work. Here are some of the key points made in this pamphlet — guidelines to keep in mind when you see advertisements for modern-day "miracle cures."

1. Does the ad promise a "quick and easy cure"?

2. Is the product advertised as effective for a wide range of ailments or for undiagnosed pain?

3. Is the product advertised available from only one source, requiring payment in advance?

4. Does the promoter use undocumented case histories that sound too good to be true?

5. Don't rely on promises of a "money-back guarantee." Many fly-by-night operators will never be there to respond to a refund request.

ACUPUNCTURE

You'd think that a therapy that consisted of sticking needles in your body would have limited appeal, but this ancient Chinese technique has become so popular in this country during the past decade that it's practically mainstream. Noted mainly as an effective treatment for pain, acupuncture has been used as an effective treatment for intestinal disorders, hiccups and ulcers and as anesthesia during major surgery (including even one case of brain surgery!). The World Health Organization has even used it to treat amoebic dysentery in countries where medicine isn't readily available.

How does it work? Acupuncturists believe that life energy (also known as "qui" or "chi") flows through specific paths in the body. When the energy is allowed to flow freely, the body is in harmony and health. Illness occurs when one of these qui pathways known as "meridians" becomes blocked. To treat illness or curb pain, an acupuncturist inserts stainless steel needles as thin as two human hairs into the patient at various points called "tsubos." Once the needles are inserted, they are twirled or connected to a weak electrical current to stimulate the qui to flow freely and bring relief.

SHIATSU

Shiatsu, which was developed in Japan, is based on many of the same theories as acupuncture. Also known as acupressure, practitioners

---

Everyday Shiatsu Remedies

You can use some of the principles of acupressure or shiatsu to feel better instantly. These quick remedies work wonders and can be done anywhere.

For headaches, grasp the webbed area between your thumb and index finger and squeeze gently until you feel your headache start to ebb.

For nausea, try pressing your thumb into the area about two inches above the crease in your wrist.

For menstrual cramps, press firmly on the spot one hand-width up from your ankle bone on the side of your calf.

use their hands to massage the patient's qui points to release the blocked qui. Like acupuncture, shiatsu is useful for relieving a variety of ailments, but it is mainly used to treat acute pain and stress. Even if you don't believe in qui and are in good health, a shiatsu massage can be a wonderful, relaxing experience. If you want to try it out, look in the Yellow Pages under "massage."

T'AI CHI

T'ai chi chuan means "supreme ultimate fist" in Chinese. While you might not have to use this most gentle of the martial arts to defend yourself from attackers, a regimen of t'ai chi may help defend your body from sickness.

The origin of t'ai chi lies far back in the mists of history. According to t'ai chi expert Cheng Tin Hung, it was developed by Taoist monks as a way to maintain good health during their wilderness meditations and as a way to protect them from attacks by wild beasts.

True to the Taoist sense of wholeness through contradiction, t'ai chi is both a fighting skill and a meditative art form. T'ai chi practitioners learn up to 100 different postures or "forms" which they perform in sequence. Watching someone practice t'ai chi is like watching a beautiful, tranquil dance as he or she finds the body's natural place of balance, builds up bodily energy and then slowly releases it.

People who practice t'ai chi are more physically fit and emotionally stable than most. They also seem to have an overall better immunity from common problems such as colds and headaches. T'ai chi is often recommended to people suffering from stress.

AKIDO

Closely related to t'ai chi, akido is a Japanese martial art that works by controlling the energy flow (called "ki") of the body.

Because akido emphasizes mental control as well as physical control and balance, it's great for reducing stress and increasing concentration. Those who practice akido every morning report that they become more focused and productive at work while maintaining a more stress-free outlook on life. Unlike t'ai chi, akido is a fast-moving workout that tones the body while it clears the mind.

YOGA

Yoga was developed in India over 5,000 years ago. Today, while saffron-robed holy men are still twisting themselves into pretzels, a lot of ordinary folks, too, are using yoga as a way to relieve stress and enhance their minds. When you practice yoga, you strive for a balance between mind and body, and achieving that balance can do wonders for your health.

Breathing is central to yoga. Practitioners of yoga believe that our life energy ("prana") flows throughout the body. Prana manifests itself in the physical world through breathing. By controlling the breathing, we can control our minds and body.

Yogis (yoga masters) can control nearly every bodily function. They can stop their breathing, withstand severe pain and even drop into such a deep trance that their hearts nearly stop. While most people never have to achieve this level of proficiency, almost everyone can use yoga to boost their energy levels and relieve stress and fatigue.

According to Dr. Robert Willix, editor of *Health & Longevity*, the series of sun salutation postures is the single best thing you can do for your back. In addition, it's a great way to deal with stress, to relax, and to achieve mind-body harmony. And it's a very effective way to warm up before you exercise.

The best time to do the sun salutation is in the morning or early evening. Start with two sets and work up to 6 to 10 sets without become fatigued or breathing heavily.

Do the positions of the exercise in one continuous, flowing motion, holding each position for 5 seconds. Your breathing should also be continuous and fluid, connecting the 12 movements — except for one brief pause in breathing when you transition between position 6 and position 7. Inhale (expanding your chest) as you extend your spine, and exhale (contracting your abdomen) as you bend or flex your spine. If you finish the inhale or exhale before you are finished holding a position for 5 seconds, hold your breath until you start to move into the next position. Be sure to breathe in and out through your nose.

1. Start in the Salutation Position, looking straight ahead and standing straight and tall, with your feet shoulder width apart and your palms together in front of your chest.

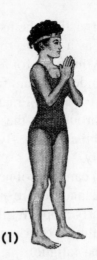

(1)

2. Inhale as you slowly raise your arms up and slightly back in a wide circle, extending your spine and looking up at your hands in the Raised Arm Position. Hold for 5 seconds.

(2)

3. Exhale as you bend forward as far as you can into the Hand to Foot Position — knees, elbows and shoulders relaxed, and hands flat on the floor or at your ankles (depending on your degree of flexibility). Hold for 5 seconds.

(3)

4. Inhale as you slowly lunge forward with your right leg, lifting your head and spine as you bend your right knee between your arms and extend your left leg back with the left knee touching the floor in the Equestrian Position. Hold for 5 seconds.

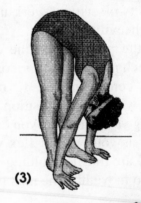

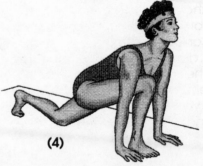

(4)

5. Exhale and bring your left leg forward to meet your right leg as you lift your hips and buttocks into the Mountain Position, releasing your spine as you press down with your hands, stretch your heels to the floor (feeling the stretch in the backs of your legs), and relax your head and neck. Hold for 5 seconds.

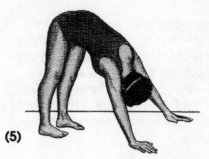

(5)

6. Without breathing, bend your knees and elbows and slowly slide your body down, touching your toes, knees, chest, hands and chin to the floor in the Eight Limbs Position. Hold briefly.

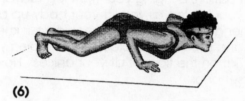

(6)

7. Inhale as you lift your head and chest, pressing down with your hands as you arch your back and bring your shoulders down into the Cobra Position. Hold for 5 seconds.

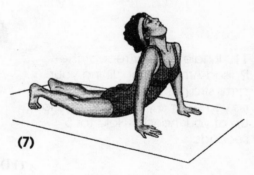

(7)

8. Exhale as you repeat the Mountain Position, raising your buttocks and hips, and releasing your spine as you press down with your hands. Stretch your heels to the floor (feeling the stretch in the backs of your legs), and relax your head and neck. Hold for 5 seconds.

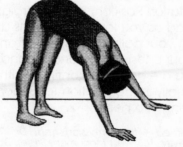

(8)

9

9. Inhale as you repeat the Equestrian Position, this time lifting your head and spine as you bring your left leg forward to bend it between your arms, and extending your right leg back with the right knee touching the floor. Hold for 5 seconds.

(9)

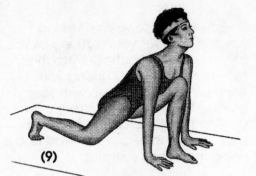

10. Exhale as you repeat the Hand to Foot Position, bringing your right leg forward to meet your left leg as you lift your body up and lengthen your spine, keeping your knees, elbows and shoulders relaxed, and keeping your hands flat on the floor or at your ankles. Hold for 5 seconds.

(10)

11. Inhale as your repeat the Raised Arm Position, lifting your arms straight up and slightly back as you extend your spine and look up at your hands. Hold for 5 seconds.

(11)

12. Exhale as you return to the Salutation Position, looking straight ahead as you lower your arms and bring your palms together in front of your chest. Hold for 5 seconds.
If you are going to continue with another set, breathe normally in the position for 5 more seconds before moving into position 2.

(12)

(Reprinted with permission from Dr. Robert D. Willix Jr.'s Health & Longevity, *105 West Monument Street, Baltimore, MD 21201.)*

10

AYURVEDA

Ayurveda ("the art and science of living") is still a relatively unknown alternative medical system that is slowly gaining popularity in the U.S. Some people claim that Ayurveda is the oldest recorded system of medicine in the world, tracing its roots back to a book called the Rig Veda published in India in 1,500 B.C. From India, some of Ayurveda's tenets spread to China in 700 A.D. through Buddhist missionaries. About 100 years later, Ayurvedic books were translated into Arabic, and Islamic teachers later spread Ayurveda's teachings to Europe in the 1500s.

Modern-day Ayurveda concentrates on maintaining health through a balance between the body (shira), mind (manas) and self (atman). Ayurvedic doctors examine their patients to determine where the problem is, and then use natural herbs, foods, spices and meditation to bring the body back into balance — preventing, as well as curing, disease.

To find an Ayurvedic practitioner in your area, call (800)843-8332.

WESTERN ALTERNATIVE THERAPIES: THE NEW TRADITIONS

For many years, the American Medical Association turned a skeptical eye to anything outside their traditional medical boundaries. Recently, however, there's been a growing acceptance of nontraditional techniques such as chiropracty, homeopathy, vitamin therapy, visualization and aromatherapy.

CHIROPRACTY

Once regarded as quacks and charlatans, chiropractors are now considered leading practitioners in the growing field of physical therapy. These days, if you suffer from neck or back pain, your doctor is nearly as likely to send you to a chiropractor as to a physical therapist, after serious problems such as meningitis or spinal cord tumors have been ruled out.

Chiropractors believe that the spine is the seat of good health and that many physical ailments are manifestations of spinal misalignment. Through touch and "manipulation" techniques, they "adjust" the patient's spinal column back into healthy alignment. Many patients have found that this therapy goes far beyond easing the aches and pains of neck and back injuries. Allergies, asthma, stomach pains and menstrual disorders all seem to be helped by chiropractic adjustment. And, recent studies have shown that it can lower blood pressure and improve agility, speed and balance.

Sweat It Out!

Many naturopaths believe that accumulated body toxins are a major cause of illness. One of the ways they help cleanse the body of toxic materials is with a sweat-wrap. By wrapping the body in materials that retain body heat and retard evaporation (such as plastic wrap or non-porous banana leaves), a patient with a build-up of sweat-excreted toxins can be purified.

If you are in basically good shape, you can try this at home. Turn on the hot water in your shower full blast. Don't try to stand in the stream — you'll get burned. Instead, let the bathroom fill up with steam, and sit in it for 20 minutes or so, or as long as it takes to work up a good sweat. If you feel dizzy or light-headed, stop.

People who try this "sweat therapy" often report feeling refreshed or rested when it's over. Steam heat is also good because it unclogs your pores, leaving you with softer, clearer skin. Scandinavians, ancient Romans, Germans and Native Americans all use (or used) variations of the "sweat bath" over the years to purify themselves.

HOMEOPATHY

One day in the early 19th century, a healthy German doctor named Samuel Hahnemann dosed himself with cinchona, a common malaria remedy. He was instantly overcome by a fever, chills, a throbbing headache and a raging thirst — all the symptoms of malaria. Based on this, Hahnemann determined that cinchona's effectiveness in treating malaria came from its ability to cause symptoms that mimicked malaria. Homeopathy was born. Using the theory "like causes like," homeopathic doctors use extremely diluted amounts of toxic substances to treat illness.

While homeopathy does have its detractors, it seems to be effective. One reason may be because homeopaths strive to treat the whole body. They see symptoms not as problems to be covered up, but as evidence that the body is healing itself. Chronic problems such as allergies, arthritis, colitis, headaches and high blood pressure all seem to be the sort of ailments helped by the homeopathic approach.

NATUROPATHY

Doctors of naturopathic medicine must undergo a rigorous 5 to 6 year training program where they learn everything from traditional Chinese medicine to botany to psychology. Like practitioners of many other alternative therapies, they focus on the body's ability to heal itself. In the naturopathic system, a good diet and a healthy lifestyle are key to keeping us physically fit and mentally stable.

Naturopathy is reported effective in treating irritable bowel syndrome, asthma, allergies, gout, high blood pressure and eczema — all disorders associated with an unhealthy diet.

VITAMIN AND MINERAL THERAPY

If you've ever taken large doses of vitamin C to fight off a cold, you've practiced vitamin therapy. Ever since two-time Nobel Prize winner Linus Pauling reported that megadoses of vitamin C kept him healthy, using vitamins and minerals to treat illness has become a popular treatment for a variety of ailments. See chart on page 14 for vitamin treatments.

VISUALIZATION

Tapping into the power of the mind-body connection, visualization therapy teaches patients to actually visualize their immune systems attacking and destroying bad cells. Researchers have reported success in using visualization to fight cancer, alleviate some of the symptoms of AIDS, and even make warts drop off overnight.

AROMATHERAPY

If you've ever had your spirits lifted when you walked into a house where someone was baking bread, then you've experienced the power of aromatherapy. Early cave dwellers probably discovered that throwing fragrant branches on their cave fires made them feel better, but it was the ancient Egyptians who perfected the art. They had scents for nearly every occasion, using them to purify the air, and as medicines and love potions.

The Greeks, too, used aromatherapy. In fact, recipes for medicinal perfumes have been found inscribed in the temples of Aesculapius, a Greek god of healing. Centuries later, the Arabian physician Avicenna rediscovered the power of plant scents. His perfumes were brought to Europe by the crusaders — and scent has been popular in the West ever since. Today, in

Common Vitamin and Mineral Treatments

adapted from *The Reader's Digest Family Guide to Natural Medicine*

Vitamin or Mineral	Helps treat...
Vitamin B1 (Thiamin)	stress, depression, hangover, motion sickness, shingles, neuralgia
Vitamin B2 (Riboflavin)	drug-induced psychosis, eye problems
Vitamin B3 (Niacin)	high cholesterol, alcoholism, migraine, anxiety, arthritis, schizophrenia
Vitamin B5 (Panthoenic Acid)	allergies, weak adrenal glands, ulcers, anxiety, depression, hypoglycemia, eczema
Vitamin B6	PMS, acne, depression, diabetes, carpal tunnel syndrome, anemia
Vitamin B12	fatigue, anxiety, memory loss, neuritis, hepatitis, eye disorders
Biotin	eczema, diabetes, dialysis problems
Folic Acid	canker sores, heart disease, psoriasis
Vitamin A	infections, acne, excessive menstrual bleeding, ulcers, aging
Vitamin C	cancer, immune problems, cardiovascular disease, diabetes, gallstones, eye problems, allergies, asthma
Vitamin D	menopausal symptoms, poor calcium absorption
Vitamin E	cardiovascular problems, blood clotting, pregnancy problems
Vitamin K	morning sickness, nosebleed
Calcium	high blood pressure, elevated cholesterol, menstrual cramps, anxiety, insomnia
Chromium	diabetes, hypoglycemia, high cholesterol, hypertension
Iron	anemia, restless leg syndrome, excessive menstrual bleeding
Magnesium	high blood pressure, PMS, migraines, asthma, fatigue, kidney stones, anxiety, depression, hyperactivity
Selenium	arthritis, dandruff
Zinc	arthritis, boils, skin ulcers, acne, peptic ulcers, enlarged prostrate

Good Smells = Good Moods

Different scents have different effects. Here's a quick guide:

Essential Oil	
Birch	muscle tension
Chamomile	relaxation
Clary sage	stimulant
Eucalyptus	muscle soreness, congestion
Geranium	relaxation
Jasmine	aphrodisiac
Juniper	stimulant, muscle soreness
Lavender	skin toning, relaxation
Lemon grass	skin problems
Neroli	skin problems
Orange flower	mood enhancer
Peppermint	relaxation
Rose	mood enhancer
Rosemary	relaxation, muscle tension
Sage	stimulation, concentration
Sandalwood	euphoria
Ylang ylang	euphoria

France, where the term "aromatherapy" was coined by chemist Rene-Maurice Gattefosse and where perfumery is a highly regarded art, medical insurance even pays for aromatherapy treatments.

Why are smells such powerful healers? Again, it's that mind-body connection. Signals from the olfactory nerve go straight to the part of the brain responsible for memory and emotion. As a result, smells can reduce stress, help relaxation, relieve anxiety, improve productivity and ease depression.

To practice aromatherapy at home, you should buy scents in the form of essential oils. Never apply these oils directly to your skin at full strength because they can trigger an allergic reaction. Instead, add some to your bath-water, perfume your home or office with bowls of water and scented oil, or burn scented candles. Massage is another pleasant way to enjoy aromatherapy. Mix the essential oils with some walnut, almond or wheat germ oil, and massage gently into the skin.

THE BACH SYSTEM

The Bach System is another alternative therapy that's really beginning to take off. Started by Dr. Edward Bach in 1930, it uses native plants and flowers to approach illness by attacking what Bach supporters believe to be the root of all problems — mental anguish. They believe that physical complaints are manifestations of mental attitudes such as lethargy, depression, over-enthusiasm, guilt or panic. Followers of this system use 38 different dilute plant extracts, gathered from plants that still grow near Bach's house, to trigger the body's self-healing abilities. Most popular is the Rescue Remedy, composed of extracts from cherry plum, clematis, impatiens, rock rose and star of Bethlehem flowers.

ENERGY

You wake up in the morning to the jarring sound of the alarm ringing next to your bed. You're still half asleep as you roll over and fumble around on the nightstand, desperately trying to shut off the racket. You hit the snooze button for just "10 more minutes" of sleep, roll over and fall back into a fitful slumber. Ten minutes later, the alarm goes off again. You realize you have to get moving, so you struggle to sit up, shut off the alarm and try to clear your head. You look at the clock and realize you're going to be late. You jump out of bed, take a shower, get dressed (while trying not to scald yourself on your coffee), grab your things and rush out the door.

You didn't have a chance to eat breakfast, so when you get to the office, you fish around in your pocket for change and hit the vending machine in the employee lounge for a candy bar. On your way back to your desk, you make a brief stop for a cup of coffee and slug it down as you walk. You still feel kind of groggy, but the coffee seems to be working, and you manage to get through the morning.

By the time lunch rolls around, you feel like you've been dragged behind a pack of wild horses. Your back aches, your thoughts are mushy, and your stomach's grumbling like a caged animal. You dash to the deli across the street, pick up a pastrami sandwich and eat it on your way back to work. By 3 o'clock, you're dead tired. Your eyes feel like dry stones, your head aches, and you barely make it to 5 o'clock.

On the way home, as usual, you get stuck in traffic. You know yelling won't make the cars move any faster, but you do it anyway, cursing your fellow motorists while you can feel your blood pressure rise and your heart pound. When you finally walk in your front door, the idea of making dinner is beyond you — so you order a pizza and a bottle of soda. Then you plop down in front of the TV, grab the remote and channel-surf for the rest of the evening.

Is this any way to live?

Wouldn't you rather bounce out of bed in the morning — ready to conquer the world — and go all day without being bogged down by fatigue?

Wouldn't it be great to come home from work with energy to spare and be able to use every waking moment to the fullest?

WHAT SAPS YOUR ENERGY?

Too many people find their energy at the bottom of a coffee cup or a soda can. They live stress-filled lives, constantly staving off fatigue so they can get their work done, only to collapse at the end of the day, physically worn out and mentally drained. Unfortunately, when we force ourselves into sudden bursts of productivity, what we really wind up doing is steadily depleting our body's natural wellspring of healthy energy. One of the absolute laws of the physical world is, "What goes up must come down." And, this law holds for our bodies, too.

STRESS

Stress is a primary cause of fatigue. When you're under stress, your body reacts by releasing a hormone called adrenaline into your bloodstream, quickening your heartbeat and breathing. Your senses improve, your mind perks up, and you get charged up and ready to act. You get a quick, short-term energy boost that dissipates just as quickly — leaving you more fatigued and worn out than you were before. This is why people often just poop out and plop down on the couch after a long, stressful day at work — their bodies are tuckered out from stress.

ARTIFICIAL STIMULANTS: CAFFEINE, NICOTINE AND SUGAR

You're tired. You want to perk up. What do you do? You drink a cup of coffee, smoke a cigarette, or grab a candy bar. Bad moves! Artificial stimulants like caffeine (found in chocolate, coffee, cola and other sodas and tea), nicotine (the stimulant in tobacco) and sugar might wake you up at first, but their longer-term effects drain you of valuable energy. Caffeine is also addictive. In fact, Dr. Andrew Weil, best-selling author of *Natural Health, Natural Medicine,* estimates that at least 80 percent of all people who drink coffee regularly are addicted to it. Once you are addicted, your body builds up a tolerance to the stimulant, and it takes more and more coffee to give you the same energy burst you used to get. At the same time, you experience mental and physical slowness, constipation, irritability and headaches when the caffeine starts to wear off. And because caffeine can interfere with your sleep, when you collapse into bed at night, you don't get a good rest. As a result, you wake up tired and begin the whole cycle over again.

Nicotine is among the strongest and most habit-forming drugs in the world. Some researchers have even said that it's at least as addictive as heroin. As most smokers will tell you, kicking a nicotine addiction can be difficult and painful.

Unless you've been living in a cave, you know that smoking is unhealthy. But you may not know that it saps energy. Like caffeine, nicotine is a strong stimulant. It makes your heart beat faster, your breathing quicken and your blood pressure rise — and when the stimulant effect dissipates, you are more tired than you were before. Smoking damages your heart and impairs your ability to get oxygen into your system. When your body is starved for oxygen, toxins accumulate in your blood stream — and you feel tired and fatigued.

Sugar is also a powerful energy-zapper. When you eat sugar, your body releases insulin from the pancreas to break down the sugar so it can be converted to energy. Sugar, especially sucrose or "white sugar," breaks down especially fast, sending your body into overdrive. And, just as with nicotine and caffeine, this quick boost is often followed by an extreme drop in energy as the sugar is metabolized by your body. This rebound effect creates a temporary state of hypoglycemia (low blood sugar). The main symptom of hypoglycemia is fatigue. In addition, it can cause nervousness, irritability, faintness, depression, drowsiness, headaches, digestive problems and many other symptoms that sap energy and make life difficult.

ENERGY FOODS

Watching your diet is the most effective thing you can do to fight fatigue. By eating foods high in fiber and low in fat and sugar, you supply your body with foods that fill you up, keep you satisfied for hours and maintain a constant supply of energy to your body.

Focus on high-carbohydrate foods like beans, whole grains, vegetables and fruits, all of which contain complex carbohydrates and high amounts of dietary fiber. Complex carbohydrates take longer for your body to break down, and so, provide sustained energy throughout the day with none of the extreme highs and lows that accompany a diet high in simple sugars. A 250 calorie donut is rapidly metabolized, gives a quick boost and causes a steep drop in energy levels once it's been used by the body. On the other hand, a 250 calorie breakfast that includes complex carbohydrates like oatmeal or bagels and fruit takes much longer to metabolize. In addition, the added bulk in these foods stays in your stomach longer and makes you feel fuller, making it less likely for you to be tempted to take a mid-morning candy break.

The following foods are especially helpful to sustain energy throughout the day. They all contain substances that keep your body charged and your mind alert.

BLUEBERRIES

Recently, doctors in Paris and Budapest isolated chemicals in blueberries called anthrocyanosides. In tests on rabbits, they found that these chemicals were effective in reducing the damage caused to brain blood vessels from a high-cholesterol diet. The anthrocyanosides helped block cholesterol from penetrating into the brain blood vessels. And since proper blood flow to the brain is essential for mental energy and health, it looks like blueberries may very well help improve brain function.

CHILI PEPPERS

Naturally low in fat, high in fiber and packed with vitamin C, peppers are a flavorful addition to a low-salt, low-fat diet. The active ingredient in hot peppers (capsaicin) is also an effective stimulant and energy booster. "Chili-heads" sing the praises of the "pepper-rush" they get from hot foods. This euphoric reaction results because pepper causes your brain to secrete pain-killing chemicals called endorphins. Many times stronger than morphine, the endorphins get your blood flowing and your sweat glands working (great for detoxifying your body) — and give you a rush that lasts for 30 minutes or more.

If you're not used to eating hot peppers, start slowly. After eating them for a while, you'll find your tolerance increasing, along with your energy levels. Remember that most of the heat is in the seeds and the white pith, so if you want pepper taste but less fire, discard the seeds. A word of caution: The capsaicin in peppers can burn. So you may want to wear rubber gloves when preparing them — and don't touch your eyes.

FISH

Increase your intake of fish, especially cold-water ocean fish. Not only are fish a lower-fat source of complete protein, but the omega-3 fatty acids so prevalent in northern fish (such as mackerel) can help lower your blood pressure and regulate your cholesterol levels — two healthy benefits that can make you feel a lot better and help you live a lot longer.

Besides the overall health benefits of fish, researchers are now discovering that this food can be an effective brain booster. Dr. Judith Wutman, a researcher at the Massachusetts Institute of Technology, has found that an amino acid (tyrosine) found in high levels in fish can rev up the brain. Tyrosine seems to stimulate the production of the neurotransmitters norepinephrine and dopamine. These brain chemicals are often depleted during strenuous mental activity — and eating fish can boost them right up again.

OATS

Grandma was right — oatmeal really is good for you. Not only have oats been shown to be a cholesterol lowering food — lowering blood cholesterol in patients by over 20 percent — but the fiber and complex carbohydrates in this grain can keep you going. One of the main causes of a mid-morning slump is that your body just runs out of fuel a few hours after breakfast. When your morning begins with high-calorie junk food, you can really feel your energy lag after the sugar has been metabolized. But oats are different. The complex

---

Brain Break Sandwich

This recipe combines the healthy goodness of whole grain bread with the brain-pumping power of fish and milk, the stimulating zip of hot peppers and the soothing effects of lettuce.

- ½ cup white albacore tuna
- 2 slices whole grain bread
- several pieces of lettuce
- 2-5 pepperoncini (to taste)
- 1 slice of low-fat cheese

Layer all the ingredients on the bread and enjoy yogurt or an apple for dessert.

carbohydrates in a bowl of oatmeal or a low-fat oat-bran muffin fill you up and are metabolized slowly, releasing controlled energy throughout the morning. So, by the time you get to lunch, you'll still be going strong.

OYSTERS

According to Jean Carper, author of *The Food Pharmacy*, as little as 3 to 4 ounces of shellfish — that's just 3 to 6 oysters — can deliver enough energizing chemicals to wake up your brain and body. That's pretty good stuff. That's because oysters are almost pure protein, and your body metabolizes this low-fat, high protein into a variety of amino acids, including tyrosine. The tyrosine goes right to your brain, boosting the neurotransmitters responsible for brain function. Your thought processes speed up, your attention span increases, and your mental energy reserves become recharged.

SEAWEED

Though seaweed is just starting to enter the American diet, the Japanese have used this vitamin- and mineral-rich sea vegetable for years. Not only has seaweed been shown to reduce the risk of cancer, help prevent blood clots and lower blood pressure, but Japanese scientists have discovered that it can also help detoxify the blood and maintain energy levels. How? Recent Japanese research on a kind of seaweed called spirulina

Seaweed in your salad

Spirulina and other algaes can be purchased in powdered form and added to dressings or sprinkled directly on salad. Other types of seaweed such as Hikiki (a dark, spaghetti-looking seaweed) and Wakame and Nori (two other types of leafy seaweeds) are becoming more available through ethnic food stores and health food shops. Their crunchy, briny taste will add an interesting texture and flavor to an ordinary everyday meal.

indicated that it helps regulate blood sugar levels. By taking spirulina, people are able to maintain consistent energy levels. In addition, because spirulina is so high in protein, minerals and essential fatty acids, it is a healthy energy food that is especially useful for people on low-calorie diets. Kelp is another seaweed that is an energy-booster.

Yogurt "cheese" for lower fat snacking

Yogurt is a versatile food that can be used as a fat substitute and as a creamy no-fat spread, if you know how.

Here's how to make a yogurt cheese that resembles cream cheese and can be used in dips, spreads and dishes where cream cheese is usually used. Start with low- or no-fat plain yogurt, about 16 to 20 ounces. Line a colander or strainer with a few layers of cheesecloth and place the strainer over a bowl. Dump your plain yogurt in the strainer, cover with a plate or some plastic wrap, and leave in the refrigerator overnight. If you don't have a strainer or cheesecloth, try a coffee filter. Your yogurt cheese spread is what's remaining in the strainer.

YOGURT

From the steppes of Russia to the hills of Bulgaria to the sun-kissed shores of the Mediterranean, yogurt have been a diet staple for centuries. The main medicinal uses of yogurt have been to treat ulcers, indigestion and diarrhea. Recently though, research at the Massachusetts Institute of Technology has shown that yogurt (and other milk products) can serve as brain food as well. Like fish and shellfish, yogurt contains a large amount of protein, which the body readily assimilates and breaks down into energizing amino acids.

ENERGY HERBS

From native South Americans who chew cocoa leaves to stay alert during long mountain journeys to Africans who chew kola nut and khat leaves to keep awake, herbs have been popular energy-boosters around the world for centuries. And today, many of the herbs that used to be available only in one region can be found in your local health food store. Here are some of the most popular of the energy herbs.

EPHEDRA

The Chinese use a plant called ma huang (or ephedra) as a stimulant. Ma huang contains ephedrine, a decongestant and bronchodialator with a healthy kick. A tea made from the powdered or cut root can keep you going for the long haul. But, use this herb with caution — ephedrine is an extremely powerful stimulant, and long-term use can be harmful. It should never be used by pregnant women or by people with elevated blood pressure.

GINKGO

Ginkgo trees have been around for over 200 million years. They are so old that many botanists consider them "living fossils," nearly unchanged since they first sprouted up during the time of the dinosaurs. These hardy trees originally were native to the Far East, but their ability to withstand adverse conditions has made them popular in many cities in the eastern U.S.

Ginkgo has been said to be effective in the treatment of senility, memory loss and mental fatigue. It does its work by helping to dilate the body's blood vessels, thereby causing increased blood flow to the brain and making the brain function more efficiently.

The active ingredient in ginkgo is in the leaves, and extracts made from them are readily available at health food stores. These extracts contain flavonoids, diterpenese and substances unique to ginkgo plants called ginkgolides.

GINSENG

For thousands of years, the Chinese have used ginseng as the cornerstone of their herbal pharmacy. More recently, scientists have been proving that ginseng really does live up to many of the claims the Chinese have been making about it. It helps people live longer, lowers high blood pressure, reduces the likelihood of stroke and generally helps overall physical health. Plus, ginseng is an effective energy-booster.

In trials in Russia and China, doctors found that ginseng can help athletes run faster and compete more efficiently. The athletes who were given ginseng increased their normal running speeds and lifted more weight. Swiss studies have shown that these remarkable effects are caused by ginseng's ability to increase the amount of oxygen in the blood — and this boosts the body's ability to release the energy in food.

PEPPERMINT

The icy taste of mint stimulates more than your mouth — it can pep you up and give you more energy as well. The people of Iceland chew mint leaves, and many truckers use peppermint lozenges to keep themselves awake. You

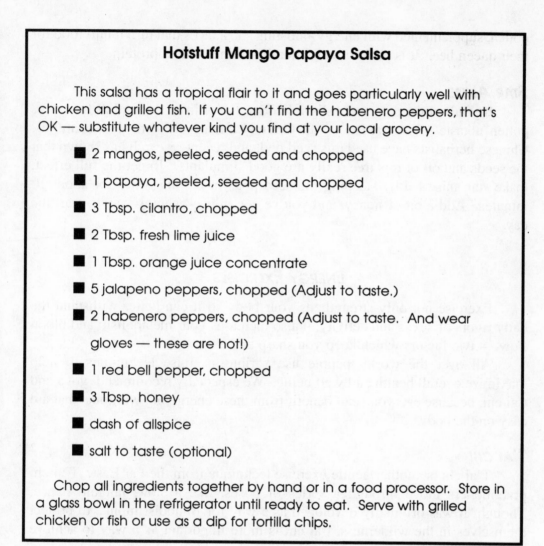

Hotstuff Mango Papaya Salsa

This salsa has a tropical flair to it and goes particularly well with chicken and grilled fish. If you can't find the habenero peppers, that's OK — substitute whatever kind you find at your local grocery.

- 2 mangos, peeled, seeded and chopped
- 1 papaya, peeled, seeded and chopped
- 3 Tbsp. cilantro, chopped
- 2 Tbsp. fresh lime juice
- 1 Tbsp. orange juice concentrate
- 5 jalapeno peppers, chopped (Adjust to taste.)
- 2 habenero peppers, chopped (Adjust to taste. And wear gloves — these are hot!)
- 1 red bell pepper, chopped
- 3 Tbsp. honey
- dash of allspice
- salt to taste (optional)

Chop all ingredients together by hand or in a food processor. Store in a glass bowl in the refrigerator until ready to eat. Serve with grilled chicken or fish or use as a dip for tortilla chips.

can also pep yourself up with peppermint by brewing it into a tea. Or, if you're doing some heavy yard work or working out, try adding a few peppermint leaves to your drinking water.

ROYAL JELLY

Though it is not really an herb, many athletes swear by this bee product. It is becoming increasingly popular with athletes competing in high-endurance sports such as marathons or triathlons. Royal jelly is produced by bees from pollen, supplemented with energy-boosting substances that turn it into food for their queen bee. It is packed with vitamins, minerals and protein.

STAR ANISE

If you've ever detected a slight licorice flavor in an oriental dish, you've gotten a taste of star anise — an Oriental energy-booster. For centuries, Chinese herbalists have used this seed pod, and recent research has shown that the seeds and oil of this tree really are good stimulants. To get the full effect, make star anise tea by steeping the seed pods in boiling water for about 10 minutes. Add a bit of honey, and you've got an eye-opening way to start the day.

ENERGY EXERCISES

Exercise not only strengthens your body so it can better withstand the daily rigors of stress and activity, it also increases your metabolism and blood flow — two factors which keep you sharp and alert.

All over the world, people use various exercise techniques to help maximize overall health and well being. We especially recommend yoga and t'ai chi, because everyone can benefit from these energizing workouts that are easy on the body.

T'AI CHI

T'ai chi is another gentle exercise technique from the Far East. T'ai chi practitioners move through a series of poses, like a slow, languid dance. Though it was originally developed as a way for Bhuddist monks to protect themselves in the wilderness, t'ai chi is more important as a way to achieve mental peace and inner focus.

Like yoga, t'ai chi strives to balance the energy flow in the body. And, indeed, studies done in China report that people who practice this ancient martial art have increased resistance to stress, greater mental acuity and better physical conditioning.

YOGA

The first recorded mention of yoga dates back to the second century B.C. in the Yoga Sutras, writings attributed to an Indian scholar and physician named Patanjali. Since then, this combination of breath control, meditation and gentle exercise has helped people worldwide attain greater peace, increased energy and physical strength.

Yoga is based on the premise that prana (life energy) flows through the body. By controlling the physical manifestation of prana — breathing — you can control your energy.

Here's a simple yoga breathing exercise that can show you just how energizing breath control can be: Sit in a relaxed position, letting your arms dangle at your sides. Close your eyes. Now, breathe in through your nose for a count of 4. Breathe deeply, trying to fill your lungs. Hold that breath for a count of 7. Then, exhale loudly through your mouth, pursing your lips and blowing for a count of 8. You'll feel a brief "high" as your body floods with oxygen. We go into greater detail about yoga on page 6.

LONGEVITY

History and legend are full of tales of great adventurers and leaders who searched for eternal youth. As far back as 2000 B.C., the Babylonian epic of Gilgamesh tells the story of a great hero who searched the world for the secret of immortality. An ancient Sumerian story tells the tale of Adapa, a fisherman who gained wisdom from Ea, the God of Water who discovered the "bread and water" of life during his travels. About a thousand years later in far off China, the great emperor Ch'in Shih Huang Ti (the same ruler who ordered the building of the Great Wall) nearly ruined his empire while he searched in vain for immortality. Alexander the Great was said to have searched for the River of Immortality in India. And when Ponce de Leon came to the Americas and settled in what was to become Puerto Rico, he searched far and wide for the legendary Fountain of Youth, a miraculous spring said to be hidden in the hills of Bimini.

Obviously, all these quests have one thing in common — they failed. If there's one thing that we can learn from history it's that there is no one secret to long life and good health. Longevity doesn't come from some magic herb, hidden spring, or secret substance but from a combination of a healthy diet, mental and physical exercise, and a lifestyle free of age-accelerating habits. In this chapter, we'll examine some of the steps you can take to live longer — and better. Remember, the search for the secret to longevity has never been a search simply for eternal life. It has been the search for eternal, vigorous, healthy youth.

LIVING LONGER, FEELING BETTER

Whatever the reason, Americans are living longer. During the 1980s, the number of centenarians (people over 100 years old) grew 160 percent from the previous decade. Experts predict that this trend will continue — that by 2040, there will be 20 to 40 million people in the U.S. older than 85, and 500,000 to

1 million people over 100 years old by the year 2050.

Why are we living longer? One of the biggest reasons is that we are taking better care of ourselves when we are well, and medical science is taking better care of us when we are sick. In the past when somebody died, it was often said that they died of "old age." Now we know that many of those deaths were caused by killers like cancer, heart disease and stroke. Knowing what's killing us is half the battle — once we know how we die, we can figure out what we have to do to live longer.

We are also feeling and looking better as we get older. The exercise craze of the past couple of decades hasn't just affected younger people — older folks are getting into fitness as well. These days you're just as likely to see seniors exercising as twenty- and thirty-somethings — a trend that is keeping us healthy longer. Also, we are learning more about how to look healthier by using a variety of natural treatments that keep our skin fresh, our hair healthy and our smiles bright!

EAT YOURSELF YOUNG

In his book, *Complete Nutrition*, Israeli doctor Michael Sharon says it best: "Good eating habits ... improve health and slow down the aging process." Every day, new medical findings agree that the biggest factor for longevity is a good, healthy diet.

One of the best ways to find out how to use diet to live longer is to look at societies where longevity is common. The Hunza of the Himalayas, the Vilabamba of Ecuador, the Mayan Indians of the Yucatan, and people from remote regions of Bulgaria all have more than their fair share of members who live beyond 100 years old. Not only do natives of these cultures live longer, most of them are free from many of the ailments that plague more industrialized societies — cancer, ulcers, indigestion, tooth decay and senility.

What's their secret? It looks like a high-fiber, low-fat diet that's short on calories and long on nutrition is what we need to live longer. Eating for longevity is easy as long as you load up on fresh fruits and vegetables, eat lots of grains, a good amount of non-meat proteins (including tofu, beans and fish), and supplement your diet with some of nature's youth-boosters.

NATURE'S YOUTH-BOOSTER FOODS

While a good diet is essential to maintain good health, there are some super age-fighter foods that you can add to your diet to further reduce the effects of aging. Some work because they're high in essential nutrients which battle age-related diseases like cancer and high blood pressure. Others work because they contain amino acids which boost mental and metabolic function. And still others are good because they contain substances to boost the immune system and help eliminate dangerous free radical molecules linked to aging.

VEGETABLES

Naturapathic doctors, health specialists and longevity experts all agree that a diet high in veggies can keep you young by supplying vitamins, minerals and fiber in tasty packages. One word of caution, though. Make sure that the vegetables you buy are fresh and that you wash them thoroughly before eating to eliminate any pesticide residue. Whenever possible, buy organically grown produce.

BEANS

A staple of many indigenous peoples around the world, beans are not only good for your heart, they help provide much-needed fiber, protein and complex carbohydrates for general nutrition. As an added bonus, beans are a leading source of phytochemicals and protease inhibitors — high-powered anti-cancer agents.

If one particular organ can really benefit from the addition of beans to your diet, it is your colon. In studies at the University of California, Berkeley, Dr. Sharon Fleming, called by some the "dean of bean researchers," found that beans stimulated colon bacteria to give off volatile short-chain fatty acids which lower cholesterol, reduce blood pressure and lessen the risk of colon cancer.

BROCCOLI

Fresh, raw broccoli is a great source of sulforaphane, a substance that's been shown to reduce the growth of breast tumors in mice. If you prefer not to eat your broccoli raw, microwave it with a bit of water to retain the maximum amount of sulforaphane. There's not much sulforophane left in steamed, boiled or frozen broccoli.

Another super benefit of broccoli is that it's loaded with beta-carotene, as well as vitamins A and C. Beta-carotene (also found in carrots and other orange or dark-green vegetables) helps fight cancer while warding off the effects of ultra-violet radiation. The A and C vitamins also help fight cancer and infections. If your're a smoker (and we sincerely hope you're not), eat lots of broccoli — beta-carotene and vitamin A have both been shown to help your body resist lung cancer.

BRUSSELS SPROUTS

Looking like little cabbages, these tasty vegetables pack a big punch against cancer. Dr. Lee Wattenberg, a professor at the University of Minnesota Medical School, was the first to discover that Brussels sprouts, along with cabbage and broccoli, are chock-full of substances called indoles — potent preventers of cancer. These vegetables put your body's natural detoxification mechanisms into high gear, helping to clean out the toxic substances that accumulate and cause cancer. In seven of the largest-scale cancer studies done in Greece, Norway, Japan, Israel and the U.S., Brussels sprouts were shown again and again to fight colon cancer, a leading cause of death in older men.

GARLIC

Garlic is a real wonder. Not only can you use it to flavor nearly every food (some people even make garlic ice cream!) it can add years to your life because it fights infection, reduces the risk of cancer, thins the blood, stimulates the immune system and even reduces blood pressure.

At the Bombay Hospital Research Center in India, doctors found that patients who ate large amounts of garlic had reduced rates of blood clotting. Additional tests in India revealed that garlic could drop blood cholesterol levels by almost 100 points in 2 months! And in Bulgaria, researchers found that garlic can lower blood pressure by over 20 points when eaten regularly.

Both Chinese and Japanese doctors regularly prescribe garlic to reduce blood pressure. Cancer also seems to bow down before the power of garlic. Back in 1952, Russian scientists found that garlic was a potent tumor-fighter. More recently, Japanese researchers found that when mice with breast cancer were injected with garlic extracts, their cancer was reduced.

ONION

The humble onion is an excellent age-fighter. Studies done on Bulgarians (who consume some of the highest quantities of onions in the world) show onions can lower cholesterol, thin the blood and reduce blood pressure. One of the keys to a healthy life is a healthy heart, and onions lead the way.

ORIENTAL MUSHROOMS:
SHIITAKE, OYSTER, STRAW, ENOKI AND TREE-EAR

The Chinese symbol for Shoulau, the god of longevity, is a walking stick with a mushroom on the top. And they couldn't have picked a better symbol — more and more evidence shows that Oriental mushrooms, particularly the shiitake, are a real boon to longevity. Japanese studies, along with American know-how, have shown that shiitake mushrooms contain a substance called lentinan, a long-chain sugar that prevents viral infections. Lentinan stimulates the immune system to pump out interferon, a substance which works wonders against cancer and infections. On top of that, shiitake mushrooms have been shown to lower blood cholesterol by over 30 percent.

Other Oriental mushrooms — the tree ear, enoki, oyster and straw mushrooms — also have beneficial effects. Tree ear mushrooms have been shown to fight heart disease and stroke by reducing the threat of blood clots. Enoki mushrooms, a stringy mushroom that looks like a strand of spaghetti with a little cap, seems to stimulate the immune system. And, when combined with oyster and straw mushrooms, tree ears and enokis reduced the rate of tumor growth in laboratory rats.

FRUITS

When it comes to taste and health benefits, few foods can top fruits. Fresh oranges, lemons, mangos, papayas and bananas are loaded with vitamin C and other nutrients which help keep you young. On top of that, the fiber in fruit can help lower your cholesterol and strengthen your immune system. The best thing is, because they're so sweet and taste so good, fruits are one natural "medicine" you won't mind taking.

CITRUS

The biggest claim to fame for citrus is that it's got lots of vitamin C, an antioxidant vitamin that's been shown to fight off colds and ward off cancer, as well as protect against the ravages of alcoholism and smoking. Discovered by Hungarian scientist Albert Szent-Gyorgi in 1936, this vitamin is an invaluable part of the diet. Citrus fruits are also loaded with bioflavonoids —

cancer fighting chemicals that are concentrated in the peel and white "pith" of these fruits.

PAPAYAS, MANGOS, BANANAS

Exotic and super-sweet, tropical fruits have many anti-aging benefits. Bananas are full of magnesium, a compound shown to protect circulatory function. Eating a banana a day is also a great way to get pectin, a water-soluble fiber which can help prevent hypoglycemia and blood-sugar swings.

Papayas are loaded with enzymes which can help increase the rate of metabolic action in the body. These enzymes help the body fight off infections, while strengthening the immune system and reducing the effects of allergies.

Mangos are also high in enzymes, and they've got something else that papayas don't — high quantities of phytochemical bioflavonoids. Produced when the plant grabs energy from the sun, phytochemicals act as antioxidants and immune system boosters.

SEAWEED

Once thought of as a strange ingredient in Japanese food or as a nuisance to avoid while beachcombing, seaweed is now coming into its own as a youth tonic. Not only is it effective for fighting the ravages of time on the human body, but as seaweed works its way into the western diet, it is becoming appreciated for its good taste.

KUMBU, HIJIKI, ARAME, WAKAME

These seaweeds are staples of the Japanese diet. Even though they all may look different, they've got one thing in common — they're great sources of alginic acid. Studies at the Montreal Children's Hospital in Canada have shown that this naturally occurring polymer binds toxic heavy metals accumulated in the colon and helps eliminate them from the body.

LAMINARIA

The brown seaweed called laminaria has been a long-time staple of Japanese folk medicine with good reason. In Japanese studies during the 1960s, when laboratory rabbits were fed extracts from this seaweed, their blood pressure went down.

CARRAGEENAN

This is one type of seaweed that you've probably eaten. You don't eat seaweed, you say? Read your labels — carrageenan is commonly used as a thickening agent in ice cream and other foods. While you probably won't be doing yourself any favors by loading up on ice cream, eating carrageenan by itself has been shown to work against ulcers and as an anti-coagulant.

SPIRULINA

A spirulina algae plant is barely large enough to be seen with the naked eye — but put a few million of them together in a pond and you've got a ready food source. Spirulina was discovered by Belgian botanist Jean Leonard when he noticed that African tribesmen were gathering and eating it from Lake Chad. Later investigation revealed that this "pond scum" called spirulina is high in nutrients and rich in protein.

According to Japanese studies, spirulina is a wonderful rejuvenator and a potent energy-booster. It can stabilize blood sugar, help fight hepatitis, and even soothe ulcers. And if you are hoping to prolong your life by shedding a few pounds, spirulina capsules taken before meals will help trigger your body's "full" mechanism, making you want to eat less.

YOGURT

Probably one of the best-known age-busters on the planet, yogurt has been with us for thousands of years. Legend has it that it was discovered by the Old Testament prophet Abraham, who received the secret of yogurt making from an angel.

One of yogurt's main benefits is that it helps replensih normal colon flora, restoring digestive function and normalizing bowel action. This does wonders for both constipation and diarrhea — something few commercial stomach remedies can claim. In addition, yogurt is loaded with seven natural antibiotic substances, which help ward off infection and disease.

French studies have revealed that yogurt can also help protect against cancer. One 1986 study showed that women who ate yogurt had a much lower rate of breast cancer than women who ate large quantities of other dairy products.

To make sure the yogurt you buy is healthful, look for evidence on the label that it contains active acidophilus cultures, not just that it was made with them. Some yogurt is heated after packaging, and this heat kills the very bacteria that makes it beneficial.

TOFU & OTHER SOYBEAN PRODUCTS

Once thought of just as a meat substitute, tofu is gaining acceptance as a warrior in the battle for longevity. A cheese-like substance made from the curd of processed soybeans, tofu is not only a low-fat meat substitute, it also helps lower cholesterol levels in the blood while supplying copious amounts of bioflavonoids, which protect against cancer. Miso, a paste made from soybeans that is eaten frequently in Japan, has been shown to reduce the stomach cancer rates in Japanese women by over 30 percent. As an added benefit, soybeans have been shown to replace estrogen, an important consideration for older women going though menopause.

FISH

As little as 1 ounce of fish per day can lower your risk of heart disease by over half! Long recognized as a healthy source of protein, fish really can help lengthen your life. Studies on the diets of Eskimos found that the omega-3 fatty acids found in the fish they eat helps keep their rates of heart disease far below what it might otherwise be.

These fatty acids also do wonders for people suffering from arthritis. Dr. Joel M. Kremer, a professor at New York Medical College, found that daily doses of fish oil helped lessen the joint pain and fatigue of his arthritis patients. It turns out that fish oils interfere with the body's production of leukotriene B4, an agent which triggers swelling and pain.

Studies at the Massachusetts Institute of Technology indicate that fish can help keep you mentally alert as you age because it contains large amounts of the amino acid called tyrosine. This substance really helps kick your brain into high gear because it triggers the production of norepinephine and dopamine.

OATS

You have no doubt heard a lot of hype over the past few years concerning the benefits of oat-bran in your diet, but you may not know why oats are good for you. Not only do they provide water-soluble fiber that can help lower cholesterol, but they are also a great source of fiber for fighting intestinal problems, regulating blood sugar, and even reducing the incidence of cancer.

OLIVE OIL

The health of the people in Mediterranean countries is a great testament to the heart-smart benefits of olive oil. People have been using olive oil for so long, no one knows exactly where or when they first began. However records show that as long ago as 1200 B.C., King Ramsees II of Egypt used it to heal almost everything. Ramsees may have gone a little overboard, but he was on the right track.

People in Crete eat more olive oil than any others in the world. And they also have one of the world's lowest incidences of heart disease and cancer. You don't have to be a Nobel prize-winning scientist to see the connection. Olive oil is so good, in fact, that a recent study at the University of Minnesota showed that in a sample of over 2,300 men from around the world, those that consumed olive oil as their main source of fat had much lower rates of death by heart disease.

Olive oil's main benefit is that it lowers "bad" LDL cholesterol, while raising the blood levels of "good" HDL cholesterol. It also thins the blood, reducing the risk of clots and strokes. In addition, the 1,000 plus chemical compounds found in olive oil have been shown to reduce many of the effects of a high-fat diet. Dr. Bruno Berra, a professor at the University of Milan in Italy found that one olive oil chemical called cycloarthanol neutralizes the absorption of cholesterol in the bloodstream — so much so that 1 tablespoon of olive oil negated the cholesterol-raising effects of 2 whole eggs.

GINKGO

Ginkgo biloba is a tree that has existed for over 200 million years — a "living fossil." Buddhists used to consider it holy, and for good reason — recent research has discovered that ginkgo extracts really do help reduce the effects of aging on the brain.

Discovered by German Engelbert Kaempfer in 1690 and later exported to Europe, ginkgo is one longevity secret that seems to grow almost everywhere. In fact, it's become a common plant on many city streets because its hardiness allows it to grow under very adverse conditions.

What's the secret? Ginkgo contains the substances ginkgohereroside and proanthocyanidine, substances that are powerful free-radical scavengers which protect brain cell membranes. In a recent German study, patients suffering from chronic cerebral insufficiency were given ginkgo for a year. At the end of the trial, it was found that symptoms such as short-term memory loss, insomnia and headaches had been reduced substantially. If you want to try it for yourself, ginkgo extract capsules are now available in many health food stores.

BREWER'S YEAST

This isn't the same yeast that makes your bread fluffy. Brewer's yeast is a by-product of brewing that is a great source of B vitamins, which have been shown to combat many of the problems of aging by helping to strengthen the body and quicken the mind. It's especially useful for liver problems, particularly cirrhosis of the liver brought on by alcoholism. In addition, brewer's yeast can help perk you up, often relieving fatigue, depression, constipation and irritability — symptoms suffered by many older people. Brewer's yeast is also very high in protein, a big plus for bedridden or sickly folks.

TEA

For at least 4,000 years, the people of China have been using tea as a medicine. Tea was also used by the Greeks as a cure for colds and bronchitis. And both the Russians and the French dosed themselves with tea to treat headaches, digestive problems and high blood pressure.

What can it do for you? In India, scientists have found that tannin, the bitter substance in tea, kills both herpes and polio, and doctors in Russia often prescribe tea for hepatitis and dysentery.

In 1985, Japanese scientists announced the exciting news that epigallo-catechin gallate, one of the tannins in tea, helps protect against cell mutation and cancer. Of all the teas, Japanese green tea seems to be the most effective against cancer. In a Canadian study, researchers found that the anti-cancer properties stem from the fact that tea can stop the formation of nitrosamines, a group of powerful cancer-causing chemicals.

WORK THOSE YEARS OFF

Aside from watching your diet, leading an active life is the next most important factor for longevity. Regular exercise, be it a 10-mile run or just a daily stroll in the park, will keep your body going for many, many years.

Exercise makes you feel years younger by speeding up your metabolism, lowering your weight and your blood pressure, and making your heart stronger. Once you've strengthened your heart with exercise, it doesn't have to work as hard to pump blood. Since your heart is the main "machine" in your body, by reducing the wear and tear on it, you add years to your life. A healthy heart that beats 60 to 70 times per minute is far less likely to wear out as one which has to work at 85 to 90 beats per minute.

Since study after study has shown that heart disease and high blood pressure are the leading causes of death in the U.S., it's obvious that with a stronger heart you'll live longer.

Regular exercise is good for your head, too. It lowers stress and prevents depression — common problems among older people. Stress itself can wreak physical havoc on the body (see the chapter on relaxation, page 73), and depression can dramatically reduce the quality of your life. Exercise releases endorphins, your brain's natural painkillers, that give you a lift you just can't get any other way. It raises your spirits, clears your head and boosts your mental functioning.

Adult-onset diabetes is a common problem in older people — a problem that can shorten your life. Here, too, regular exercise can help. Studies among diabetics or people with a pre-diabetic disorder have shown that exercise can improve the body's efficient use of insulin.

It can also help prevent many of the aches and pains that come with aging. By strengthening your musculature, you also strengthen your body's resistance to gravity, which can really take the strain off of your joints and back. In addition, studies have shown that regular exercise can be helpful for people with arthritis by reducing joint pain and swelling.

ESTABLISH GOOD HABITS FOR A LONG, HAPPY LIFE

To extend your life "to the max," follow our diet and exercise recommendations and reduce stress, either by changing your lifestyle or by taking up a meditative exercise such as yoga or t'ai chi. The effects of stress on your body can shorten your life. In addition, when you're stressed out, your body releases hormones called glucocorticoids, which we know play a big role in the aging process. Cushing's disease, one example of a problem that results from excess glucocorticoids, causes aging problems such as osteoporosis to appear early in life.

If you smoke, stop. There's nothing worse. Not only does smoking wreck your lungs, it also strains your heart and your immune system, making you more susceptible to disease.

Finally, drink alcohol in moderation. Many studies have shown that drinking a glass of wine a day has great benefits for your heart. However, too much alcohol, especially in women, is a major source of liver damage, cancer and vitamin deficiencies. That's all there is to it!

So, start now — today — to establish these good health habits that really will help you live longer, better and happier.

Nutrition

The human body is an extremely complex but resilient machine that can function for a long time on just about anything it can digest. However, to be truly healthy, the body needs to be fed a wide variety of the right foods. Good nutrition can mean the difference between an unnaturally short life filled with health problems — and a long life filled with energy and vitality.

The best way to understand the hows and whys of good eating is to examine what nutritionists call the macronutrients. These substances are the main building blocks of the body

Protein

Protein is the stuff that holds us together. Structurally, proteins form your muscles, your skin tissues and your ligaments. Internally, proteins make up your hormones, antibodies, blood and enzymes. Every tissue that breaks down and needs repair needs protein — and since the body is constantly in need of repair and raw materials for growth, protein is essential to good health. In fact, within a year, 98 percent of all the atoms in your body are replaced.

Proteins are constructed of amino acids, complex molecules essential for nearly every body function. To work properly, proteins must be "complete," containing all eight essential amino acids. Most complete proteins come from animals — meat, fish, eggs and dairy products. However, to make complete proteins from plant materials, you need to eat them in combination. Beans and rice or beans and corn are classics, and versions of these complete protein dishes can be found in nearly every culture — Latin America, China and the Middle East for example.

Carbohydrates

To produce energy, the body must burn carbohydrates. Simple carbohydrates (like sugar) are burned up quickly, because the body can metabolize them into energy almost immediately. That's where the "rush" in a "sugar rush" comes from — that quick, intense burst of energy is the sugar being burned off in the body. Unfortunately, as you know if you've ever experienced a "sugar rush," that energy is quickly depleted. On the other hand, complex carbohydrates — bread, pasta, potatoes and grains — metabolize more slowly than their sugary counterparts, making them long-term sources of energy.

That's why it's so important to eat a big breakfast that's loaded with carbohydrates. Not only do whole grains and cereals give you a wake-up boost in the morning, they stick with you until lunch, breaking down slowly and keeping your blood sugar on an even keel.

FATS

Fat is the most concentrated source of food energy available, packing in 8 calories per gram — twice the amount of energy in carbohydrates or proteins. Fats, which stimulate the gallbladder, are essential to hormone production and act as a transport mechanism for vitamins throughout the body. When fats are broken down in the body, they produce glycerol and fatty acids that prevent blood clots, regulate metabolism and control hormone action.

So what's so bad about fats? It's not that fats are bad — the problem is that we eat too many of the wrong kinds of fats. Fats basically come in two forms — saturated and unsaturated. Saturated fats — lard, butter and tallow, for example — come mainly from animals and are less easily metabolized by the body. Unsaturated fats — like olive oil, canola oil and corn oil — come from plant sources and are more readily processed. Because unsaturated fats are so easily broken down and used by the body, they're not as likely to be stored as body fat.

You need fat for your body to function. On the other hand, increased fat intake can cause obesity, heart disease and cancer. So use all fats in moderation, sticking to unsaturated vegetable oils whenever possible. Canola and olive oil are two of the healthiest, and olive oil has the added benefit of helping to reduce blood cholesterol and blood pressure.

FOODS FOR HEALTHY LIVING

A balanced, low-fat, high-fiber diet can do more for you than provide nourishment for your body. Around the world, many foods have been used for centuries as medicines, both to treat acute symptoms and to help stave off illness and disease.

Cancer-Reducing Foods

Some of the most exciting research in food is being done in the realm of cancer-reducing nutrition. Scientists are learning that by eating foods high in phytochemicals and beta-carotene, we can substantially reduce the risk of this killer disease.

Broccoli

Broccoli is the rising star on the cancer front. Studies done at the Roswell Park Memorial Institute in Buffalo, New York have shown that eating lots of broccoli can substantially lower the risk of cervical cancer in women. Additional research has shown that men who smoke and eat dark-green vegetables (like broccoli) have half the lung cancer risk of smokers who don't eat this edible flower.

Spinach

A study by Dr. Richard Shekelle, a scientist at the University of Texas, showed that smokers can really benefit from eating spinach. His research found that people who eat spinach (and other foods high in beta-carotene) have eight times less chance of developing lung cancer as people who don't eat these foods. In a more recent study, Italian researchers found that spinach can block the formation of nitrosamines — some of the most potent cancer-causing chemicals. Even back in 1969, spinach was found to be good stuff. Japanese scientists discovered that spinach could lower blood cholesterol by converting it into a substance called coprostanol, which the body easily eliminates.

Cabbage

In 1931, German scientists discovered that rabbits fed cabbage could survive lethal doses of radiation by helping them resist toxins that ordinarily cause cells to go from healthy to cancerous. In the 1950s, scientists in France replicated the earlier research of the Germans, and during the U.S. government's extensive nuclear experimentation in the late 1950s, they too found that cabbage could help animals survive otherwise deadly radiation exposure.

In studies in Japan, Greece and the U.S., cabbage has also been shown to fight off colon cancer. The Japanese discovered that people who eat large portions of cabbage every day have the lowest overall death rate, and Greek research has indicated that adding vegetables like cabbage to your diet can reduce your risk of colon cancer by over 800 percent.

KALE

Kale is a potent source of beta-carotene and chlorophyll — two of the best cancer-reducing substances available in food. As little as ½ cup of kale a day can reduce your risk of cancer.

BRUSSELS SPROUTS

Of all the cancer-reducing foods, Brussels sprouts are probably the most effective. They are loaded with beta-carotene and chlorophyll. In a recent study, animals who ate Brussels sprouts and were then given massive doses of cancer-causing chemicals were far less likely to develop cancer than animals who weren't fed the sprouts.

And in Greece, Norway and Japan, studies have shown that people who eat the most green vegetables (including Brussels sprouts) have lower incidence of cancer. Scientists don't know exactly why Brussels sprouts are so effective, but they suspect chemicals called glucosinolates, found in high levels in this vegetable, are responsible.

CARROTS

In studies done by Dr. Richard Shekelle and epidemiologist Regina Ziegler, carrots were shown to not only help reduce the lung-cancer risk of smokers, but to reduce the risk of cancer in ex-smokers and people exposed to cigarette smoke as well. Beta-carotene seems to be the key. Found in high concentrations in carrots, this nutrient seems to stop the formation of cancer in its later stages. That's why carrots are so good for ex-smokers — the beta-carotene keeps cancers that may have started from developing into full-blown tumors.

YOGURT

At the turn of the century, Russian biologist Ilich Metchnikoff asserted that the secret to long life enjoyed by rural Bulgarians (some of the longest-lived people in the world) is that they eat large amounts of yogurt. More recently, research in France has shown that women who eat yogurt (with live yogurt cultures) are much less likely to develop breast cancer than women who don't eat yogurt. And in studies conducted all over the world — Japan, Italy,

Switzerland and Poland — people who eat yogurt show less incidence of disease and infection.

Yogurt may help lower the risk of cancer by boosting the immune system, the body's natural defense against disease.

HEART SMART FOODS

Reducing fat and increasing fiber can help lower cholesterol, reduce blood pressure and keep blood clots from forming. And, there are some foods that you can add to your diet to further reduce your risk of heart disease.

FISH

Fish is so good for your heart that some people have called it an "ocean-going aspirin" because of its anticoagulant effect on the blood.

The important ingredients in fish are omega-3 fatty acids, substances found in great abundance in fatty, cold-water fish. These fatty acids help reduce your body's production of prostaglandins and leukotrienes, two hormone-like chemicals which can trigger blood clots, immune reactions and inflammation. In addition, these same fatty acids can reduce the formation of arterial plaques — deposits of cholesterol on the walls of the arteries that can lead to high blood pressure, strokes and heart attacks. Fish oil also thins the blood to protect against potentially harmful blood clots.

GARLIC

Many studies have shown that garlic can significantly lower blood pressure. For example, research carried out in California showed that garlic extracts can lower bad LDL cholesterol and raise good HDL cholesterol. And studies on the Jain vegetarians in India showed that their

While raw garlic is definitely better for you than cooked garlic, garlic that has been cooked still maintains many of its health benefits. Try roasting garlic with olive oil to turn the pungent garlic cloves into a mellow spread for toasted bread.

By the way, eating garlic doesn't have to give you bad breath. Many people report that eating parsley with their garlic helps. One reason may be that parsley is high in chlorophyll, a natural odor-fighter. You can also take garlic in tablet form.

Rancid Oils: An Overlooked Danger

Rancid oil not only looks and smells bad, it's potentially toxic. Among other things, it can cause:

- vitamin E deficiency
- stomach ulcers
- intestinal ulcers
- digestive tract damage

Oxygen and light break down oil. So, store your cooking oils in a cool, dark place. And, if you must fry your food, don't reuse the oil. Heat makes it become more saturated, reducing the health benefits even of unsaturated vegetable oils. Even worse, some studies have shown that when heated, cooking oil can degrade into cancer-causing compounds.

high consumption of garlic keeps their blood cholesterol levels over 75 points below those of people who don't eat garlic.

OLIVE OIL

Recent research has shown that people who eat olive oil as their main source of fat have a much lower incidence of heart disease than people who don't use olive oil. This is one of the most unsaturated oils you can buy. That's why it is less likely to bring on many of the problems that saturated fats can, including obesity, high blood pressure and high cholesterol. In fact, olive oil does the exact opposite. In study after study, it has been shown to actually lower blood cholesterol levels, lower blood pressure and thin the blood to prevent clots and strokes.

KELP & OTHER SEAWEED

Doctors in Japan have long used an extract of the Laminaria seaweed called Kombu to lower blood pressure. And recent studies have confirmed this wisdom by showing that seaweed extracts contain histamines, substances which have been shown to be anti-hypertensive (blood pressure lowering). During the mid-1980s, scientists also discovered that seaweed can help protect against excess sodium, a leading cause of high blood pressure.

DIGESTIVE SYSTEM HELPERS

Digestion begins when you take a bite. As you chew, saliva is released in your mouth, softening the food and beginning to break it down with enzymes. Then, when you swallow, the chewed food travels through the esophagus into your stomach, where your body begins the real work of extracting nutrients. In the stomach, gastric juices consisting of pepsin and hydrochloric acid break down complex foods into simpler compounds. At the same time, your stomach muscles begin to pump, mixing the food with gastric juice and moving it toward the small intestine. This process usually takes 3 to 5 hours.

In the small intestine, bile is secreted from the gallbladder, and pancreatic liquids are secreted from the pancreas, mixing with the partially digested food. Fats and sugars are extracted and allowed to absorb into the bloodstream.

Finally, after most of the nutrients are extracted in the small intestine, what's left of your meal moves on to the colon or large intestine, where water is absorbed, and the solid waste is eventually eliminated.

A diet high in fiber and low in fat keeps the digestive system moving by speeding absorption and quickening the rate at which wastes and toxins are removed from your body.

YOGURT

Yogurt is loaded with prostaglandins — natural ulcer antacids. In fact, prostaglandins are so effective against ulcers that a substance called Prostaglandin E has been used as an anti-ulcer drug by many orthodox doctors. Eating yogurt containing active cultures can also help restore your intestine's balance of healthy bacteria that prevent diarrhea.

BRAN

From ancient times up until recently, most people got their bran naturally from the foods they ate. Grains were rarely milled to the point of eliminating the bran. In fact, the refining process that got rid of the fibrous outer husk was so complex only royalty and the very rich (often one and the same) could afford white flour. The common people had to subsist on brown bread made from whole grains. (Little did they know they were getting the better end of the health bargain.)

Bran contains complex carbohydrates, protein, fats, vitamins and (most important for digestive health) some forms of cellulose. Because cellulose is indigestible by the body, when you eat it, it moves through you, taking waste along with it. Indeed, rural Africans, who eat a particularly high amount of cellulose and other fibers, have a much lower rate of degenerative diseases than Americans. Fiber helps prevent hemorrhoids, varicose veins, constipation, diverticulosis, high blood pressure, colon cancer and heart disease — and it has been shown to help assuage the effects of diabetes.

BEANS

In research carried out at the University of California, Berkeley, scientist Sharon Fleming found out that men who were fed large quantities of beans were less susceptible to diseases of the colon, including cancer. Not only did the fiber in the beans help the digestive system, but the vegetable also seemed to stimulate the colon to produce substances that help lower cholesterol and reduce blood pressure.

Beans don't have to be a gas

Many people avoid beans because they tend to produce so much intestinal gas. However, when properly prepared, beans can be as gas-free as any other vegetable.

The secret to gasless beans is to soak them for a long time before cooking. Put dry beans in enough water to cover and let them sit overnight. In the morning, you'll have soft beans — ready to cook and free of undesirable flatulence-producing side effects.

ESSENTIAL EXTRAS: VITAMINS & MINERALS

As foods become more processed, they often become stripped of many of the naturally occurring nutrients our ancestors were able to get from their food. In addition, even though we may boost our intake of fresh fruits and vegetables, more and more of them are being grown synthetically in over-farmed soil that just doesn't contain enough minerals. As a result, many people these days suffer from vitamin and mineral deficiencies that they may not even be aware of. Please refer to the chart on page 50 for food sources of vitamins and minerals.

VITAMINS: THE BIG FOUR

Vitamins help produce enzymes, and enzymes help our bodies convert food to energy and carry out vital biological processes. Without the proper amount of these essential nutrients, we cannot be nourished by our food. Vitamins also help regulate how the body maintains itself and keeps on running. And some vitamins have been shown to be helpful in fighting serious disease.

VITAMIN A

Vitamin A was discovered by American scientist Elmer McCollum in 1913. This was one of the landmarks in modern nutritional science. For the first time, researchers made a link between diet and health.

Vitamin A is fat-soluble, which means it builds up in the fatty tissues of the body and is not readily excreted. In nature, vitamin A can be found in fish oils and liver (in the form of retinol) and in yams, leafy vegetables and yellow fruits (as carotene).

Vitamin A is important for fighting infections, boosting your immune system and maintaining healthy skin. It is also essential for maintaining good night vision.

B VITAMINS

So far, scientists have discovered 16 B vitamins, nutrients that help convert carbohydrates into energy. If you have a vitamin B deficiency, your body cannot process food effectively and you tend to be tired, constipated and sick to your stomach. In addition, vitamin B is essential for healthy skin and hair.

The B vitamins occur naturally in liver, wheat germ, bran and brewer's yeast. Green and yellow vegetables high in B vitamins are best eaten raw, because these vitamins are water-soluble, which means they are easily dissolved when boiled or steamed.

Vitamin B1, also called thiamin, can help lift your mood and stimulate your appetite. Vitamin B3 (niacin) can help maintain a strong constitution by boosting blood circulation, thinning the blood and lowering cholesterol while strengthening digestion. In fact, niacin acts so quickly on the circulatory system, that many people report a prickly flush that quickly spreads over the body and then subsides as the niacin is metabolized. Vitamin B5, also known as pantothenic acid, is known as the "longevity vitamin." An important

Vitamin Chart
Natural Health Secrets from Around the World

Vitamin or Nutrient	Benefits	Sources
Vitamin A	Reduces risk of measles; boosts immune system; helps wound healing; fights skin diseases	Apricots, asparagus, beans, carrots, cheddar cheese, citrus fruits, eggs, organ meats, peas, squash, yogurt
Vitamin B1 (Thiamin)	Maintains normal nervous system function; helps metabolize carbohydrates; protects against effects of alcoholism, depression, anxiety, stress	Beans, cold-water fish, corn, figs, grains, meat, nuts, pasta, peas, poultry, rice bran
Vitamin B2 (Riboflavin)	Helps protein metabolism; can relieve depression, anxiety, and stress disorders; helps maintain eyesight and healthy skin; may help heal carpal tunnel syndrome	Almonds, broccoli, cheese, fish, green leafy vegetables, meat, milk, potatoes, poultry, wheat germ, yogurt
Vitamin B3 (Niacin)	Lowers blood fat levels; helps maintain healthy nervous system	Brewer's yeast, fish, lean meat, nuts, organ meats, poultry
Vitamin B6	Used in most bodily functions; essential for forming prostaglandins (regulators of body processes); functions as a neurotransmitter, assisting nervous system and brain function; boosts immunity and cancer resistance; helps reduce side effects from oral contraceptives	Avocados, bananas, beans, bran, liver, poultry, salmon, shrimp, sunflower seeds, tuna, wheat germ, whole grain breads
Vitamin B12	Energizes the body; protects against cancer; helps various nervous disorders; keeps brain functioning at top condition	Beef, clams, cold-water fish, crabs, milk, liver, poultry, seafood
Vitamin B15	Helps eliminate body toxins; antioxidant action protects against cancer; lowers cholesterol; reduces hangover	Bran, brewer's yeast, brown rice, pumpkin seeds, sesame seeds, whole grains
Beta-carotene	Increases ability of immune system to fight disease; may reduce the risk of cancer (especially lung cancer)	Broccoli, brussels sprouts, carrots, grapefruit, green leafy vegetables, mango, papaya, squash

Vitamin Chart
Natural Health Secrets from Around the World

Vitamin or Nutrient	Benefits	Sources
Biotin	Good for skin; protects against eczema and dermatitis; helps hair growth and muscle strain	Brewer's yeast, brown rice, eggs, fruit, liver, milk, nuts
Vitamin C	Antioxidant; protects against cancer; may help kill viruses and colds; anti-histamine action helps allergies; helps build collagen to prevent wrinkles; boosts immune system; lowers cholesterol	Broccoli, cabbage, cantaloupe, citrus fruit, green leafy vegetables, peas, peppers, potatoes, strawberries, sweet potatoes, tomatoes, yams
Calcium	Builds bones; protects against osteoporosis; lowers blood pressure; reduces risk of heart disease; helps soothe leg cramps; good for skin tone	Beans, collards, figs, mackerel, milk and milk products, okra, sardines, soybeans, spinach, tofu, yogurt
Choline	Reduces cholesterol; improves neuro-transmitter activity; promotes memory and learning; good for kidney, liver, and heart; reduces symptoms of menopause; increases adrenaline synthesis	Bran, brewer's yeast, green leafy vegetables, organ meats, wheat germ
Chromium	Maintains blood sugar levels; helps sugar metabolism; helps burn fat; lowers high blood pressure; helps people lose weight	Meat, molasses, rice bran, shellfish, wheat germ
Copper	Prevents anemia; antihistamine; helps in the metabolism of Vitamin C; good for hair and skin	Legumes, molasses, prunes, seafood, soybeans
Vitamin D	Boosts immunity and helps protect against cancer; assists in the healing of psoriasis and osteoporosis	Herring, mackerel, milk, sardines, tuna

Vitamin Chart
Natural Health Secrets from Around the World

Vitamin or Nutrient	Benefits	Sources
Vitamin E	Helps treat neurological disorders, heart disease, breast disease, and pre-menstrual syndrome; may be useful in fighting the effects of aging	Green leafy vegetables, lima beans, nuts, rice bran, salmon, shrimp, soybeans, sunflower seeds, wheat bran, wheat germ
Folic Acid	Helps prevent birth defects; reduces cervical dysplasia in women who take oral contraceptives; improves mental function; stimulates the formation of red blood cells	Avocado, beans, cantaloupe, carrots, egg yolks, green leafy vegetables, liver, pumpkin, Torula yeast
Inositol	Aids nerve transmission; regulates enzyme activity in the body; good for skin tone; helps induce sleep and relieve anxiety	Brewer's yeast, cantaloupe, fruits, grains, molasses, organ meats, peanuts
Iodine	Reduces body fat; relieves anxiety and nervousness; increases energy; helps skin and hair; boosts immune system	Iodized salt, onions, seaweed
Vitamin K	Helps prevent bleeding; reduces risk of cancer; helps ward off osteoporosis	Broccoli, cabbage, green leafy vegetables, romaine lettuce, turnip greens
Pantothenic Acid	Prevents graying of hair; assists in the synthesis of important steroids and cholesterols; helps body metabolize nutrients; good for immune system	Beans, brewer's yeast, cod's roe, meat, molasses, nuts, organ meats, royal jelly, wheat germ, whole grains
Selenium	Works best in combination with Vitamin E; increases immune response; boosts energy and sex drive; helps protect against arthritis and multiple sclerosis; may prevent cancer	Brewer's yeast, nuts, onions, tuna, wheat germ
Zinc	Helps wounds heal; assists in the formation of blood; important for many metabolic functions which use enzymes; may prevent cancer and blindness; can help with arthritis	Beef, crab, dark poultry, fish, organ meats, oysters, pumpkin and squash seeds, wheat germ, yogurt

ingredient in that most famous of bee products, royal jelly, it is particularly good for the liver, kidney and adrenal glands.

One of the most important B vitamins is B12, first isolated in 1926 as a cure for anemia, but later found to be helpful for brain function, iron assimilation and childhood growth.

VITAMIN C

Vitamin C was first isolated in 1936 by Hungarian Albert Szent-Gyorgyi and was later championed by two-time Nobel Prize winner Linus Pauling. In addition to being an antioxidant, vitamin C boosts our immune system by increasing antibody function and raising levels of interferon, a substance that's been shown to reduce cancer risk. Megadoses of vitamin C (over 2,000 mg per day) can lower cholesterol by catalyzing the reaction that turns fats into bile acids.

Vitamin C supplements are readily available in the form of ascorbic acid tablets. You can also load up on vitamin C by increasing your intake of citrus fruits, especially oranges and limes. And when you do, be sure to eat some of the white pith that lines the rind. It's bitter, but it contains high levels of bioflavonoids, substances that can help reduce your cancer risk and increase the effects of vitamin C on your body.

VITAMIN E

Vitamin C is a good antioxidant, but research at the Shute Institute in Canada has indicated that vitamin E is three times better. By preventing the formation of damaging free radicals in your body, vitamin E can help protect against brain cell damage, anemia, immune diseases and DNA damage that leads to cancer or premature aging. Women going through menopause can especially benefit from vitamin E supplements because estrogen, often taken to lessen the symptoms of menopause, can cause vitamin E deficiencies.

Wheat germ is one of the best natural sources of this important vitamin. Available in most health food stores and supermarkets (in the cereal aisle), wheat germ can be sprinkled on food, baked into breads and cakes, and even eaten like breakfast cereal with milk. Other natural sources of vitamin E are green vegetables, whole grains, eggs and soybeans.

MINERALS: JUST A TRACE

Minerals help vitamins do their work in breaking down food. In addition, many of the basic chemical reactions that make our bodies run are dependent on these nutrients. While many fruits and vegetables grown today have lower amounts of minerals than the ones our grandparents ate, you can still get much of what you need by eating foods like wheat germ, brewer's yeast, alfalfa sprouts, bee pollen, seaweed, molasses and nuts. And, in fact, this is better than taking mineral supplements, because your body doesn't seem to absorb minerals taken in pill form as readily as minerals that you get in foods.

IRON

Iron is the most common trace mineral found in your body. It makes up the most important part of your red blood cells — hemoglobin, which transports oxygen around your system. Without iron, fatigue sets in, because your body processes "smother" from a lack of oxygen.

Iron supplements really can boost energy, especially in menstruating women who often lose as much as 10 to 15 mgs. of this mineral per day. Unfortunately, some of the best natural food sources of iron are organ meats (liver and kidneys), which can contain high levels of fats and contaminants. However, oats, peaches, raisins, molasses, beans and green leafy vegetables also provide needed iron — and extra fiber.

COPPER

Copper helps your system absorb iron while forming hemoglobin to oxygenate the body. In addition, copper aids in the production of enzymes, substances essential for food absorption and metabolic function.

Use copper supplements carefully, because slightly elevated amounts can cause a variety of illnesses. Depression, anxiety, high blood pressure and arthritis are common symptoms of excess copper. People who are especially susceptible to this condition are women taking birth control pills, smokers and people in areas with a lot of pollution. If you are in one of these high-risk groups, take zinc to help reduce your risk.

ZINC

Zinc is the second most abundant trace mineral in the body. Essential for growth and fertility, it is found in high amounts in raw oysters, fish, wheat germ, brewer's yeast, milk and beans.

Oysters have long been praised as an aphrodisiac, and because of their high zinc content, they may well be. Zinc is perhaps the most important mineral for sexual function, especially in men, where zinc is essential for proper prostate function. Just a 35 percent reduction in zinc levels can cause enlargement of the prostate — and a 66 percent reduction can lead to prostate cancer, one of the leading causes of cancer among men.

CHROMIUM

Until recently, few people knew about the need for chromium in the diet. Chromium is essential for the metabolism of glucose, and is also necessary for the metabolism and production of fatty acids and cholesterols. Recent studies have shown that diabetics and people with hypoglycemia are in dire need of chromium in their diets. And, in fact, the rise of adult-onset diabetes and hypoglycemia has been traced by some to the rising popularity of processed foods. When raw cane sugar is refined into white sugar, almost 93 percent of the chromium is removed. And when whole wheat flour is turned into white flour, almost 75 percent of the chromium is removed.

That's why it's important to eat a variety of whole, unrefined foods including molasses, wheat germ and "raw" sugar.

PANACEAS

History is filled with stories about the search for a magical cure. The ancient Greeks prayed to Panacea, the mythical daughter of the god of medicine, believing her touch could cure anything. During the Crusades, the great knight Fierabras was said to possess a soothing balsam which would heal all wounds. And, even up until a few hundred years ago, European alchemists searched for the Philosopher's Stone, which they believed would not only heal any ailment, but would also turn lead into gold. Although Panacea remains as mythical today as she was for the ancient Greeks, nature has provided us with some remarkable "cure-alls," that add considerably to our overall health and well-being.

Today, you don't have to look far to find the secret to health and longevity. Chances are you have some of the main ingredients in your own refrigerator. Garlic, onions, honey (and other bee products), ginger, ginseng, fish oils and aloe show up over and over again in folk remedies from all over the world and throughout history.

GARLIC AND ONIONS: ANCIENT CURES FOR TODAY'S ILLS

Cut into an onion or crush a clove of garlic. That pungent odor is allicin, the main chemical ingredient that makes these two humble roots such effective medicine. But allicin isn't the only beneficial substance in garlic and onions. Both contain thousands of healthy components that make them among the most valuable plants in the world.

A Call for Healing: The Garlic Hotline

If you want to find out more about what garlic can do for you, pick up the phone and call the Garlic Hotline at (800)330-5922. It was established by the Medical and Nutrition Information Center at Cornell University in New York.

A Recipe Against Infection

Using garlic to retard infection can be a safe and natural alternative to harsh chemical antiseptics. Here's how to make it:

With a sharp knife (or a garlic press), crush or finely mince several cloves of garlic into a bowl. Add 2 tablespoons of olive oil and stir. Cover the bowl and set aside to let the essence of garlic infuse the oil. When you're ready, strain the oil to remove the garlic bits and apply with an eyedropper to the infected area, or rub gently on a cut to promote healing.

CAUTION: *Make only enough garlic oil to use right away. Garlic loses its effectiveness if left sitting for too long.*

Babylonians first used garlic over 4,000 years ago, and knowledge of its healing powers quickly spread all over the ancient world. Greek Olympic athletes used it for quick energy, the Chinese prescribed it to lower blood pressure, and the Roman legions munched on it to sustain them over their long marches and to heal their battle wounds. In this century, French doctors during World War II used garlic on the battlefield to bandage injured soldiers and treat tuberculosis.

First and foremost, garlic is a strong antiseptic. Louis Pasteur, the 19th century French chemist known as one of the father's of modern medicine, reported that when he dropped a clove of garlic onto a plate of bacteria, the

What's a Clove of Garlic?

When we talk about garlic cloves, we're referring to the individual segments that make up a garlic bulb. Dr. Andrew Weil, author of the book *Natural Health, Natural Medicine,* tells the story of one of his patients who got "clove" and "bulb" confused:

I once told a patient with a sore throat to eat 2 cloves of raw garlic. He called me several days later to say that he had been cured, but that the treatment had been one of the hardest things he'd ever done. It turned out that he thought 'clove' meant the entire head.

deadly germs were inhibited. Since then, research has discovered that garlic also can retard harmful fungi, viruses and parasites.

Garlic can also help your blood by lowering your cholesterol. In 1990, Dr. Robert I-San Lin, one of the world's experts on the medical uses of garlic, reported this finding at the First World Congress on the Health Significance of Garlic and Garlic Constituents. Since then, other researchers have agreed with Dr. Lin's findings and have gone on to discover that garlic can lower blood triglyceride levels, too.

Onions, garlic's bigger cousins, have also been used since the dawn of time to fight colds, heal wounds, kill germs, and relieve intestinal disorders. Because they contain substances that draw out fluid and inhibit bacteria, they're great for burns, cuts and scrapes. And that's not all. Like garlic, onions have anti-oxidant qualities that can fight the cancer-causing free radicals in your

Bacteria, Smothered in Onions!

Since the 1500s, when onions were a primary treatment for burns and gunshot wounds, onion poultices have been used to promote healing and to protect against infection. If you burn yourself in the kitchen, why not just reach in the fridge and grab an onion for a soothing poultice?

To make an onion poultice, chop an onion very fine or grind it up in a food processor. Apply the chopped onion directly to the affected area, holding it in place with a soft cotton bandage. Every hour or so, chop some more onion and reapply, changing the bandage each time. Keep this up as long as you need relief.

Why does this work? Two reasons: The onion draws water away from the wound, which helps retard bacteria. Also, onions, like garlic, contain antiseptic compounds that inhibit germs on contact.

system. In fact, in Georgia, where more Vidalia onions are eaten than anywhere else in the U.S., researchers found a 65 percent lower rate of stomach cancer.

The same vapors that make you cry when you slice into an onion can soothe your sore throat and cough. So when you feel that first tickle of a sore throat coming on, chew an onion. If you've got a cough, try mixing some onion juice with honey — another one of our seven panaceas. This powerful combination acts as an expectorant.

Finally, onions are mild stimulants. Eating an onion can give you a burst of energy when you're feeling groggy by acting as a gentle stimulant — and onions have been used through the ages to restore sexual potency.

"BEE" HEALTHY WITH HONEY

Ever since the first caveman got up the courage to raid a swarming hive to gather honey, bees have helped us try to be healthier. Ancient literature is packed with passages praising the power of this liquid gold. The Bible, the Talmud and the Koran all mention honey, as do age-old writings from the Greeks, Romans and Slavs. And the benefit from bees doesn't stop with honey. Beehives are a veritable cornucopia of healing substances: bee pollen, royal jelly and bee propolis. While these products don't taste as good as honey, their healing properties are just as sweet.

HONEY

Until several hundred years ago, the only sweeteners used in Europe were honey and fruit juice. Then, when explorers discovered the New World, they also discovered sugar cane and began to refine sugar. Because sugar is easier to store, easier to ship, and doesn't spoil as quickly, it quickly pushed honey (with all its health benefits) to the back of the cupboard. Today, sugar is everywhere in the food we eat.

What's so bad about sugar? Everyone knows that too much sugar can make you fat and decay your teeth, but that may be the least of it. Recent research shows that when you eat sugar, it causes your pancreas to go into overdrive, pumping out insulin as a way of balancing the sugar in your bloodstream.

Is honey better? Bee-lieve it! Honey's sweetness comes from glycogen, which our bodies process much more slowly than regular table sugar. Honey is also loaded with nutrients: potassium, sulfur, sodium, phosphorus, magnesium, silica, copper, iron, maganese, enzymes, amino acids, B vitamins,

---

Honey Hotline

More information about the healing benefits of honey is just a (free!) phone call away. The National Honey Board Food Technology Program sponsors the Honey Hotline to answer all your questions. Call the hotline at (800)356-5941 or write to: National Honey Board Food Technology Program, P.O. Box 281525, San Francisco, CA 94128-1525.

vitamin C and nucleic acids. And, if you take calcium supplements, honey can help your body to absorb the calcium 25 percent more quickly — great for strong bones and teeth.

Honey is much more than a healthy sweetener. For thousands of years, it has been used as a soothing, antibacterial salve for wounds, sores and skin ulcers. During wartime, Greek, Roman, Assyrian, Chinese and Egyptian doctors took pots of honey with them to the battlefield to spread on wounded warriors' injuries. It turns out these ancient healers were right. Research shows that honey stops bacteria by drawing water out of damaged tissue. Honey also helps healing by promoting cell growth on the edges of a cut and by working with the body's cells to generate hydrogen peroxide, an antiseptic. Recent experiments have also proved that honey can stop even the nasty *Staphlococcus aureus* bacteria, a frequent cause of infection.

Honey is good for more than cuts. Hippocrates, the "father of medicine," routinely prescribed honey mixtures as a treatment for fever. Many folk remedies rely on honey's ability to relieve sore throats, insomnia, snake bites and upset stomachs. And, the Greek physician Galen even used honey mixed with powdered bees to cure baldness.

POLLEN

When bees leave the hive to look for flowers, they're seeking more than nectar. The second most important "food" for the hive is pollen, a powder gathered from the inner parts of flowers. Bees collect this powder, moisten it with nectar, and pack it into special sacs on their bodies called *corbicula,* or pollen baskets. Once they get back to the hive, these busy bees unpack their sacs and hand over their load to special "nurse bees," who synthesize the pollen into "royal jelly" and feed it to the young, developing bee larvae.

Unlike adult bees who exist almost entirely on nectar and honey, growing bees need extra protein, and pollen provides it. In fact, pollen is

---

Raw Or Processed?

The best honey is raw, not processed. Raw honey is loaded with bee pollen, enzymes and nutrients, all of which are destroyed when it is processed with high heat and filtration. In fact, once honey is processed, all you're really left with is the sugars. So, for maximum health benefits, stick to raw, unprocessed honey, which is available in most health food stores.

Two Pollen Panaceas

Beekeepers gather pollen from bees in two ways, each yielding a different type of pollen.

"Pellet pollen" is the easiest to collect. Beekeepers simply put a piece of screen over the front of the hive. When a bee comes home loaded with pollen and tries to squeeze through the screen, her (all worker bees are female) pollen is knocked off into a collecting tray. This pellet pollen is so named because it looks like little yellow-brown pellets. Because it's so easy to get, pellet pollen is relatively inexpensive and widely available.

"Bee bread" is rarer and more expensive. When a bee comes back to the hive with her load of pollen, whatever isn't used immediately is stored away in the cells of the hive. Before sealing each pollen-packed cell, worker bees preserve the pollen by mixing it with diluted honey. This special pollen-honey mixture then ferments, preserving its nutritional value. To harvest the bee bread, beekeepers must remove the comb, freeze it, and then use a sharp knife to carefully extract the mixture — a long, painstaking process.

The jury is still out on whether bee bread is better than pellet pollen, though many experts think bee bread is more readily absorbed by the digestive system.

almost 25 percent protein, and contains 18 amino acids, over a dozen vitamins, 28 minerals, 11 enzymes and carbohydrates, and 14 fatty acids. With all this goodness, it's no wonder pollen has been called nature's most prefect food.

Many athletes take pollen to boost strength and endurance during intense competition. Even athletes that many people would consider to be "past their prime" have used pollen to boost their strength beyond that of most young athletes. Seniors like Harry Sittonen and Noel Johnson take bee pollen every day with amazing results. Sittonen regularly competes in 75-mile ultramarathons, and Noel Johnson, who holds the 1991 World Senior Boxing championship title, also has the honor of being the oldest living finisher of the 1979 New York Marathon at 82 years old!

Pollen may be a "perfect food," but science is just starting to discover its value in preventing disease. Pollen helps protect the body against cancer, pollution and radiation. According to the New York Cancer Research Group, beekeepers as a group have a low rate of cancer compared to the other occupations studied, a finding that attests to pollen's powers.

Royal Jelly

No, this isn't what Britain's Royal Family spreads on their scones. Royal jelly is the super-nutrient-rich glandular nectar produced by worker bees to feed their queen. Like pollen, royal jelly is bursting with nutrients: flavonoids, amino acids, trace minerals, pantothenic acid and vitamins B1, B2, B6 and B12. People around the world use it because it helps trigger the brain chemical called serotonin, a substance which boosts energy and concentration, curbs the appetite, and helps produce sound, restful sleep. Research shows that royal jelly can even alleviate certain kinds of depression brought on by low serotonin levels.

Propolis

The ancient Greeks were the first to identify this brown, waxy, resinous substance used by bees to guard the entrances to their hives. The word means "before the city" in Greek, and the same substance that protects bees from intruders has been shown to be one of nature's greatest natural remedies.

Propolis: The Bee's Knees in Hive Protection

Bees search far and wide to collect the sticky sap from balsam poplars, pines and other cone-bearing trees to make propolis, which they carry home to their hives in baskets on their hind legs. Once they're back at the hive, they mix the resin with wax secreted from the underside of their abdomens, producing the substance we know as propolis.

Because propolis hardens into a tough surface, bees use it to narrow the entrance of their hive to protect against predators that might try to invade the nest. The stickiness of propolis makes a great sealer. If an intruder makes it past the entrance, bees sting it to death and cover it with propolis. Finally, bees use this substance as a lining for their queen's egg chamber. Because it does such a great job of inhibiting microorganisms, propolis keeps the birthing area sterile and germ-free.

Asians, Arabs and other people around the world use propolis to treat everything from bad breath to colds, migraines, hearing loss and other serious ailments. The Russians have even been using it to stimulate the body's white blood cells to prevent infections both before and after surgery. Research in Poland has confirmed the antibiotic qualities of propolis. In a recent study that pitted bee propolis against an array of conventional antibiotics, propolis prevented the growth of over 56 types of staphylococci bacteria. The conventional germ killers — ampicillin, penicillin, streptomycin and others — failed the test. Further study has even shown that while microorganisms typically "learn" to resist modern antibiotics, they never learn to resist the power of propolis.

Most health food stores now carry a variety of propolis preparations, including toothpaste (for sore gums), ointments (for bad knees and tennis elbow) and salves (for rashes, cuts and blisters).

GINSENG: HEALTH RICHES FROM THE EAST

Chinese herbalists have always said, "A person would rather take a handful of ginseng than a whole cartload of gold and jewels." Today, as we find out more and more about the beneficial effects of ginseng, this old saying begins to make that look like quite a bargain! Sometimes called the "most heavily studied herb in the world," ginseng has been shown to cure, prevent or assist in the healing of over 20 major ailments, including stress problems, diabetes, tumors, depression, anxiety, high blood pressure, impotence, fatigue and even radiation sickness.

This wonder root has a long and fascinating history. The ancient Chinese gave it the name "jen shen," which mean's "man root" because it resembles a gnarled human. They believed that ginseng was a gift from heaven, only growing where lightning struck clear water. Because of its body-like shape, the Chinese consider ginseng to be a whole-body tonic, a health "normalizer" that works to harmonize the workings of the entire body. For at least 5,000 years, the Chinese have based a major part of their system of medicine around ginseng. At one point in time, ginseng was held in such high esteem that only the Emperor was deemed worthy enough to pick it.

On the other side of the world, Native American Hopi and Papago tribes have been using ginseng for thousands of years to calm colds and soothe sore throats. Closely related to Chinese ginseng (Panax), wild American ginseng

(Panax quinquefolius) once grew from southern Canada all the way down though the Appalachian Mountains to Tennessee. In the 18th century, a Jesuit priest returned to Paris with a sample. Knowing the Chinese would pay a premium for ginseng, Jesuit missionaries quickly began combing the hills of the New World, touching off a frenzy that many historians compare to the California Gold Rush. Even Daniel Boone and Davy Crockett got into the act and made their fortunes as ginseng dealers.

By the turn of the century, most wild American ginseng had been wiped out by over-harvesting. Today, most of the ginseng in the world is cultivated in the U.S. and exported to China — where it is considered superior to the native healing root.

In recent laboratory studies, researchers have found that ginseng can improve memory and increase learning. It can also play a significant part in lowering levels of "bad" (LDL) cholesterol and increasing the levels of "good" (HDL) cholesterol,

> ### French "Love Wine"
>
> Because ginseng increases physical endurance, strengthens the sex drive, and heightens our senses of touch, taste and smell, it may indeed be the food of love.
>
> So if you want a little something extra to get you (or that special someone) in the mood, try sipping on this traditional herbal preparation called French "Love Wine."
>
> Pour 2 parts good Chablis into a container with a lid and add the following:
>
> - ■ 1 oz. vanilla bean, crushed
> - ■ 1 oz. cinnamon chips or broken cinnamon sticks
> - ■ 1 oz. dried rhubarb
> - ■ 1 oz. dried ginseng
>
> Mix well and put in a cool, dark place for 2 weeks, remembering to stir it once a day. Serve chilled, after straining through a piece of cheesecloth to remove the bits of herbs and spices.

reducing the risk of heart disease. Ginseng also contains saponins, which can reduce hardening of the arteries.

Like garlic, both American and Chinese ginseng act as antioxidants, releasing compounds that reduce cancer-causing "free radical" molecules. In fact, Japanese researchers have found that ginseng's antioxidant powers are so strong that laboratory-grown cancer cells revert back to normal, healthy cells when treated with ginseng extracts.

Siberian ginseng (Eleutherococcus senticosus) is a close cousin to

Chinese and American ginseng. Discovered in the 1960s by Russian botanists searching for a cheap, native substitute for expensive Chinese and American plants, Siberian ginseng has proved to be an athletic stamina booster. Further research has revealed that Siberian ginseng reduces stress reactions, protects the body against extremes of heat and cold, increases sexual drive and removes toxins from the body.

GINGER: A SNAPPY PANACEA

Ginger's main claim to fame is that it's great for stomach and intestinal problems. Over 2,500 years ago, doctors in China discovered ginger's healing powers when they discovered that dosing victims of seafood poisoning with gingerroot helped stop the nausea, vomiting and diarrhea. Today, it is especially effective when used to neutralize the negative effects of stress on our digestive systems.

When you are stressed out, your body responds by releasing adrenaline (a powerful stimulant) and by lowering your blood sugar. When the adrenaline hits, your digestive system shuts down, often causing nausea and stomach upset. Ginger counteracts the effects of adrenaline on your body, stimulates your digestive system and helps normalize your blood sugar.

For people convalescing from a long illness, ginger is a great healing tonic. In fact, Tibetans have used ginger preparations for thousands of years to help those recuperating from severe illness. Ginger helps stimulate the appetite, something that is very important for patients who have lost the urge to eat. Additionally, ginger contains compounds called gingerols which can strengthen the heart and boost circulation.

Recent research has shown that ginger is effective for treating premenstrual syndrome (PMS), as well as menstrual cramps, irregular or painful menstruation, and migraine headaches. Pregnant women can benefit from ginger's ability to soothe nausea, and studies have shown that ginger helped 75 percent of the women who took it for morning sickness.

Ginger is heart-smart, too. Russian and Japanese studies have shown that ginger's active ingredients (the gingerols we talked about earlier) strengthen the heart muscle. Additionally, ginger can lower your cholesterol and thin your blood, two things that can do wonders for your heart health. In fact, ginger is so good for the heart that it's come to be known as a "cardiotonic!"

Stomachache Tea

Ginger is a tasty remedy for stomachaches, nausea and diarrhea. You can get ginger capsules at your local health food store — or you can mix up a batch of homemade "Stomachache Tea."

Peel and chop about 2 tablespoons of fresh gingerroot. Don't use the powdered ginger that you may have in your spice cabinet. It's good for cooking, but the drying process destroys ginger's medicinal effects.

Place the chopped ginger into a mug and add enough boiling water to fill. Put a plate over the top of the cup and let the tea steep for at least 5 minutes.

After your tea has steeped, take off the cover, add some honey (another great stomach remedy), stir and enjoy. Your stomachache will be gone in nothing flat.

Ginger also has healing properties when applied topically. In Japan, massage therapists often use an oil infused with gingerroot as a rub-down to heal joint and spinal problems. And because ginger's heat boosts blood circulation wherever you rub it on, it can be a useful treatment for minor arthritis and muscle pain. It is also an excellent treatment for burns. For generations, mashed ginger has been used to treat burns and ease pain. In fact, some people say that mashed ginger applied to a burn is so effective that the pain goes away instantly, and the burn heals quicker.

FISH AND FISH OILS: OCEANGOING TONICS

For centuries, Eskimos have lived on a diet that at first glance looks like a one-way ticket to the hospital. Instead of a low-fat, high-fiber diet, the Eskimos subsist mainly on whale blubber and fatty fish such as mackerel and cod. With all that fat, you would think the Eskimo population would be filled with cases of high blood pressure, skyrocketing cholesterol levels, heart disease and arterial sclerosis (hardening of the arteries). In fact, the opposite is true. Even with their high-fat diets, Eskimos enjoy a remarkably low rate of heart disease. Though they eat almost no whole grains or fresh fruit, they have one of the lowest rates of heart disease in the world. Why? Scientists in the

1970s found the answer in the wonderful effects of fish and fish oils.

It turns out that many of the cold-water fish the Eskimos eat contain extremely high quantities of omega-3 poly-unsaturated fatty acids. These substances, found in the greatest concentrations in the oil and fat of the fish, have the remarkable ability to prevent blood platelets from sticking together and forming deadly clots. On top of their blood-thinning effects, omega-3 poly-unsaturated fatty acids have also been shown to have a positive effect on cholesterol, lowering blood levels of LDL and VLDL cholesterol, which can clog arteries and cause heart attacks.

You, too, can benefit from this Eskimo health secret. A study published in the prestigious American journal *Therapeutics* showed that people who take fish oil can reduce their chances of artery re-blockage after angioplasty surgery. Angioplasty is often a last-ditch effort to clear blocked arteries by stretching them out, and the cholesterol lowering effects of fish oil can keep arteries from clogging up again, lowering the chance of later heart attacks.

Some of the biggest names in health medicine agree. Studies conducted by the Johns Hopkins School of Medicine, the Harvard School of Public Health, the Rockefeller Foundation and the National Institutes of Health all found that eating moderate amounts of fatty fish such as mackerel or sardines at least twice a week can reduce deaths from heart disease by nearly one third! And studies conducted in the early 1980s at the Bowman Grey Medical School showed that cod-liver oil works twice as well as aspirin to reduce the risk of blood clots, a leading cause of heart attack and stroke. This is good news for people with stomach problems, because fish is much, much easier on your stomach than aspirin.

Your heart isn't the only part of your body that can benefit from fish and their oils. Many vitamin and mineral therapists have found that eliminating red meat and eating fish instead can bring relief to arthritis sufferers. Fish oil is also an excellent source of vitamins A and D, two nutrients that help your body absorb calcium. This is especially important for women suffering from or worried about osteoporosis, which can be aggravated by a lack of calcium in the diet. (And, the vitamin A in fish oil helps strengthen and beautify hair — a double bonus!)

Though the evidence is strong that eating more fish and fish oil is good for your health, many people find the smell and taste to be offensive. However, because people all over the world have started to demand fish oil (for the omega-3 fatty acids), the market has responded with a variety of easy-to-take oil products. Cod-liver oil capsules are fast becoming the most popular form of fish oil — you can even find it flavored with mint, orange or cherry.

ALOE VERA: A GROW-AT-HOME MIRACLE

You've probably used aloe — which Italians call the "miracle plant" — many times. Its healing and strengthening properties have made it an essential ingredient for many modern skin lotions, hand creams, hair products and sunburn preparations. What you might not know is that aloe is an ancient remedy, used for thousands of years by many different cultures from the Africans, Egyptians, Chinese and Europeans to the natives of both North and South America. Aloe vera is so useful that health expert Dr. Andrew Weil

---

Grow Your Own Medicine

Sure, you can buy aloe at the drug store, but why spend the money when you can grow your own medicine at home.

Aloe is a succulent plant that resembles a cactus and needs very little care to thrive as a houseplant. It can even go several months without light or water, making it a great plant for those of us who weren't blessed with a green thumb.

You can get aloe vera plants at most nurseries. Make sure that your get aloe vera (*A. barbadensis*). Some nurseries carry other varieties such as lace aloe (*A. aristata*), which might look pretty, but have no medicinal value.

Once you get your plant home, it's very easy to care for. If you live in a warm climate where it rarely freezes, you can leave your aloe outside year-round. If you live in a cooler locale, let your aloe plant enjoy the spring and summer outside, but make sure to take it in before the first freeze. Keep it out of direct sunlight (which will turn its leaves brown) and let the soil dry out between waterings.

To use it, slit open one of the leaves and apply the gel that oozes out directly to the affected area. It may sting for a bit, but that will pass quickly as the healing properties of the plant go to work. If you have a burn, bandage the slit leaf on your finger and leave on for about 24 hours. The burn will heal quickly.

---

recommends that every home have a plant growing on the kitchen windowsill.

Egyptian doctors as long ago as 5,000 B.C. recommended the gelatinous sap of the aloe plant for burns and wounds. As a member of the family of plants known as the "vulneraries" (or wound healers), aloe heals for a variety of reasons. First, it contains large amounts of water, which can keep wounds sterile by depriving harmful bacteria of the air they need to grow. Additionally, it contains high levels of magnesium compounds, which are effective natural painkillers. Finally, aloe contains several important vitamins and a substance called "allatonin," which has been shown to nourish tissue and speed cell repair.

Besides healing minor burns and scrapes, aloe may help heal more serious conditions. In tests with laboratory mice, researchers at Texas A&M University have shown that acemannan (aloe's active ingredient) can be effective in inhibiting cancerous tumors. Aloe's immune-boosting effects might even make it an effective tool in the battle against AIDS. Scientists at the University of Texas Southwestern Medical Center are looking into this possibility. Other research has already shown that the acemannan in aloe stimulates T-cells, one of the body's immune system watchdogs.

While research continues on aloe as a cure for serious illness, you can use it at home for a variety of everyday problems. It's available in many drug stores as a 99 percent pure gel that can be applied directly on scrapes, cuts, burns, rashes, acne and eczema. Aloe's high water content makes it a great sunburn remedy. Keep a bottle of gel in the refrigerator. Cool aloe not only soothes the pain of sunburn, its healing effects can even help stop peeling and blistering. In fact, aloe is such an effective burn medication, it can heal radiation skin burns.

You can also use aloe on muscle strains and aches. Just crush a few aspirin, mix the powder with some aloe vera gel, and rub into your sore spots. The aloe will carry the aspirin tablets straight to your bloodstream, bringing relief directly where you need it.

Like the other "panaceas" we've talked about, aloe is good for your insides as well as for your outsides. For hundreds of years people in the rural U.S. have used a tonic brewed from aloe to relieve the symptoms of arthritis. Aloe is great for the digestive system, too. Many health food stores carry aloe vera juice — as little as 1 teaspoonful after meals can soothe your stomach. The same African tribes that discovered aloe's external healing properties thousands of years ago also use it internally as a cure for menstrual problems, flu, snake bite, muscular dystrophy, meningitis, intestinal parasites and constipation. And Dr. Andrew Weil, in his book *Natural Health, Natural Medicine,* recommends aloe as a remedy for stomach ulcers, ulcerative colitis and constipation, as well as an internal and external remedy for hemorrhoids.

PANACEAS VS. PLACEBOS

Garlic, ginseng, onions, fish oil, aloe, ginger and honey — they're all easy to get and they all have been proven to be effective remedies for many ailments. But do they *really* work? Or do they work just because we *believe* they will work? The answer is "yes" — to both questions.

All of these so-called panaceas have legitimate medical effects on our bodies. And when we expect them to work — because we have evidence that they have worked for our ancestors for thousands of years — those effects are greatly enhanced. This is proof of the importance of the mind-body connection, an influence so powerful it can heal even when a patient is treated with a placebo — a "sugar pill" with no inherent medical value.

In Latin, the word "placebo" means "I will please," and in the medical world, studies have shown that inert placebos do work over 30 percent of the time. Psycho-immunology may hold the key to this phenomenon. Pyscho-immunologists, who study the way our brains affect our immune systems, have found that if you believe you will be healthy, chances are you will be healthy. On the other hand, if you're stressed out, unhappy or expect to get sick, you often do get sick because these feelings depress the immune system, preventing your body from fighting off disease.

So, if garlic, ginseng, onions, fish oil, aloe, ginger and honey — and all the alternative treatments you'll find in this book — really work, that's great. And, if they work because you *believe* they will work, that's even better. Remember, above all else, you carry the greatest cure of all within you — your brain — the one true proven panacea!

RELAXATION

Feeling tense? Stop what you're doing. Place the middle finger and thumb of your right hand over your nostrils, resting your index finger on the bridge of your nose. Pinch one nostril closed and inhale deeply through the other one. Try to visualize the air filling every inch of your lungs. Now, close that nostril, open the other one, and exhale completely, imagining that you are emptying every bit of air from your lungs. Continue inhaling and exhaling through alternate nostrils for a minute or so. Feel the tension leave your body every time you exhale, relaxing you completely.

Feel better? You've just used a yoga technique called *pranayama*, one of the many secrets that folks all over the world use to relax. There's no mystical secret why it works — deep, slow yoga breathing is the exact opposite of short, shallow, stressful breathing. It boosts circulation and triggers the body's relaxation mechanism, calming you down and clearing your head.

But using yoga is just one of many ways to relax and relieve stress. All over the world, people have developed safe, natural ways to relieve tension, including breathing techniques like the one you just tried, body-calming exercises, meditation, herbs and diet. Every society has its own forms of stress, and over the ages they've all developed ways of coping.

How can relaxation help you? What can you do to become more relaxed? To answer these questions, let's first take a look at the opposite of relaxation — stress — and see what it is and how it can affect your body.

THE DAMAGING EFFECTS OF STRESS

Sweaty palms, rapid heartbeat, "butterflies in the stomach," shortness of breath, a stiff neck — we all know what stress *feels* like. In fact, in today's busy world, many of us may have forgotten what it feels like not to be stressed out!

In his book *The Wisdom of the Body*, Harvard researcher Walter B.

Cannon first described the body's reaction to stress as the "fight or flight" response. This involuntary response developed in our ancient ancestors as a way to help them stay alive. When faced with danger, early man's metabolism sped up, shutting down the digestive tract, making the senses more acute, and making him better able to survive as a hunter (and sometimes as the hunted!). In those days, the stress was short-lived, and once the immediate danger was passed, the body returned to normal. The difference today is that we don't have an occasional saber-toothed tiger to run from, but a regular series of daily stresses that never seem to stop. Rather than being able to release the stress and relax, we just keep going, our bodies constantly on edge. The result of chronic stress reads like a laundry list of our most common health problems: fatigue, muscle aches, headaches, high blood pressure, ulcers, digestive problems and even cancer.

Why does the body do this to itself? It seems strange that a reaction originally developed to keep us alive now contributes to making us sick. Dr. Peter Chanson, author of the best-selling book, *The Joy of Stress,* may have the answer. He points out that many of the "original benefits" of stress reactions have become "today's drawbacks" if left unchecked. (See chart on page 75.) The reactions that once kept our ancestors from getting eaten are now eating us!

It would be nice if we could just eliminate or avoid all the things that cause stress in our lives, but for most of us, moving to the top of a mountain isn't an option. Instead, learning to cope with stress can help us gain control of the stress reactions in our bodies.

When your body is relaxed, you breathe more deeply and slowly. Your mind clears, your blood pressure declines, and your body begins to heal itself. A relaxed state can even help you achieve greater concentration and make tough mental jobs easier.

But how do you relax? For many of us with hectic schedules, pressures at work, and obligations at home, relaxing doesn't come easy. Far too often, we deal with stress by turning to quick fixes that actually make the problem worse. Smoking, drinking and excessive eating may initially make us feel better, but usually end up damaging our health and putting us under more stress. In addition, people who are stressed often turn to drugs to make them feel calmer. But these offer only short-term relief and do more harm than good.

The most successful relaxation methods take a holistic approach,

adapted from Dr. Peter G. Hanson's The Joy of Stress		
Natural Response to Stress	**Original Benefit**	**Today's Drawback**
Release cortisone	Protected us from allergic reactions to dust in a fight	Damages immune system, leaving us more open to cancer and infection
Increased thyroid hormones	Speeded up body metabolism for extra energy	Shaky nerves, weight loss (or gain), insomnia, exhaustion
Increased endorphins	Painkiller to help during battles	Chronic headaches, backaches, increased sensitivity to pain
Decreased sex hormones	Decreased fertility to keep population down during droughts, famine, long journeys	Premature ejaculation and impotence (in men); decreased ability to reach orgasm (in women)
Shutdown digestive tract	Rerouted blood away from digestive tract to the muscles and heart for greater endurance and strength	Dry mouth, digestive problems, weight gain, bloating, nausea, cramps, diarrhea
Increased blood sugar and insulin	Quick energy boost for running and strenuous activity	Diabetes, hypoglycemia
Increased blood cholesterol	Increased fuel for endurance	Hardening of the arteries, heart attack, other forms of heart disease
Rapid heartbeat	More blood to the muscles and lungs for increased strength	High blood pressure, which can lead to heart attack
Quick, deep breathing	Provided more oxygen for the muscles, increased strength	Can aggravate breathing problems and increase damage done by smoking
Thicker blood	Increased the blood's ability to carry more oxygen and fuel to the muscles, helped stop bleeding	Strokes (from blood clots), heart attacks, and other circulatory problems
Skin "goosebumps" & sweats	Helped increase sensitivity of touch, helped cool down body during battle	Perspiration problems and odor
Heightened senses	Eyes dilated for better night vision, hearing, touch, smell, and taste (greater warning of danger)	Can become "burnt-out" after excessive stimulation, increased accidents and fatigue

addressing not only the needs of the body, but the needs of the mind and spirit as well. For thousands of years, people around the world have relied on a combination of exercise, diet and mental discipline to treat the acute, immediate effects of stress, and to build strong bodies and minds that can withstand constant day-to-day pressures.

While many people practice one discipline (such as yoga or t'ai chi) exclusively, there's no reason why you can't mix and match techniques to find the combination that works best to help you achieve total relaxation naturally.

Take a 10-Minute "Meditation Vacation"

If you're having a hectic day at work or at home, try a 10-minute "meditation vacation" to calm yourself. Here's how:

1) Find a comfortable chair in a quiet space and dim the lights. If you're at work and share an office, try getting away to a vacant office.
2) Next, close your eyes and let your mind wander. Don't try to control your thoughts — just go with the flow.
3) Just continue to drift. After a minute or so, slowly open and close your eyes, taking deep breaths and letting them out slowly.
4) After another minute, open your eyes, wait 30 seconds, and slowly close them.
5) Now, begin to concentrate on a pleasant thought. Some people find that it helps to repeat a positive word or phrase (called a mantra) to focus their thoughts. Others concentrate on a peaceful sound or image. It doesn't matter what you use. If it works for you, do it.
6) Keeping your eyes closed, repeat your mantra (or continue to focus on a pleasing sound) until you feel yourself slipping into a comfortable rhythm.
7) Feel your tension slipping away. Continue focusing on your thought for another 8 minutes or so. Don't worry if you have to open one eye to check the clock — it won't break your meditation.
8) When your time's up, slowly open your eyes, exhale and slowly stand up. You'll feel relaxed, invigorated and ready to face the world!

THE IMPORTANCE OF EXERCISE

A strong, healthy body can withstand stress much better than one that is weak and out of shape. Strengthening your heart, muscles and lungs not only helps your body resist the strain of stress, it makes you look and feel better, too. One of the best stress-busters is exercise.

Exercise doesn't have to mean running 10 miles a day or pumping iron for hours at the gym. Beneficial exercise can be as simple as taking a brisk walk around the block, swimming a few laps in the pool, or even making a habit of taking the stairs instead of the elevator whenever possible. Like they say on TV, "Just do it!" Regular exercise strengthens your body, melts off the pounds, and makes your body release endorphins — neurotransmitters that lift your mood.

One alternative form of exercise is yoga, a type of mental and physical training that's been used in India for thousands of years. While there are many dimensions to yoga, much of it has to do with controlling your breathing while you strengthen your body. Turn to page 8 for some helpful, stress-reducing yoga exercises you can begin to use now.

T'ai chi is another ancient technique that is becoming more popular in this country. Practiced by Taoist monks and Chinese citizens for over 5,000 years, t'ai chi is both a self-defense system and a meditative exercise that consists of a series of postures called "forms." Because of its subtlety and gracefulness, it takes a long time to master. But once you do, you will be rewarded by excellent muscle tone, flexibility, balance and coordination. It is also an excellent way to manage stress. In fact, some therapists have used t'ai chi to treat stress-related diseases like ulcers and gastrointestinal disorders.

Proper breathing is another way that you can alleviate your body's reactions to stress. One of the secrets of t'ai chi, yoga and other meditative exercises is that they emphasize deep, slow breathing. This triggers what Harvard doctor Herbert Benson calls the "Relaxation Response" — a state of heightened alertness and peacefulness during which your heart rate slows down, and your blood becomes more oxygenated.

HELP FROM NATURE'S PHARMACY

No matter what kind of regular exercise you do, there still may come a time when you need a little extra help to get relaxed. Rather than turning to harmful substances such as alcohol, tobacco and synthetic tranquilizers, try nature's pharmacy. For ages, people have been using the healing properties of herbs to relieve tension and help heal physical and emotional ailments caused by stressful living. The most common way is to ingest them, usually in the form of a tea made by steeping an herb (such as chamomile or valerian root) in hot water. However, as anyone who's ever visited a spa knows, herbal wraps, masks and baths also can be very relaxing (and good for the complexion!).

Foods can also be great stress-reducers. Did you know that lettuce contains a substance called lactucarium which functions as a gentle calming agent? In fact, many common plants such as mint, onions and even oats can help you calm down after a stressful day. The best thing about using nature's remedies is that they are almost always very gentle, non habit-forming and free of many of the side effects too often found with chemical tranquilizers. (Learn more about using herbs and foods as natural stress remedies in the stress section beginning on page 467.)

Simple Self-Hypnosis

Self-hypnosis is a great way to relieve the stress of everyday life.

1. Find a comfortable chair, close your eyes and breathe slowly and deeply.

2. Focus your concentration on a single spot or object in front of you. Some people find that gazing at a beautiful crystal or a flickering candle works well.

3. Continuing to breathe rhythmically, focusing your concentration, tell yourself that you are relaxed and at peace. Feel your arms and legs get heavier and warmer as your relaxation grows.

4. As you become completely relaxed, visualize a beautiful scene or focus on a calming thought. Let that pleasant thought fill your mind, expanding and crowding out unpleasant, stressful feelings.

5. Continue for as long as you feel you need to. When you are ready to end your session, just allow your attention to expand.

CALMING THE MIND AND SPIRIT

Calming your body is only half the equation. To achieve total relaxation, you must also calm your mind and spirit. Meditation — a cornerstone of Japanese Zen, yoga and many of the martial arts such as aikido and t'ai chi — is one of the best ways to do this. Unfortunately, many people have the impression that meditation has to involve a mystical state that only shamans, yogis and Oriental wise men can achieve. In reality, there's nothing mystical about meditation — it's just a way of training yourself to turn your concentration inward, away from the pressures of the outside world while focusing on peaceful, calming thoughts.

In the late 18th century, the Austrian doctor Franz Mesmer discovered that he could bring people into a trance-like state by helping them focus their concentration. When Mesmer realized that people in a hypnotic trance were more susceptible to suggestion, he found that if he told people they felt better, they did. He not only used hypnosis (or Mesmerism as it was called then) to cure a variety of disease, he used it to help his patients relax.

Even though Mesmer's original theory (that his technique worked by controlling "animal magnetism") has been disproven, hypnosis has been proven very effective for treating everything from ulcers to overeating to stress. You don't have to consult a professional to benefit from Mesmer's discovery. Self-hypnosis is easy to learn and practice at home. See box on page 78.

While meditation and self hypnosis are two of the more popular ways to relax your mind and spirit, other techniques such as visualization, lucid dreaming and artistic meditation have been very helpful for many people. Australian Aborigines have used their dreams as a way of interpreting and controlling their daily lives for thousands of years, and the people of Tibet have been using drawings to focus and relax throughout their history. All of these methods work by focusing concentration inward, away from the immediate pressures of the outside world. And all of these methods — in conjunction with a healthy diet and regular exercise — will protect you from the unavoidable stressors in your life.

Using Herbs: Preparing at Home

Often when you hear about natural healing with herbs, you also hear some pretty strange directions for using them. Eating herbs by adding them to foods is simple enough, but what do you do if a remedy calls for making a strange-sounding thing called a "poultice" or a "decoction?" Checking your handy kitchen cookbook won't help, and you're probably not going to have any luck looking in the dictionary or encyclopedia, either.

Never fear! We know how difficult it can be to find out how to prepare many herbal remedies, and unless you have a friendly neighborhood herbalist to consult, you've probably been confused, too. The thing is, most of these preparations are pretty easy to make and can be concocted using tools you probably already have handy in your kitchen. Let's take a look and learn how to do it!

Poultice

Though it sounds like something exotic, a "poultice" is simply a mash of herbs applied to the body. To make a poultice, add a little hot water to some dried or fresh, chopped herbs, and spread the paste on a piece of gauze. Place another piece of gauze on top and apply to the afflicted body part, holding it in place with some pieces of surgical or first-aid tape. You may want to keep the poultice warm by holding a hot water bottle on it, but this isn't absolutely necessary. Helpful poultices include comfrey for wounds and sores, papaya for insect bites, hot onions for bronchitis and dandelion for boils.

Compress

A "compress" is like a poultice except that essential oils, infusions or decoctions are used in place of the actual herbal material. To make a compress, soak a clean towel or thick piece of gauze in the essential oil, infusion or decoction, wring out, and place on the body part you are trying to heal. Compresses can be either hot or cold, depending on the application. A hot eucalyptus compress applied to the chest is often good for colds or congestion.

INFUSION

"Infusion" sounds pretty technical, but if you can boil water, you can make one. Infusions are basically just teas made from combining either 1 ounce of dried herbs or 2 ounces of fresh herbs with a pint or so of boiling water. To get the maximum effect, you should crush or finely chop the herbs before infusing.

Making an infusion is easy. Place crushed or chopped herbs in a large mug or warmed teapot. Pour in 1 pint of boiling water, cover and allow to steep for at least 10 minutes. During this time, the herb pieces should settle to the bottom of the cup or the pot. If you are bothered by pieces of herb, just place the herbs in a tea ball before adding the water. You may be able to find a pot made especially for loose tea, with an insert in which you place the herbs while steeping. Add a bit of honey or lemon to taste and drink it up.

If you want, you can even make your own tasty herbal blends by adding other herbs that you like for additional flavor. Licorice, anise, lemon balm, mint or fennel make good herbal additions.

Why don't you try your own infusions at home? Chamomile works great if you're tense, blackberry or ginger are nice if you are suffering from indigestion, and ma huang is a wonderful stimulant if you're feeling tired.

DECOCTION

Some herbs need a little extra help before they'll release their good stuff. That's where decoctions come in. Much like an infusion, a "decoction" is made by steeping parts of plants in boiling water. However, because decoctions are made from the tougher parts of plants — stems, nuts, roots and seeds — you'll need to boil the herb for a few minutes for maximum effect.

To make a decoction, chop, crush, grate or grind the herb you want to use. Place these small pieces into a glass or stainless steel pot (never aluminum!), cover with water and simmer for at least 10 minutes or so. Allow to cool slightly and strain the mixture through a piece of cheesecloth, a sieve or even a coffee filter. Add a little extra sweetener if you want, sit back and enjoy!

Good herbs for decoctions include valerian root for tension, star anise seeds for fatigue or fenugreek for respiratory ailments.

SYRUP

More often than not, once a child hears that something's good for him, he won't want to take it. You can get around this by sweetening the deal by making a syrup.

Making a "syrup" first begins by preparing an infusion or decoction. While the mixture is still hot, add 12 ounces or so of sugar per pint of liquid and allow the mixture to cool. If you don't want to use sugar, you can even make a simple syrup by combining an infusion or decoction with ¼ of its weight of honey. Stir completely, bottle and cool in the refrigerator.

Syrups made of chamomile or valerian are a gentle sleep aid. If you've got a cold, try making a syrup of onion infusion and sugar. The French prepare a concoction similar to this and swear by it when they're sick.

CAUTION: *Honey should not be given to children under 1 year old.*

Infusions and Decoctions for Your Outsides!

You don't always have to drink your infusions or decoctions to get the most out of them. Some are good for all sorts of external uses. Try a sassafras infusion on cuts and scrapes. Or, try a mixture of lavender, comfrey, rosemary, mint and thyme in an infusion to soften your skin. If you've got skin irritation, try some burdock steeped in water and allowed to cool.

TABLET

We're all familiar with tablets and capsules, but you might not know that you can make your own at home. Many health and herbal remedy stores now sell empty gelatin capsules in either the .35 gram ("0 size") or .5 gram sizes ("00 size"). Simply fill them with finely powdered mixtures of herbs, and you've got a wonderful, portable way of taking your herbs with you wherever you go! Try not to make more than you'll use in a week, though — herbs lose their potency fairly rapidly, even when confined to a capsule. Try powdered ma huang or ginkgo for pep, pollen for overall health, or mint for heartburn or gas.

SUPPOSITORY

"Suppositories" allow quick absorption of herbal substances, because chemicals inserted in the lower intestine are absorbed more effectively. This method is particularly good for remedies intended for the entire body.

To prepare your own home-made suppositories, add powdered herbs to melted cocoa butter, pour into molds made from aluminum foil and allow to cool. Store your suppositories in the refrigerator to keep them from melting and to keep the herbs fresh and potent.

ESSENTIAL OILS

Getting essential oils out of plants requires complicated equipment, and most people aren't ready to make the investment to do this at home. However, you can purchase essential oils from health food stores and fragrance shops, and then you can add them to a base of almond, olive or sunflower seed oils to use as a massage rub.

Here is one way to make your own infused oils. Add your herbs to a bottle of olive, safflower or canola oil and allow to sit in a cool, dark place for 1-2 weeks. When you're done, strain the oil to remove the bits of herb. Not only can you do this for herbs that you want to use for medicinal purposes, but you can do it for plants you cook with such as garlic, onions, rosemary, ginger and hot peppers.

TINCTURE

Concentrated mixtures of herbs, "tinctures" are prepared by mixing herbs with water and alcohol. Tinctures are usually not consumed "straight" but are instead diluted with water and taken with meals.

To make a tincture, combine 1 part herb with 5 parts liquid (for dried herbs) or 1 part fresh herbs with 2 parts liquid. The liquid you use depends on the herbs you're using. If you're making a tincture with acidic herbs such as sassafras bark, use 1 part alcohol to 3 parts water. If you're using a resinous herb such as balsam, use a 9 to 1 water/alcohol mixture. Allow your herbal blend to sit for at least 2 weeks so that it can blend completely. When you're ready to bottle, use a French-press coffeepot or a fine sieve with cheesecloth to press the preparation so that all the liquid is squeezed from the herbs. Store in a dark place.

Tinctures are often used in herbal remedies that require mixing concentrated herbal preparations with other liquids. In particular, homeopathic and Bach System methods of healing make a wide use of tinctures.

BATH

Often herbs are most useful when you can soak in them. In particular, aromatic herbs such as lavender, chamomile or rosemary are great soaks to relieve tension and muscle aches.

To make an herbal bath, fill a muslin bag with an herbal mixture and hang it over the bathtub faucet so that the incoming water flows through it. Or, if you like, you can add a few drops of essential herbal oils or tinctures to your bathwater. Either way, it's a soothing, relaxing soak!

Herbal baths work so well for two reasons. First, when you lie in warm water, your pores open and allow the herb to seep in. This is great if you're suffering from skin irritations, sore muscles or arthritis. In addition, the warm water of the bath vaporizes the essential oils of the herbs. As you soak in your bath, you breathe in these oils, which quickly go to work.

Finally, you don't have to immerse yourself completely in order to get the maximum benefit from an herbal bath. Sitz baths, where you merely cover the lower portion of your body in the water, are great remedies for cystitis, prostrate problems or hemorrhoids. If you want something extra special, add some Epsom salts for added benefits.

CREAM

Creams and salves are made by heating herbs and oils together in a pot for a few minutes. Once the herbs have had a chance to infuse themselves into the oil, add a few ounces of beeswax, pour into a jar and allow to cool. Take care to heat the herb/oil mixture slowly — a few hours at least — and allow to cool completely before using. If kitchen work isn't your strong suit, try heating the herb/oil mixture in a double boiler over a low flame or even in a crockpot on low overnight. This will keep the mixture from burning and reduce the chances of your ending up with fried herbs!

You can even jazz up your usual cold cream or hand lotion by adding a few drops of herbal tincture or essential oils. Mix thoroughly and store in a closed container.

LINEAMENT

If you've got some sore muscles after a tough workout or are suffering from swollen, arthritic joints, lineaments may be the way to go. Lineaments work because they contain highly volatile essential oils in an oil or alcohol base and are absorbed through the skin quickly.

You can make a lineament much like an infusion or a tincture, by allowing the herb to propagate through the oil and sit for a few weeks. Some good lineaments to try are eucalyptus or menthol lineaments for muscle aches, hot-pepper lineaments for arthritis (take care not to make them too concentrated or you could burn your skin), or invigorating ginger lineaments for fatigued, tired muscles.

A Little Goes a Long Way: Herbal Remedies for Children

Children aren't just little adults — their bodies have different requirements and often don't need the same dosages of medications for effective treatments. This applies to herbal remedies, too. The good thing about herbs is that they are far more gentle than even over-the-counter remedies, but you should still take care to give the right dosage and watch for any side effects. Here are some handy rules for determining herbal dosages for children.

- **Weight Rule:** Divide the child's weight by 150 to determine dosage. For example, if a child weighs 75 pounds, divide 75/150 to get 0.5, or ½ the adult dosage.

- **Cowling's Rule:** Divide the age that the child will be on his or her next birthday by 24. For example, if a child is 2, divide 3 by 24 to get .125 or ⅛ the adult dose.

- **Young's Rule:** Add 12 to your child's age. Then divide your child's age by that number. For example, if a child is 8, the formula would be 8/(12+8)=.4. The child would get ⅖ of an adult dosage.

ACNE

If you were like most adolescents, your teenage years were like a roller coaster ride. Attending proms and driving dad's car were definite "ups" — dealing with acne was a "down."

Acne blemishes are the result of overactive oil glands, which don't always calm down after high-school graduation. Although most people see their acne clear up in their mid-twenties, some face adult acne well into their thirties.

Several factors may influence the development of acne and other skin eruptions — such as blackheads, whiteheads, cysts and blemishes in general — including family history, lack of sleep (which interferes with the body's natural renewal process), foods rich in iodine or preservatives (such as lunch meats and fast food), and hormone production.

Contrary to popular belief, acne is not caused by chocolate, sugar or soaps, all of which have little to do with the onset or course of this condition.

Here are several tips from around the world to help you put your best face forward.

ALOE Oily skin and acne have been effectively treated by many dermatologists with the versatile aloe plant. Look for a gel mixed with some vitamin E or moisturizer.

CHAMOMILE A European-style chamomile facial is used in many fine salons in the United States. To make one at home, steep chamomile flowers in boiling water. Then, covering your head with a large towel, bend over the hot fragrant water. Keeping your eyes closed, allow the chamomile steam to open the pores of your face. Lavender, lady's mantle or elder flowers can be used in place of chamomile. Be sure to cleanse your face immediately after the facial. Embedded dirt and blackheads will wash away easily.

CHINESE ANGELICA Acne is often worse when your body's hormones are changing — for example, during menstruation or puberty. To help control hormonal excesses, the Chinese take Chinese angelica, which is frequently used in Oriental herbal remedies. You can eat it raw or cooked, or take it as a tincture.

CUCUMBER To the Chinese, acne is a "hot" skin condition. So, they eat fresh, cool cucumber to treat it. The vegetable is sometimes preserved and eaten for its cooling action on all the body's organs.

ECHINACEA This natural antiseptic is also called purple coneflower and Sampson root. Native American Indians used this helpful herb to treat skin problems like acne and boils. They applied an echinacea tincture directly on the blemishes.

ESSENTIAL OILS Dab pure essential oil of lavender or castor oil directly on blemishes.

HONEY Warm honey will help bring spots to a head, and you can get the job done quicker if you add a little wheat germ. Dab each blemish at night and in the morning, leaving the preparation on for 15 minutes before rinsing with lukewarm water.

ICE When the first sign of a blemish appears, apply ice at least twice daily, hourly if possible. Wrap the cube in a soft piece of cloth, and then gently roll it over the inflammation for a minute or two. This not only reduces the redness, it lessens the inflammation and helps the skin heal.

LEMON BALM The Greeks, Romans and Arabs were all very fond of using the lemon balm plant for skin care. This natural antibacterial is a member of the mint family. If you break the leaves between your fingers, you will smell lemon with a hint of mint. Lemon balm compresses can soften skin and draw out impurities. The herb has a cleansing effect, which may help you if you have acne.

LEMON JUICE Lemon juice is a natural astringent that can be used in many ways and in many combinations. If your skin is "greasy," after washing, try swabbing with equal parts of fresh lemon juice and rose water, elderflower water or distilled witch hazel.

Residents of the English countryside preserve their healthy, wholesome appearance with the help of lemon juice. They slice a lemon and rub it over blackheads and acne once a day until the condition improves. This treatment is especially effective around the nose.

Try a mixture of egg whites and lemon juice to control blackheads and tone oily skin. Simply heat up the juice of a lemon and whip in a couple of egg whites until the concoction thickens. Refrigerate until needed, then apply with a cotton swab.

Another topical remedy for cleansing and healing calls for a mixture of blended cabbage leaves, distilled witch hazel and lemon juice.

OATMEAL Oatmeal mixed with buttermilk is a gentle natural cleanser.

PAPAYA Ayurvedic practitioners believe that a mask of mashed papaya may help with acne. After applying the fruit, rinse with warm water followed by cool water.

SLEEP Although each person

For most women between the ages of 20 and 40, the primary causes of acne are:

■ **Stress**, which causes your oil glands to overproduce and to release hormones like cortisone and testosterone.

■ **Hormonal changes**, such as those caused by menstruation and pregnancy, which create increased progesterone levels.

■ **Medications**, especially birth control pills (which are high in progesterone), and drugs that contain iodine.

■ **Oil-rich make-up** which can clog pores, especially when overused or used on oily skin. If you must wear make-up, stick with oil-free cosmetics and make sure you meticulously remove it at the end of every day.

■ **Inadequate skin care**. Your twice-daily regimen should include cleansing and toning.

varies as to the number of hours of sleep he or she needs, if you don't get enough rest, it is harder for your skin to rejuvenate. Sleep is the time when your body revitalizes and repairs itself.

SOAPWORT Since medieval times, Arabs, Chinese and Indians have been using soapwort as a skin treatment. Juice extracted from the leaves and roots of the plant apparently stops the itching and irritation that accompanies acne. The juice is mixed with water to form a sudsy lather that is used as a soap to cleanse the skin.

VINEGAR After cleansing, wipe your face with a cotton ball soaked in a solution made of equal parts of vinegar and water, and then rinse with hot water. This will help restore proper skin pH acidity.

VITAMIN A Vitamin A (as beta carotene) is a proven remedy for acne. Many expensive skin care creams containing retinal (a form of vitamin A) are currently on the market, but you don't have to run out and buy any of them. Good food sources of beta-carotene include carrots, pumpkins and sweet potatoes. Fresh carrot juice is a tasty alternative. The carrot juice can be mixed with apple and beetroot juice, all of which are good for the skin. If you don't have a juicer, there are many fruit and vegetable juice "bars" where you can buy these healthy mixtures, freshly squeezed.

VITAMIN B Stress can do a lot of physical damage to your body. To minimize the harm that stressors can do to your skin (for instance, causing a breakout of acne or other types of blemishes), take vitamin B. A good multi-B tablet taken daily is helpful not only to diffuse skin problems, but also to promote overall health.

WATER Drink water to flush impurities out of your system. If you can't finish 8 full glasses a day, drink as much as you can. (Other liquids don't count.)

ZINC Zinc reduces the painful inflammation that often accompanies acne flare-ups. You can take 25-50 milligrams of zinc each day, or eat pumpkin seeds, which are rich in this mineral.

Turn to page 439 for more skin care tips.

AGING

When the Spanish explorer Ponce de Leon set out for the New World, he wasn't looking for gold or silver, or even a new trade route to India. He was looking for the Fountain of Youth. As things turned out, he discovered Florida instead.

The Fountain of Youth does exist, however, and we are discovering more of its magic every day. Scientists say that the human body was designed to last well over 100 years, and longevity rates are getting closer and closer to that figure. The average life expectancy in the United States is currently about 76, which is a lot better than it was in ancient Rome, where the average person lived for only 22 years.

Even as late as the beginning of this century, the typical American lived only to age 48. Better nutrition, medical advances, and improved lifestyle have helped to prolong the average lifespan. Still, most of us succumb to heart disease, stroke, Alzheimer's disease or some other ailment generally associated with old age. And while we age, our quality of life usually goes downhill. We ache in the joints, don't see well and generally can't do the things we used to do.

Although people age in a similar manner everywhere on earth, in some countries and in certain cultures centenarians are far more common, and many of the ailments of age are less pronounced. We can learn many lessons from them.

BLACK CURRANTS Researchers in Wales significantly prolonged the life of aging female mice by feeding them black currant juice concentrate. The currant is very high in vitamin C — 400 milligrams in 3½ ounces of the fruit. It also contains flavonoids. Both of these nutrients protect blood vessels and improve eyesight.

According to Chinese legend, some Orientals have lived to be over 200 years old. Although this amazing claim is difficult to substantiate, the Chinese have always had a lot of wise advice for those who want to protract the aging process.

The Chinese philosopher Confucius recommended eating and drinking in moderation, being especially careful to eat only foods that have been finely chopped. Shi Chengjing of the Qing Dynasty advised that the longest life is the one that has been fully enjoyed, which ties in with the Chinese proverb, "An ounce of mirth is worth a pound of sorrow."(One sure way to remain happy, suggest the Chinese, is to adhere to a regular schedule of sleeping and eating.) This advice is not all that radical. In fact, contemporary medicine has repeated most of it exactly. But there are a couple Chinese secrets that are slightly more unusual:

■ The Chinese believe that one way to prolong life is to include a daily portion of grapes in your diet. They often eat grapes plain or, as a special treat, steeped in wine.

■ Another Chinese secret is the peach, which they believe to be the ultimate symbol of longevity. Belief in the powers of the peach to give fertility and immortality is incredibly strong. Chinese tradition holds that peaches should be exchanged between friends and lovers as a sign of the highest affection.

The benefits of the peach were not lost on traders who visited China. They brought the fruit to the Americas, where it gained immediate popularity with native tribes. Much later, the peach was such a favorite with Thomas Jefferson that he had peach trees planted at his home in Monticello.

Black currants can be made into jam or jelly, or brewed into a healthy tea that can be taken several times a day.

_____ **COCONUT** A traditional Chinese remedy to prevent premature aging is made from the coconut. They place freshly cut cubes of coconut meat into a jar and cover them with sugar. Then they store the jar for 2 weeks, and eat 2 to 3 coconut sugar cubes twice a day.

_____ **EXERCISE** Perhaps our lifespans are, to some degree, genetically programmed. But environmental factors also play a significant role in determining how long we live. We don't just want to live long lives becoming weaker and feebler every day. We want to learn how to slow down or reverse the aging process. Current research indicates that we can do this by maintaining an alert mind and a healthy, active body.

According to Swedish physiologist Per-Olof Astrand, aging is associated with decreased muscle strength. Regular physical training can effectively postpone deterioration of the body for 10 to 20 years.

Your mind needs exercise as well. Keep it sharp by maintaining a lively, changing environment. See page 38 for more information about the benefits of exercise.

FO-TI-TIENG According to the Chinese government, a thorough investigation confirmed that the famous Chinese herbalist, Li Chung Yun, lived to be 256 years old. He died in 1933. Li claimed that his secret of longevity was his daily use of Fo-Ti-Tieng, an herb found in the Eastern tropics that is currently being studied by Western researchers. He used the herb to make a tea, which he mixed with ginseng root. He drank this tea, and ate only fruits and vegetables grown above the ground.

GINKGO Many people around the world believe that the ancient ginkgo biloba plant has the ability to improve memory, increase mental alertness, and lessen ringing in the ears. In Europe and Asia, over five million people take ginkgo each year to prevent the effects of aging. The usual dosage is one 40mg tablet 3 times a day.

Research conducted in France, and at several other places in Europe, indicates that the herb acts by increasing the blood flow to the brain and improving the oxygen supply to the heart and other organs.

GINSENG One of the most treasured secrets in China is the versatile ginseng root. Daily doses of the herb do seem to slow the aging process. This has been substantiated by scientific study in both China and Russia.

GOTU KOLA This plant, which grows principally in India and Africa, is said to increase the vitality of 70- or 80-year-olds, possibly by decreasing the effects of stress on the adrenal glands. Especially popular in the Philippines, it is eaten raw or cooked, in salads and curries, and is made into teas.

HONEY   The natives of the Burmese jungle live very long lives. And they remain virile, energetic and healthy. They claim that this is the result of a steady diet of honey cakes, which they make from honeycombs.

The use of honey and pollen to inhibit aging is not confined to the Burmese jungles. Many Russian people over 100 years old have claimed that pollen was a principal food in their regular diets. And ancient Babylonian, Egyptian, Persian and Chinese texts all mention bee pollen as a secret to longevity. (One tablespoon a day is recommended.)

When you eat honey, you take advantage of several medicinal herbs at once because natural, unprocessed honey contains some of the pollen collected by bees from a variety of beneficial plants and flowers.

CAUTION: *Bee pollen should not be used by asthmatics.*

ROYAL JELLY   The Mayans of Guatemala and the Toltecs of Central Mexico used royal jelly as a youth tonic.

Royal jelly, the substance set aside in active hives for the queen bee, is much rarer than regular honey. It is even richer in vitamins, and is said to be a source of relief for a number of ailments associated with old age — including everything from gray hair to arthritis, and the general aches and pains that plague every tired body.

> ## Longevity Soup
>
> The Chinese make a soup they call "longevity soup," which is appropriately named because it contains so many nutritious ingredients. They crush bones from chicken and pork legs to extract the precious marrow. Then they mix this with a sauce made from dry orange peel, star anise, cinnamon bark, cloves, scallion heads, fennel, red chili, black pepper, nutmeg and licorice. They simmer the soup over low heat with other ingredients such as peanuts, mushrooms or radishes.

VITAMIN B   To relieve deafness, traditional Chinese medicine recommends that you eat pork kidney, or small amounts of fresh peanuts on a regular basis. This remedy may work because some forms of deafness are due to problems with the optic nerve. Organ meats, like kidney and liver, are high in B vitamins, which are needed for nerve function. And peanuts contain the B vitamin, inositol, which is very important for nerve transmission.

VITAMIN C In Cuba and China, researchers found that people who take high doses of vitamin C tend to live 5 years longer than people who don't.

YERBA MATE Yerba mate (mah-tay) is a form of holly that is grown in Paraguay, where it is made into a tea that is the national beverage. Charles Darwin, the famous naturalist, called this beverage "the ideal stimulant," since it contains caffeine, but less than coffee or ordinary tea. The Paraguayans use it as a remedy for headaches and insomnia, to relieve fatigue, and to stimulate mental and physical energy.

Paraguay Tea is made from finely ground leaves of the yerba mate plant steeped in hot water. The natives drink 1 cup early in the day, served hot or cold, plain or sweetened, with lemon or cream added.

YOGURT The Tamish live in the Abkhasia region of the Caucasus Mountains. They are world famous because they often live well past 100. Intensive research suggests that their incredible health and longevity is due to diet. They eat a lot of kefir, a fermented milk product. They also eat a lot of yogurt and pickled beets. As a result, they get a great deal of lactic acid in their diets.

Yogurt has a well-known reputation for prolonging life. In Yugoslavia, there are many centenarians who have consumed higher-than-normal amounts of yogurt during their lifetimes. And in France, yogurt is often referred to as the "milk of long life."

One of the benefits of yogurt is that it contains the good acidophilus bacteria. The acidophilus bacteria live in your digestive tract — and do something very important that can prolong your life. As you age, the cells that line your digestive tract — from one end to the other end — also age. When this happens, it becomes more difficult for you to absorb important nutrients from your food. Therefore, you start to develop deficiencies in key vitamins and minerals. You eat, but your food doesn't do much for you. You don't have enough nutrients to repair cells and organs, or to make new cells. So you age faster. The acidophilus bacteria help keep down the level of harmful bacteria that release toxins that can kill or damage intestinal cells. Over the years, this protective mechanism keeps your intestines working properly. Your cells don't age as fast. So neither do you.

ALLERGIES

The human immune system is designed to kill dangerous foreign invaders — everything from common viruses to cancer cells. However, it sometimes malfunctions and attacks relatively harmless allergens (the term used to describe the source of any allergy). To destroy the presumed invader (which could be a certain food, a pollen, animal hair, dust or a chemical), the immune system produces antibodies that are released into the bloodstream. The body remembers the incident (the memory is imprinted in sensitized white blood cells called lymphocytes), and the antibodies produced by these cells stand ready to strike every time that same allergen is encountered. We call this an allergic reaction.

The trouble is, most allergy medications can be a bittersweet experience. Antihistamines block the release of (you guessed it) histamines, which can make you feel a lot better. However, too much medication can make you drowsy, and dry out your mucous membranes. Nasal decongestant sprays shrink swollen membranes in the nose and can temporarily relieve your symptoms. But doctors advise taking these sprays for no more than three days in order to prevent the rebound effect of swelling and congestion.

An allergic reaction can be extremely serious. In some cases, a single bee sting or food causes such severe swelling in the upper airway that the victim chokes. Of course, death is the exception, not the rule. Most of us simply suffer some congestion and sneezing during the spring and fall, when pollen counts are high, or a slight cough when consuming dairy products.

A few people are lucky enough to suffer no noticeable allergies at all. Immunity is not always a matter of luck, however. In some parts of the world, it is the result of health secrets passed down through generations.

BIOFLAVONOIDS Some physicians believe that bioflavonoids boost vitamin C's ability to relieve hay fever symptoms. These compounds are found in the white pulp of oranges, grapefruits, and other fruits and vegetables. You can also take bioflavonoid tablets.

BROTH Hot broth can speed up the flow of mucus, especially if your soup contains the fire power of onion, garlic, cayenne pepper or horseradish.

EPHEDRA Ephedra, or ma huang, is a potent anti-allergic herb. It contains alkaloids that help soothe bronchial spasms, making it effective against asthma.
CAUTION: *Ephedra should never be used by pregnant women or people with high blood pressure.*

EUCALYPTUS Australians ease congestion by breathing in eucalyptus vapors. To try this, put the leaves into a large pot of boiling water, and boil them for 5 minutes. Turn off the heat and, with a towel draped over your head, breathe in the steam. You can also add a few drops of lemon balm or chamomile oil. All of these will soothe mucous membranes.
CAUTION: *Don't get too close to the steam — you could burn your face.*

EXERCISE Many allergy sufferers have found that exercise, such as running, walking or bicycling, helps to clear their congested noses.

If outdoor allergens and pollens are a concern for you, become a mall-walker. Many shopping malls open early to accommodate walkers. Or, stay indoors and work out at a home gym, skip rope or join an aerobics class.

You might try to walk in the evening, since pollen counts are the lowest then. Pollen levels are also lowest after it rains, and near lakes, ponds and other large bodies of water.

GINKGO For centuries, the Chinese have been using ginkgo biloba to treat allergies. Both its bark and its leaves provide effective remedies. Ginkgo treatment is also popular with other Asians, the Germans and the French. Ginkgo contains ginkgolides, which are compounds that smooth and soothe lung tissue and relax constricted bronchial tubes.

HERBAL TEA Fenugreek is full of calcium and other minerals and has a soothing effect on the respiratory system. If you suffer from hay fever, drinking 1 cup of fenugreek seed tea a day may help. This remedy dates back to the ancient Egyptians who drank a cup before each meal to clear and stimulate their senses of smell and taste.

Other herbal teas that act as decongestants are made from anise, echinacea, peppermint and chamomile.

HONEY The rich Greek dessert baklava, generously laced with honey, might add a few pounds to your middle, but it also might prevent you from sneezing your way through springtime. Honey has long been used by Greeks, Asians, Italians and Hungarians to prevent hay fever. The small amounts of pollen from the flowers that are found in the honey desensitize the honey eater to the allergic effects of these flowers. For this reason, it is best to eat honey that has been gathered in the area where you live.

HORSERADISH The Japanese have a passion for washabi, a potent form of

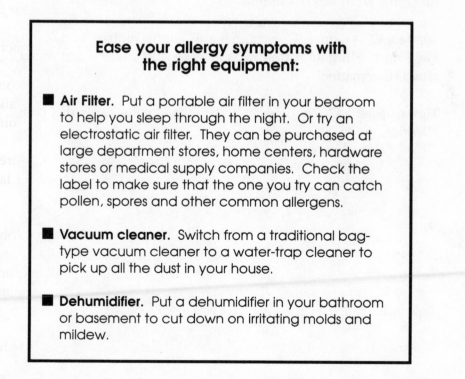

Ease your allergy symptoms with the right equipment:

■ **Air Filter.** Put a portable air filter in your bedroom to help you sleep through the night. Or try an electrostatic air filter. They can be purchased at large department stores, home centers, hardware stores or medical supply companies. Check the label to make sure that the one you try can catch pollen, spores and other common allergens.

■ **Vacuum cleaner.** Switch from a traditional bag-type vacuum cleaner to a water-trap cleaner to pick up all the dust in your house.

■ **Dehumidifier.** Put a dehumidifier in your bathroom or basement to cut down on irritating molds and mildew.

horseradish eaten with sushi that can make your eyes water and clear your sinuses. Japanese allergy sufferers take a spoonful a day as a preventive, especially for hay fever. Once the symptoms subside, a few teaspoons of horseradish each month are all that are needed.

☛ **NOTE:** If your grocery store doesn't carry washabi, substitute regular horseradish.

NETTLE The stinging nettle plant is common throughout the world. Fresh plants irritate the skin. When dried or cooked, however, they lose their sting and are safe and non-toxic. Some allergy sufferers take stinging nettle capsules to relieve their itching eyes.

PANTOTHENIC ACID Sandra Stewart, M.D., former assistant director of the Outpatient Department of Children's Hospital in Columbus, Ohio, takes a 100-milligram tablet of panothenic acid to relieve congestion. According to her article in "Annals of Allergy," many of her patients also find relief from this B vitamin.

VITAMIN C Vitamin C is a natural antihistamine, and can reduce swelling and inflammation in your nose and sinuses and speed repair after inflammation.

Turn to page 243 for remedies to fight the "itchy" eyes that come from allergies.

APHRODISIACS

    True aphrodisiacs! Few treasures have been so eagerly sought. Almost every ancient culture claims to have discovered at least one love potion, and even advanced modern societies have joined the quest. Indeed, who hasn't had occasion to yearn for a little help to fan the flames of passion? Or, a bit of magic to improve real or perceived physical limitations?

    Since people are so different in this intimate aspect of their lives, it is not surprising that no single aphrodisiac can claim to be universally effective. Yet, people in all corners of the world continue to hope — and have fun experimenting with — new (and ancient) ways to enhance sexuality. And, since "variety is the spice of life," we offer you a smorgasbord of possibilities.

ARTICHOKES The French, famous around the world for their gourmet cuisine and their romantic spirits, use the artichoke to inspire romance. They steam an artichoke and then dip the leaves in melted butter and Dijon mustard. They believe that the most powerful part of the vegetable is the soft artichoke heart. If you've ever sucked sensuously on artichoke leaves, you probably understand their aphrodisiac quality.

ASPARAGUS This vegetable is loaded with nutrients essential for energy, including potassium, phosphorous and calcium. Go light on the cream sauce and you have a delicious, healthy aphrodisiac.

CHASTE BERRIES The berries of the Agnus castus are considered to be a powerful sexual stimulant by Arabs and Egyptians.

    Generally, these berries are eaten by sexually active men interested in improving their sexual prowess — especially when they have worn themselves out by overindulging.

Chaste berries are said to restore the sex drive and to dramatically enhance performance. Research in Germany indicates that they can affect reproductive hormone levels.

CHIVES This syrup recipe of unknown origin is reported to be effective against frigidity. Boil 1 cup of finely minced chive leaves and roots with 2 cups of champagne. Simmer and drink unstrained. Chives, like garlic and onions, are rich in the minerals that are needed to make sex hormones. (And the champagne reduces stress.)

CHOCOLATE No discussion of aphrodisiacs would be complete without a mention of chocolate. Since its introduction to Europe in the early 16th century, chocolate has been regarded as one of the world's most exotic and sensual foods.

The scientific community has not yet reached a conclusion about the effects of chocolate on the libido — however, it does contain caffeine (a stimulant) and magnesium. One historical persona whose sex drive appears to have been affected by this rumored aphrodisiac was the chocoholic Montezuma. He reportedly drank 50 cups of chocolate a day before visiting his harem of 600 women.

Indeed, many people around the world are convinced that chocolate increases sexual vigor. This belief is particularly strong among the French, Swiss, Italians, English and Belgians. Perhaps that's why these countries are the world's top producers of chocolate.

CLAMS The Japanese eat clams (which, like oysters, contain zinc) for sexual vitality. After baking for about 2 hours at 400 degrees, the clams are cooled and crushed into a powder. The Japanese recommend taking ½ teaspoon of the clam powder with water, 2 hours before bedtime, for 1 week.

DAMIANA The damiana shrub grows in abundance along the dry, brushy hillsides of the Rio Grande. Also common to California, Mexico and the Antilles, damiana acts as a powerful aphrodisiac because it is a stimulating nerve tonic that relieves debility, depression and lethargy.

In Mexico, the leaves are used to make tea and are added to liqueurs to enhance the flavor.

DATES Men in Saudi Arabia, Iran and Egypt know what to do with a date — eat it. Dates, sweet Middle Eastern fruits that resemble figs, are highly prized for their ability to stimulate the libido — possibly because they are a good source of minerals.

FENUGREEK In Turkey, fenugreek is eaten in powdered form mixed with honey. Turkish men say that it increases their sexual potency — and Turkish women claim that it strengthens their sexual energy and appeal. Fenugreek contains oils with a high concentration of vitamins A and D, which are often lacking in people with weak sexual desire or impotence.

As an added — and often related — benefit, eating fenugreek, or drinking fenugreek tea, sweetens the breath, helps eliminate perspiration, and gives the body a perfumed aroma. To make a fenugreek tea: Pour 1 cup of boiling water over 2 teaspoons of fenugreek seeds. Steep for 5 minutes, stir, strain, add honey and lemon, and drink a cup a day.

> ## Curiosity Box
>
> *Anthony and Cleopatra munched halvah, a sweet Middle East treat — to increase their sexual stamina. Make halvah at home by grinding up a cup of sesame seeds and mixing in raw honey until it has the consistency of dough. Then break off bite-sized pieces and enjoy.*

HONEY The term "honeymoon" comes from a common practice of brides in ancient Celtic tribes. To stimulate sexuality, they drank honey-beer for a month following the wedding ceremony. Honey contains aspartic acid, vitamin E and traces of hormones. (The hops in the beer also contain traces of hormones.)

Here's one recipe we found for honey-beer: Place 1 ounce of hops in a porcelain or Pyrex container. Cover the hops with 1 pint of boiling water. Let stand for 15 minutes, and then strain. Add a teaspoon of raw honey to a wineglass full of the brew and drink an hour before each meal.

HOPS Most aphrodisiacs are meant for impotent men. The English, however, have an aphrodisiac that is especially for women — hops tea. Hops contain the female hormone estrogen, which is the scientific basis for its use as a female sexual tonic.

Hops are also the main flavoring agent in beer. The English used hops to brew beer — starting in the ninth or tenth century. They learned that the aromatic, bitter tasting resin in the hops acted as a preservative. It is lupulin, a bitter yellow extract of hops, that appears to have a stimulating effect on women. Unfortunately, in men lupulin has a sedative and depressant effect (which may be why some men fall asleep after a few beers).

JASMINE Among herbalists, jasmine is known to have a calming effect on the nerves. However, in India, the scent is thought to arouse erotic notions, acting as a powerful aphrodisiac. Centuries ago, lovers would bathe in moonlight near a garden containing jasmine plants.

Try massaging your body with oil of jasmine to help overcome frigidity.

CAUTION: *The essential oil should only be used externally.*

KINO GUM The kino tree, widely used in India as the source of a treatment for minor cuts, is known in Africa as the source of a pleasant aphrodisiac.

LAVENDER The delicate aroma of lavender was considered to be an aphrodisiac by Europeans during the Middle Ages. Lavender has sedative properties, and is good for calming anxiety and tension. A massage with lavender oil relaxes muscles, eases pain — and sometimes arouses passion.

To make an alluring body powder, mix equal parts of dried lavender and rose petals. Crush the blossoms finely with a mortar and pestle. Then pour the mixture into a container and stir in an equal amount of cornstarch.

LICORICE Many consider the women of France to be the most sensual in the world. Perhaps this secret aphrodisiac is the source of their reputation. To enhance their love lives, French women drink anisette or licorice water. (Licorice is another natural substance that has been found to contain hormones.)

MAGNOLIA The magnolia tree is well-known for the sweet perfume of its large, beautiful flowers. It has another quality, however, for which it is renowned among the Chinese. They boil the blossoms to make a tea that stimulates the libido. Today, magnolia blossom tea is commonly found in supermarkets and health food stores.

OYSTERS For hundreds of years, oysters have been regarded as potent aphrodisiacs. While this may be part mental imagery — on the half-shell it is said to resemble a women's genitalia — there is also a scientific reason. Oysters are an excellent source of zinc, a mineral known to be important for the health of the reproductive system. For men with low sperm counts, zinc is often recommended by doctors.

PEPPERS Throughout history, and all over the world, hot spicy peppers have been known as aphrodisiacs. Most plants belonging to the pepper family contain a substance called capsaicin, a stimulant.

RICE BRAN OIL A common ingredient in Japanese food, rice-bran oil is said to stimulate activity of the pituitary gland. Because the pituitary gland controls the production of male and female hormones, the Japanese consider the oil to be an effective aphrodisiac.

ROSES During Rome's most decadent era, huge quantities of rose petals, fragrant and smooth to the touch, were piled high in festive arenas, on streets — and in bedrooms.

In the United States, roses are a favorite flower to indicate love. The aroma has a very strong romantic effect on women. Enhance your sexuality by sprinkling some fresh rose petals in your bath and wearing rose-scented perfume.

SAW PALMETTO The berries of the saw palmetto were eaten by several American Indian tribes to stimulate sexuality. Four to five berries a day was the recommended dosage. The berries contain steroidal saponins that are often used today to treat atrophy of the testes and prostate inflammation.

Some Ancient tribes discovered that women who ate the berries firmed up their breasts. And, for women who are lactating, saponins also stimulate the production of milk.

SESAME SEEDS In ancient Babylon, women cooked up a sesame seed and honey concoction to boost their husbands' sexual vitality. Although the recipe was intended for Babylonian men, the women occasionally indulged in the tonic themselves.

Sesame seeds and raw honey contain powerful stamina-enhancing substances, such as magnesium, calcium, potassium, bee pollen and more. These nutrients stimulate the adrenal gland, which makes the sex hormones.

SOYBEANS Here's another recipe to remedy frigidity. Steam soybeans (black soybeans, which are rich in protein) and dry them in the sun. Grind the dried beans into a powder, then add ground sesame seeds (rich in minerals) and honey. Drink with warm water.

WARNING: Avoid alcohol. Although a drink may loosen up your inhibitions, too much alcohol depresses the nervous system.

APPETITE STIMULANTS

Food is the fuel that keeps your body going and your energy levels high — which is the reason a healthy appetite is so important for overall wellness. While vitamin and mineral supplements can help, there is no substitute for eating complete, well-balanced meals.

Lack of appetite can sometimes be a symptom of a serious underlying physical or emotional illness. However, in today's hustle-bustle world, it is more often the result of worry, anxiety or a high-stress lifestyle. No matter what the cause, if you have lost interest in eating, we have some time-honored suggestions to stimulate your appetite and get those digestive juices flowing again.

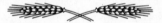

ALFALFA Alfalfa is widely touted as an appetite stimulant. The little legumes are an excellent source of vitamin E and beta-carotene, and alfalfa sprouts make a great topping for any salad or sandwich. To make your own sprouts, follow these easy directions:

1. Put 1 tablespoon of alfalfa seeds in a jar and soak in warm water overnight.

2. Cover the top of the jar with a piece of cheesecloth (or nylon stocking) and drain off the water.

3. Rinse the seeds with warm water, and drain again — then store the jar on its side in a dark place.

4. Rinse and drain the seeds 2 or 3 times a day for 3 or 4 days. When 2 small leaves develop, the sprouts are ready to eat.

CAFFEINE Caffeine is a well-known appetite stimulant that's found in coffee, tea, cola drinks and chocolate.

CARAWAY SEEDS We don't know how long people have been using this herb as a treatment for appetite disorders, but we do know it has been around for a very long time. Scientists have found fossilized caraway seeds that are 5,000 years old. To make a therapeutic tea, grind or crush 1 teaspoon of caraway seeds, and steep them in 1 cup of boiling water.

DANDELION Dandelions grow wild in just about every part of the world. The nutritious greens contain vitamins A and C, calcium and iron. Use the pungent young leaves in your salad to perk up your taste buds.

DILL People back in colonial times took fresh dill leaves with them to church to munch on during long, boring sermons. This may have kept them awake — but it also may have made them hungry, since dill is an appetite stimulant.

GINGER In France, ginger oil is placed on a sugar cube which is then sucked on to increase appetite.

ARTHRITIS

Arthritis strikes the fingers, knees, elbows, hips, jaw — any place in the body where there is a joint between the bones. The most common form of arthritis, called osteoarthritis, is characterized by pain (especially after exercise), bony swelling of one or more joints, and stiffness. Although it is usually associated with the wear and tear on joints that comes with aging, it can be aggravated by repetitive stress to a joint and/or obesity.

Gout, another form of arthritis, usually affects the toe joints, causing "podagra" (or classic great toe pain). You'll find remedies for gout on pages 269-272.

Rheumatoid arthritis, an inflammatory form of joint disease, is considered an autoimmune disease — one in which the body's immune system attacks itself. It most frequently occurs in women between the ages of 20 and 35 and affects approximately 6.5 million Americans every year. The symptoms of rheumatoid arthritis — which may come and go, or even disappear completely — include tenderness in almost all joints, a lack of flexibility, soft tissue swelling (the joint feels puffy to the touch), body aches, and fatigue. See pages 431-443 for more information about rheumatism.

For all forms of arthritis, the common treatments are similar: aspirin, warm compresses, mentholated ointments and gentle exercise. These therapies often work, but are they the only ways to treat arthritis? "No!" say healers from across the centuries and around the world. We searched for more, and here is what we found.

ALFALFA Appalachian mountain people make alfalfa leaves and seeds into tea as a remedy for arthritis — probably because of the plant's anti-inflammatory properties. Because it reduces knuckle swelling and joint pain, alfalfa is often recommended for people who spend much of their time at the typewriter or computer keyboard. (Health food stores carry alfalfa tablets, if you'd rather skip the tea.)

BLACKSTRAP MOLASSES The British, known for their fondness for sweets, swear by crude blackstrap molasses dissolved in water. When taken every morning, they say this preparation eases and even eliminates pain in the joints. Molasses is an excellent source of minerals, including iron, potassium and magnesium. Since it's also a concentrated sweet, rinse out your mouth or brush your teeth after using this treatment. Otherwise, you may be trading one pain (arthritis) for another — a toothache!

CELERY An old German folk remedy has people with joint pain slowly chew 1 to 3 teaspoons of celery seed powder mixed with spices such as rue, cloves and saxifrage. Celery is a diuretic, and the loss of excess fluid can reduce the inflammation associated with arthritis. And rue contains rutin, which can strengthen blood vessels, preventing them from leaking fluid into tissues and thus preventing inflammation.
CAUTION: *Rue should not be used during pregnancy.*

CHERRIES To alleviate pain form arthritis, the Japanese eat 6 to 8 cherries a day (canned, frozen or fresh). This centuries-old remedy not only relieves pain in the joints — it also tastes delicious! Cherries are good sources of minerals like magnesium (a natural painkiller) and potassium, which acts as a diuretic, reducing inflammation by ridding tissue of excess fluid.

COPPER Until recently, all Western doctors dismissed as folklore the idea of wearing copper bracelets to treat arthritis. Indeed, there are many, probably most, doctors who are still skeptical. Researchers in Australia, however, have found that people who wear copper and take aspirin experience more effective athritis pain relief than those who treat their pain with aspirin only.

DANDELION One of the best remedies for treating arthritic conditions probably grows right in your backyard — fresh young dandelion leaves. Because of the high vitamin A and C content, these greens help your body repair damaged tissues and help your liver clear toxins out of the blood.

European herbalists have used these anti-pain dandelion recipes for many years:

- ■ Steam or sauté the leaves, adding a touch of garlic and olive oil for flavor.

- ■ Steep 3 teaspoons of fresh leaves in 1 cup of boiling water for dandelion tea.

- ■ Make a coffee-like beverage by boiling 4 ounces of fresh dandelion root in 2 pints of water.

DEVIL'S CLAW An ominous-sounding plant, devil's claw comes from the Kalahari Desert of South Africa where it has been used for over 250 years to treat arthritis pain. Recent French and German studies found that the therapeutic action of devil's claw is similar to that of cortisone. The root acts mainly as an anti-inflammatory thanks to its active ingredient, harpagoside.

FEVERFEW Dr. Andrew Weil, a Harvard-trained physician and natural health expert, recommends freeze-dried feverfew leaves to ease the pain of arthritis. Compounds in the plant suppress the release of prostaglandins and histamines, chemicals that produce inflammation.

FISH OILS Fish oils, especially those from fatty fish (herring, salmon, mackerel, tuna and sardines) are good sources of omega-3 fatty acids. These fatty acids interfere with the formation of prostaglandins that can lead to inflammation. A daily serving of fresh fish (or fish oil capsules if you don't like fish) should produce positive results.

GARLIC Because of its ability to reduce inflammation, garlic may well ward off the pain and discomfort felt by those with arthritis.

GINGER The traditional Ayurvedic medical system of India holds that ginger is very effective in the treatment of arthritis and a host of other ailments. Recent medical research in Holland has also indicated that eating ginger really does help alleviate arthritis pain. Ginger, because of its ability to increase blood circulation, carries away inflammatory substances from the affected joint and warms the area.

Here is a Chinese arthritis remedy that uses ginger: boil 2 ounces of cinnamon twigs with 3 ounces of fresh ginger in enough water to cover the spices. Boil until the water is reduced by half. Drink a cupful 3 times a day.

GOLDENROD British herbalists recommend goldenrod tea as a remedy for the painful effects of arthritis. Because it stimulates the elimination of waste by the kidneys, goldenrod helps rid the body of toxins produced during inflammation — and so reduces arthritis pain. Goldenrod tea can be found in grocery stores and health food stores along with other herbal teas.

HERBAL BATHS Hot baths may temporarily relieve arthritic pain, since lying in the tub takes weight off of aching joints. Certain herbs, such as dried rosemary, peppermint or chamomile, when added to the hot water, make for an even more relaxing, fragrant experience. (Use a tea ball to avoid clogging the drain.)

NETTLE In Germany, vitamin C-

NATURE'S MEDICINE CABINET

Capsaicin is a natural chemical that is found in hot chili peppers and jalapeno peppers. Research has shown you can block the pain of osteoarthritis by rubbing the painful joint with capsaicin cream.

According to a study headed at the Miami Veterans Affairs Medical Center, nearly 70 percent of the study patients who used hot pepper cream reported pain relief. The cream works by interfering with the release of Substance P., a chemical in nerve endings which transmits the sensation of pain. The study found that capsaicin cream works best on aching knees and fingers, as opposed to hip joints, which are much deeper.

It takes 1-2 weeks for the cream to work. Normal application is 3-4 times daily. As for side effects, a burning sensation may occur, which usually disappears after several days of continued use. People with sensitive skin should apply it only 1-2 times daily. Be sure and wash your hands after use.

rich nettle tea is sipped to relieve arthritis.

QUINCE In the 12th century, in Bingen, Germany, a mystic named Saint Hildegard used her knowledge of natural medicine to treat arthritis. Her words of wisdom still hold today: "Detoxify, purify, and regenerate the whole organism."

To get rid of the rheumatic toxins that cause pain, Hildegard prescribed eating fragrant, raw quince. The fruit, which can be found seasonably in most grocery stores, can be cooked in water or wine, baked in a cake or pie, or made into jellies and candy.

ST. JOHN'S WORT The oil form of an herb known as St. John's Wort has been used by people with arthritis to lessen the pain of this affliction, as well as that of rheumatism.

SPIKENARD The Cherokee Indians make the powdered root of the Aralia racemosa ("spikenard" — also called "Indian root" and "life-of-man") into a tea to treat rheumatoid arthritis. They also pound the root and apply it as a poultice to painful areas of the body.

WILLOW For thousands of years, the bark of the willow tree has been used to treat arthritis. In fact, Dioscorides, the ancient Greek physician, probably deserves as much credit as Bayer, the German who first marketed aspirin, for bringing pain relief to the people. The bark, leaves, and buds of the willow contain salicin, which is converted to salicylic acid in the body. Salicyclic acid is almost identical to the synthetic pain reliever, aspirin (acetyl salicylic acid). In Dioscorides' day, patients chewed the bark of the willow tree. Today, willow tree bark is available in powdered form.

WINTERGREEN Oil of wintergreen is a source of salicin (natural aspirin).

YOGA This ancient remedy has countless useful applications — and seems to be especially effective in treating arthritis. Classes are offered in most areas of the country, and tapes are available if you prefer to practice yoga at home. Turn to page 6 for more information about yoga.

EXERCISE!

Arthritis is one of the many ailments that are helped by exercise. Movement noticeably improves with exercise. If lifting light weights or walking is too difficult, try other exercises that are even gentler on painful joints.

■ If you have arthritis in your lower body, get into a heated pool as often as you can, daily if possible. Then walk back and forth across the shallow end until you begin to tire.

■ For arthritis flare-ups in your hands, squeeze a soft rubber ball or twist a large rubber band, and gently spread the fingers apart, using the rubber band as resistance. Exercise your hands in the sink or in a pot of warm water while you're watching TV.

The American Arthritis Foundation recommends a balanced exercise program for arthritis sufferers that includes exercises for flexibility, strength and endurance. Here is a sampling:

The Shoulder Turn (to improve movement in your shoulders):
Start with your hands locked behind your neck or head, elbows pointing straight ahead (A). Slowly bring your elbows out sideways as far as you can and hold for 5 seconds (B). Bring your elbows forward as if to touch them together and hold for 5 seconds. Repeat from the beginning. (This exercise can also be done lying down.)

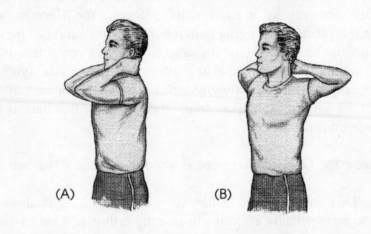

(A)   (B)

For more information, contact the Arthritis Foundation, P.O. Box 19000, Atlanta, GA 30326

The Toe-Heel Life
(to maintain flexibility in swollen ankles):

Sit in a chair with your feet flat on the floor (A). Keeping our heels on the floor, raise your toes and the front of your feet as high as you can (B). Move them to the right (C). Bring

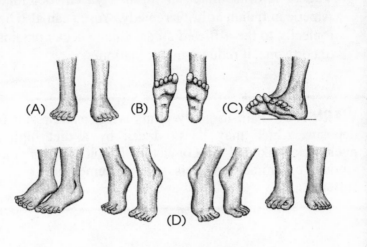

your toes back to the floor, and raise your heels as high as you can (D). Move your heels back down to the floor and repeat the same movements to the left. Repeat from the beginning.

The Hip and Knee Bend (to maintain strength and motion in swollen knees and hips):

Lie on your back, knees bent with feet flat on the floor (A). Bring one leg up and grab behind the thigh, pulling toward you (B). Hold for 5 seconds. Slowly return to starting position and repeat the same movements with the other leg. Repeat from the beginning.

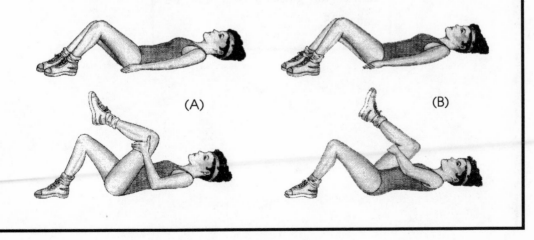

YUCCA A drink made of mashed yucca root mixed with water is an American Indian arthritis remedy. Yucca can also be mashed and applied topically to the afflicted area. Since yucca contains a substance similar to cortisone, it reduces inflammation.

WARNING: Pain in gouty joints is often the result of uric acid crystal deposits, which may be produced by a diet high in animal fat (or nucleotides) like red meat or caviar. Eliminating, or at least decreasing, the amount of animal products you consume may be helpful for arthritis sufferers.

For information on where to purchase any of the items listed, turn to the glossary beginning on page 523.

ASTHMA

Asthma, a respiratory ailment not yet completely understood, afflicts millions of people in the United States. During an attack, the upper airways become constricted, causing the sufferer to wheeze and have a hard time breathing. In severe cases, the victim feels that he or she is suffocating, since the trapped air cannot be exhaled. Attacks can be triggered by many things, environmental pollutants, allergens, cold, damp weather — and even exercise.

Western medicine generally relies on inhalants to prevent or alleviate asthma attacks. But many people around the world deal with asthma in other ways. Here are details on some alternative remedies.

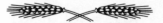

AMBRETTE SEEDS People in Trinidad steep musky-smelling ambrette seeds (musk okra) in rum or water and then chew the seeds to relieve asthma or chest congestion.

AMMI SEEDS The Bedouins are members of a nomadic desert tribe that travels throughout Arabia, Syria and West Africa. To treat asthma, they chew ammi seeds, which are native to these regions.

COFFEE How does strong coffee, black mocha coffee in particular, relieve asthma? Coffee contains caffeine, a methylated xanthine related to theophylline, a substance that relaxes the smooth muscle of constricted bronchial tubes to make breathing easier. Methylated xanthines are also found in tea and chocolate, and are diuretics as well as bronchodilators.

In Europe and Canada, drinking two 8-ounce cups of strong brewed coffee is a common remedy for asthma. This should provide relief within an hour or 2 and should last for up to 6 hours.
CAUTION: *Coffee should be used only occasionally to prevent or*

alleviate an attack. If you drink it every day, you may develop an insensitivity to its effects.

EUCALYPTUS If you have ever been near koala bears, you may have noticed that they smell like cough drops. This is because the principal ingredient in most cough drops comes from a staple of the koala's diet: eucalyptus leaves. Eucalyptus trees are native to Australia and Malaysia, where they are referred to as blue-gum trees, or Australian fever trees. The oil is widely used for respiratory ailments, such as asthma. The leaves contain rutin, a bioflavonoid, that can reduce inflammation in bronchial tubes.

At home, you can make a simple eucalyptus infusion by steeping a handful of fresh or dried leaves for 20 minutes in a quart of boiling water. Breathe in the vapors of the steaming tea, or drink the infusion in small doses. Always dilute eucalyptus oil in water before using.

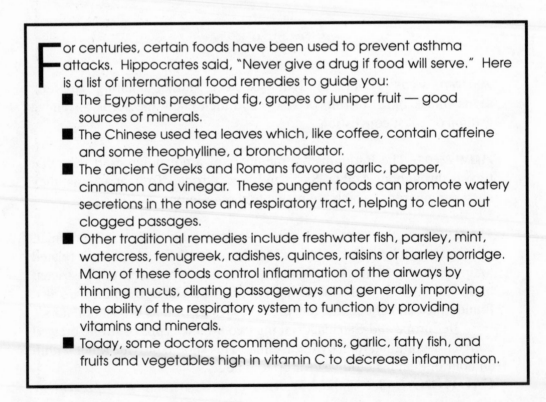

For centuries, certain foods have been used to prevent asthma attacks. Hippocrates said, "Never give a drug if food will serve." Here is a list of international food remedies to guide you:
- The Egyptians prescribed fig, grapes or juniper fruit — good sources of minerals.
- The Chinese used tea leaves which, like coffee, contain caffeine and some theophylline, a bronchodilator.
- The ancient Greeks and Romans favored garlic, pepper, cinnamon and vinegar. These pungent foods can promote watery secretions in the nose and respiratory tract, helping to clean out clogged passages.
- Other traditional remedies include freshwater fish, parsley, mint, watercress, fenugreek, radishes, quinces, raisins or barley porridge. Many of these foods control inflammation of the airways by thinning mucus, dilating passageways and generally improving the ability of the respiratory system to function by providing vitamins and minerals.
- Today, some doctors recommend onions, garlic, fatty fish, and fruits and vegetables high in vitamin C to decrease inflammation.

FENNEL In the United States, fennel is most commonly found sitting unopened in the back of a spice rack, behind the marjoram and the sage. But not in Greece. If you suffer from asthma, follow the Greek example and put your fennel to good use. The Greeks have discovered that fennel seed tea provides relief not only from the symptoms of asthma but also from many other respiratory ailments. Fennel contains rutin, and beneficial vitamins and minerals including calcium and potassium.

To make fennel seed tea, add 2 teaspoons of lightly crushed fennel seeds in 1 cup of hot water for 10 minutes. Strain before drinking.

GINGER Ginger figures prominently in Chinese medicine, and ginger tea is a popular Chinese treatment for asthma. You can find ginger tea in grocery stores and health food stores, or you can make it yourself. Press fresh ginger to extract the juice, and then use 1 teaspoon of the liquid to 1 cup of hot water.

GINKGO Ginkgo contains ginkgolides, which are compounds that smooth lung tissue and relax constricted bronchial tubes. The Chinese often use parts of the gingko tree to treat allergic sneezing.

The bark and leaves of this tree are also effective in the treatment of asthma. As the Chinese discovered before the advent of modern medicine, many asthma attacks are caused by the same allergic reactions that trigger hay fever. Ginkgo seeds can be made into a decoction for asthma. Combine the seeds with other herbs, such as ma huang, elecampane or mulberry leaves to treat both asthma and coughs.

NATURE'S MEDICINE CABINET

What the Chinese call ma huang is known among scientists as ephedra. For centuries, the Chinese have been stir-frying ephedra roots in honey and mixing them with apricot kernels. They find this preparation effective to treat asthma and a host of other illnesses.

Ma huang is the source of ephedrine, an active ingredient in many of our modern allergy and cold medications. Ephedrine causes the release of epinephrine, the quickly active stimulant component of adrenaline — used today to treat asthma by relaxing smooth muscle bronchoconstriction. Ma huang is available in health food stores and Oriental markets.

CAUTION: *Ma huang should not be used by pregnant women or people suffering from hypertension.*

Breathe Deeply!

According to the American Lung Association, an estimated 4.1 million children under 18 have asthma. Even though asthma cannot be cured, it can almost always be controlled with proper treatment and education. Without this, asthma can be seriously disruptive and even fatal. For these reasons, the ALA is implementing Open Airways for Schools, its premiere asthma education program. The ALA is dedicated to establishing the program in every elementary school in the country. Below are two exercises they teach:

Belly Breathing
1. Sit up straight on a chair or lie down on the bed or floor and bend your knees.
2. Place both hands on your belly.
3. Breathe in slowly through your nose. Take the air into your belly and feel it blow up big like a balloon. Keep your chest still.
4. Blow the air slowly out of your mouth through puckered lips. Feel your belly get small.
5. Repeat this exercise slowly 10 times. It will make breathing easier and it will make you feel relaxed.

Total Mind-Body Relaxation
1. Sit up straight on a chair or lie down comfortably on a bed or on the floor.
2. Close your eyes.
3. Place you hands on the side of your legs.
4. Tense the top of your head as tight as you can. Hold; then relax it.
5. Tense, hold, and then relax your face.
   Tense, hold, and then relax your shoulders.
   Tense, hold, and then relax your arms and hands.
   Tense, hold, and then relax your stomach.
   Tense, hold, and then relax your buttocks.
   Tense, hold, and then relax your legs and feet.
6. Now think of the most beautiful place you have ever visited and picture yourself there for a few moments. Relax.
7. When you are ready, open your eyes.

For more information, contact the American Lung Association, 1740 Broadway, New York, NY 10019-4374.

HYSSOP The Cherokee Indians used hyssop to help subdue asthma attacks, as well as general congestion. The plant contains a bitter compound that works as an expectorant, and its oils are an effective treatment for all types of respiratory ailments.

MUGWORT One of the many medicinal uses of the mugwort flower is as a treatment for asthma. Popular in ancient Greece, mugwort, which is also effective in treating other respiratory ailments, is now used in Europe, North Africa, Siberia, western Asia and the Himalayas. Mugwort contains tannins, which are astringents and reduce secretions.

ONION The proper British remedy for prolonged bouts with asthma is to soak thin onion slices in honey overnight. The resulting syrup is administered 4 times a day until the condition improves.

PERU BALSAM The Indians of Peru have found a treatment for asthma in the sap of the Peruvian balsam tree. Originally from the Pacific coast of El Salvador, this tree is well-known for its valuable wood and the strong perfume of its flowers. Peruvian Indians, however, know that the reddish-brown, syrupy sap of the tree is equally valuable for its ability to relieve respiratory ailments.

ATHLETE'S FOOT

Athlete's foot (or ringworm) is not life-threatening, but it can make life miserable. Although its causes are unknown, research does show that it is not limited to athletes and it is not only contracted from public showers or locker rooms. Studies have also shown that the group most likely to be affected is adult men, especially those who have previously had this type of infection before. Commonly, athlete's foot sufferers are those whose feet perspire, and those whose immune systems have been compromised.

The most common tell-tale sign of this fungus is its itchy, scaly, smelly rash, usually between the toes. In more severe cases, the irritation may actually cause cracked skin, while bacterial infections can complicate the malady even further. Certain variations of athlete's foot involve blistering on the sides and soles of the feet, and may require professional treatment.

However, for mild cases of athlete's foot and other minor skin irritations, a visit to the doctor is not always necessary. We've collected a variety of natural remedies, which may provide effective and inexpensive at-home relief. Just remember: You have to be patient with fungal infections. Although they're easy to detect, they often take two or more weeks to clear completely.

BAKING SODA If your feet get wet, remove your shoes and socks immediately, and carefully dry your feet — especially between your toes. Then raid the kitchen cabinet for some cornstarch or baking powder. Just spread your toes with some gauze or cotton balls, sprinkle on the powder, and then relax with your toes comfortably wedged apart.

COMFREY Comfrey is one of the most soothing remedies for athlete's foot. It contains mucilage that soothes and softens, and also a compound called allantoin that helps regenerate damaged skin. Fresh comfrey leaves can be mashed with a blender and applied to the skin.

FRESH AIR Whenever possible, free your feet from bondage and skip the shoes altogether. Fresh air and sunlight promote healing. If you can't go barefoot, try sandals or some other form of open-toed footwear.

GARLIC This herb has powerful antifungal properties, and is reputed to ward off infections caused by fungi. A clove or 2 of garlic in your daily diet may help get rid of the nasty foot fungus for good. (Some people rub raw garlic directly on the infected area.)

SAGEBRUSH The Zuni Indian of New Mexico uses sagebrush, a plentiful desert plant, to prevent athlete's foot infection. They simply gather the soft aromatic leaves and put them in their shoes. You can find sagebrush leaves in most health food stores.

TEA TREE OIL The Melaleuca tree — also known as the tea tree — is indigenous to Australia and has been hailed as a successful treatment for fungal infections of the skin. This shrub-like tree, which is also found extensively throughout South Florida, is non-toxic and non-irritating to most skin types. Australians apply a tiny drop of the tea tree oil to affected areas several times a day. They continue the treatment for a couple of weeks after all visible signs of the infection has cleared to be sure all of the fungus has been destroyed.

VINEGAR If your athlete's foot isn't too severe, try washing your feet and then soaking them in a bath of white vinegar and water (7 or 8 tablespoons to a quart of water).

VITAMIN E The healing properties of vitamin E oil are effective for athlete's foot.

WEAR NATURAL MATERIALS Shoes made of vinyl, rubber or any other synthetic product — that means both the sole and the upper — aggravate, or may even cause, athlete's foot. Leather and cotton products are recommended. And choose cotton socks whenever possible.

BACKACHE

If you have a backache, you have lots of company. At any given time, more than 31 million people in the United States suffer from back pain. In fact, 80 percent of all Americans suffer back pain at some time in their lives. Backaches account for 25 percent of all sick leave and $20 billion annually in medical costs in the United States alone.

The causes of back pain are diverse, and successful treatment is elusive. Therefore, if you suffer from severe or recurring back pain, you really should seek professional medical advice.

The traditional Western treatments for back pain often involve painkillers and surgery. Sometimes these methods work. More often they don't. Common sense measures are often the best way to ward off or treat backaches. In addition, you might want to try some of the little-known, time-tested, international remedies that we have found to safely relieve mild back pain.

BIRCH BARK Native Indians knew that the birch tree has many medicinal uses. They gathered the leaves or inner bark of the black birch and steeped them in hot water to make a tea to relieve lower back pain.

BLACK BEANS An Oriental remedy for back pain is to take 2 tablespoons of black beans every day for a month. Beans are good sources of protein, which is needed for strong muscles. And back pain is often the result of poor tone in the muscles that support the spinal column.

CHINESE TIGER BALM The soothing natural salve called Chinese Tiger Balm, is effective for the relief of back and other body pains. Chinese Tiger Balm is a healing ointment which contains aromatic oils of camphor, menthol, peppermint, clove and cajeput. When massaged into a painful area, it increases blood flow to surface skin.

EXERCISE!

Prevention and treatment of back pain through exercise deserves special mention and some special attention on your part. The vast majority of back problems are caused by muscle or ligament strain. That means both prevention and cure are possible if you're willing to spend a few minutes exercising each day.

If you already have a chronic back problem (the kind that never really leaves and flares up from time to time), you need to improve your strength and flexibility. Concentrate on your lower back, both when it's extended (straight) and when it's flexed (bent), your hamstrings, and your stomach muscles.

Here are a few exercises you can easily do to prevent back injuries or pain:

1. Single knee-to-chest stretch — Lie on the floor on your back and pull one knee into your chest until a comfortable stretch is felt in your lower back and buttocks. Hold for a 10 to 15 count. Repeat with opposite knee. Repeat 2 to 5 times.

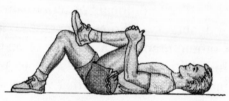

2. Angry cat stretch — Get on all fours with your back level. Slowly arch your back so you look like an angry or frightened cat. Hold for a count of 2. Repeat 5 to 10 times.

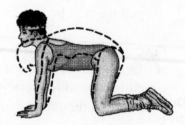

(Reprinted with permission from Dr. Robert D. Willix Jr.'s Health & Longevity, *105 West Monument Street, Baltimore, MD 21201)*

3. Pelvic tilt — Lie on your back with your knees bent and your feet flat on the floor. Using your stomach muscles, suck in your belly while you tilt your hips upward, flattening your lower back against the floor. Hold for a 10 count. Repeat 10 times.

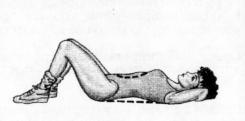

4. Mid-back stretch — Kneel on the floor. Extend your arms and torso forward, reaching as far as you can. Hold for a count of 10. Repeat 3 times.

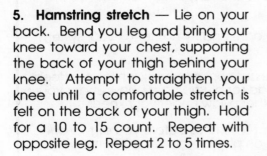

5. Hamstring stretch — Lie on your back. Bend you leg and bring your knee toward your chest, supporting the back of your thigh behind your knee. Attempt to straighten your knee until a comfortable stretch is felt on the back of your thigh. Hold for a 10 to 15 count. Repeat with opposite leg. Repeat 2 to 5 times.

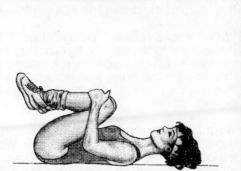

6. Double knee to chest stretch — Lie on your back. Pull both knees to your chest until a comfortable stretch is felt in your lower back. Hold for a 10 to 15 count. Repeat 2 to 5 times.

No matter how many painkillers and anti-inflammatories you stock in your medicine chest, you won't be able to eliminate back pain from your life unless you also use some good old-fashioned common sense.

Check your mattress. Make sure your mattress and box springs still have some life left in them — worn springs and soft mattresses wreak havoc on bad backs.

Drive in comfort. Lean slightly forward while you're driving. Keep your knees even with your hips (or preferably, higher than your hips). And when you're driving long distances, make regular stops so you can get out of the car and refresh your entire body with a short walk.

Lean forward. When standing, especially for long periods of time, lean forward slightly, so as to shift some of your weight away from your back. Also, try shifting your weight from one foot to the other.

Lift properly. Never, ever bend over to lift anything, even if it's relatively light. It doesn't take much to strain your back, especially as you get older. In order to lift anything without compromising your back, it's essential to do it from a squatting position (knees bent) to make sure your legs do the work. Avoid lifting heavy objects at all, whenever you can, by dividing the load or using a dolly.

Move. Try not to stay in the same position for any length of time, be it sitting, standing or lying down.

Rest. Sleep eight hours a night, if you can, and try not to tax your system by overworking or overplaying.

Sleep in an "S." In order to relieve pressure on your back while your sleep, try putting a neck roll behind your head (or plump up a pillow under your neck to get a similar effect) and another pillow under your knees.

Warm up. Be sure to stretch for at least 5 minutes before you exercise. (And when we say "exercise," we mean physical activities like mowing the lawn or cleaning the house, too.)

Watch your posture. Your mother didn't tell you not to slouch just because it looks bad — it also may injure your back. Sit up tall and straight — on a straight-back chair if possible. Be sure both feet are firmly planted on the floor, with your knees level with (or higher than) your hips. Avoid sitting on soft, mushy couches and chairs, especially for long periods of time.

Wear sensible shoes. The sturdier the shoe, the greater the support; therefore, the better for the back. Women who wear high heels are especially prone to lower back pain. They should wear low-heeled shoes, instead, as often as possible.

HEAT Backache sufferers often get relief by using a moist, hot towel or a heating pad. Lie on your stomach and have someone else put the heated pad on your back. Then cover it to keep the heat in.
CAUTION: *Heating pads should never be set on high and then placed on the skin. Use a towel in between to prevent burning.*

HYDROTHERAPY Water therapy is effective for many ailments. In the Orient, sufferers of back pain soak their feet in hot water for 20 to 30 minutes. Back pain and spasms are often relieved in this way. The nerves that go to the feet come off the lower spinal column, so warming them may do the trick.
CAUTION: *If you have ulcers, avoid this treatment. It may stimulate blood circulation, which could indirectly stimulate acid secretion in the stomach.*

ICE If your back pain is the result of a sudden strain or spasm, it's usually best to apply ice immediately. Later on, switch to moist heat.

KUNG FU In Hong Kong, back pain is treated not only by doctors, but sometimes also by masters of kung fu. The concentrated exercises and body control required to practice this martial art is an effective treatment. The inflammation that contributes to pain may be caused by noxious chemicals released by damaged cells. Movement of blood carries such toxins away from the area. So, any therapy that moves muscles and causes increased blood flow speeds recovery.

NATURAL ANTI-INFLAMMATORIES If your backache is caused by tissue inflammation, you might find relief by trying one of the natural anti-inflammatories already mentioned as a treatment for arthritis. These include cherries, devil's-claw tea, blackstrap molasses, celery, feverfew, alfalfa, ginger, yucca and fish oils.

PAPAYA Fiji Islands residents were the first to recognize the medicinal values of the fruit and bark of the papaya tree. Several other cultures have since recognized the papaya's powerful curative abilities. And research is now being done to develop the fruit's active enzyme, papain, to treat herniated (slipped) discs in the lower (lumbar) area of the back, a frequent source of severe back pain.

BAD BREATH

Bad breath can be a sign of a serious health problem like liver trouble, kidney failure, poor digestion, ulcers, sinusitis or periodontal disease. However, in most cases this malodorous malady is caused by poor dental hygiene or a diet that's heavy on pungent, spicy foods — and is easily remedied. To avoid embarrassment — and to keep yourself "kissing sweet" even while enjoying a garlic, onion, hot pepper, pepperoni pizza — try some of these natural tips we've gathered from breath-conscious cultures throughout the world.

ANISE SEEDS The Greeks chewed or sucked on anise seeds to freshen their breath. And today, it is common to see a bowl filled with breath-sweetening anise seeds as you leave an Indian restaurant. Anise seeds, which taste like licorice, also can be used to flavor baked goods.

BASIL Besides enhancing your favorite recipes, a sprig of fresh basil may sweeten your breath. It is commonly used by people in Portugal for just that purpose.

CARDAMOM In India, Guatemala, and the Orient, the perfect ending to a spicy meal is to chew on cardamom seeds to cleanse and sweeten the breath. In European cocktail lounges and bars, cardamom seeds are sometimes added to the food to cover up alcohol breath. Cardamom oil works even better, but is expensive and hard to find. Cardamom tastes like a mild ginger (it's a close relative) with a touch of pine.

CLOVES Cloves have many medicinal qualities. Besides using them as a toothache cure, the Chinese chew on 1 or 2 cloves to get rid of bad breath.

FENNEL In India, people use the fennel seed to freshen their breath by munching a handful after meals. Its licorice/lemon/pine taste is pleasing to most palates.

FENUGREEK Mistresses of the rich in ancient Athens kept their breath fresh by rolling perfumed oils around in their mouths throughout the day. It wasn't until later that the Greeks discovered fenugreek. This herb can be made into a tea to keep your breath fresh for long periods of time.

GINGER Raw and crystallized ginger are pleasant breath sweeteners.

GRAPEFRUIT Theophrastus, a Greek historian, believed that grapefruit was a good breath freshener. The vitamin C and bioflavonoids in grapefruit help make gums healthy. Other fruits that are especially recommended to counteract garlic breath are strawberries, red dates and persimmons.

MINT Another well-known folk remedy for bad breath is to chew on fresh mint leaves and stems. Mint contains menthol, which has a pleasant aroma.

PARSLEY In ancient Rome, people used parsley to cover up the smell of alcohol on their breath. And the Chinese cook coriander (Chinese parsley) with fish, pork or beef to eliminate bad breath.

Although most of us throw away this common garnish, parsley is edible. And because it has a high chlorophyll content, it is a natural breath sweetener. Chewing on a sprig of parsley can eliminate garlic breath, which may be the reason so many garlic pills are combined with parsley.

SAGE Many Arabs, American Indians and Far Eastern Indians rub their teeth with sage leaves to cleanse them and give a sweet smell to the breath.

STAR ANISE Orientals favor chewing star anise as a breath sweetener. It has an aroma and flavor similar to aniseed, but is stronger and sweeter, with just a hint of licorice. Chinese star anise — which has star-shaped fruit, aromatic leaves, and flowers that are white, pink or purple — is sometimes used as a flavoring agent in candy and chewing gum.

CAUTION: *Chinese star anise should not be confused with Japanese star anise, which is from a type of evergreen tree that is poisonous.*

BALDNESS

While it's true that many men experience some hair loss as they age, many others begin to lose their hair in their twenties or thirties. Premature baldness can be caused by nutrient deficiencies — and in these cases, it can be reversed. Usually, however, genetics is the cause for male pattern baldness.

Full baldness seems to affect only men. But thinning hair can also be a concern for women. Fortunately, except for the need for a little extra head protection during especially hot or cold weather, baldness is harmless. Nonetheless, fear of baldness has become a social obsession.

Advances made by Western medicine on this front have been negligible. One substance, minoxidil, has been proven to bring back some hair growth on the thinning, bald crown of the head, but it must be continuously applied, and is not effective on the "receding forehead" areas most characteristic of male pattern baldness. Minoxidil is also not effective for all people. So, while we cannot guarantee any of the following international alternatives, we believe they are worth considering.

BURDOCK Frequently eaten as a vegetable, burdock root is common throughout Europe. Some French people say that it also prevents hair loss, especially when the oil from the plant is rubbed into the scalp. The French also like to use a mixture made of equal quantities of burdock root, fresh burdock leaves and wine vinegar.

GINGER Ginger increases blood circulation. This nourishes hair roots and may encourage hair growth — which is probably the reason the following two Chinese remedies for growing hair back involve fresh gingerroot.

■ To try the first remedy, finely grate a chunk of ginger. Warm it slightly, spread it on the bald area, cover it with a shower cap for 30 minutes, and then wash it off. (But don't try this if there is any broken skin on the scalp.)

■ To try the second remedy, dip a cotton ball in a solution of 1 part ginger juice to 10 parts alcohol, and massage the bald area. Rinse after 30 minutes.

KELP Popular in Scottish diets, kelp helps prevent skin wrinkles. Eating kelp is also said to make your hair richer and more full-bodied. Minerals are important for hair growth — and kelp is full of minerals, particularly iodine. Hair loss is one of the earliest manifestations of hypothyroidism, which is caused by too little iodine in the body.

ONION There are many intriguing folk remedies for baldness that make use of the onion — for example, rub a little onion juice on your head and lie out in the sun.

Russian barbers sometimes recommend this hair-nourishing recipe to their balding customers: Mix 1 tablespoon of honey, 1 shot of vodka, and the juice of one onion. Rub into the scalp every night, cover, and then rinse off in the morning.

VITAMIN B Many Europeans — particularly the English, French and Germans — use organ meats in their cuisines. They also eat tongue and foods made with yeast. As a result, they get an ample supply of B vitamins, including vitamin B2, which could be effective against hair loss.

Vitamin B6 is found in yeast, bananas, pears, liver and salmon. And biotin is another B vitamin to consider. It is found in some special shampoos and lotions.

BLISTERS

Blisters are generally found on the feet, hands, knees and elbows, but may occur on other parts of the body as well. A blister is a watery swelling of fluids or blood just underneath the surface of the skin. It is caused by continuous rubbing or any other source of consistent irritation. Also, certain skin diseases and rashes (like poison ivy or poison oak) may cause blistering, as will severe burns and frostbite.

If you have a blister, your best bet is to leave it alone. Put a clean bandage on it once or twice daily, and allow the wound to heal itself. Usually, the swelling goes down and the water or blood is reabsorbed into the body.

Sometimes a blister breaks on its own, in which case you should carefully wash it with plain soap and water, and apply a bandage. Change the dressing several times a day. Since infection may be a complication with an open blister, check it regularly for signs of pus, unusual redness, or excessive swelling.

Here are a few natural blister care remedies.

CABBAGE In England, cabbage — high in vitamin C and minerals good for the skin — is used to soothe blisters. They boil the cabbage leaves in milk, which is also soothing, and apply when cool.

FIGS For minor blisters, Italians take a couple of mashed figs and mix them with a tablespoon of honey. Then they apply it to the blister.

LICORICE ROOT Finely powdered licorice root is used by people in the Middle East to dry up blisters.

General Blister Care

Your best course of action when treating a blister is to leave it alone. Don't break it. The fluid inside the bubble will be naturally reabsorbed causing the blister to disappear.

It's best to keep the blister covered with a Band-Aid to avoid irritation. If the blister does pop, clean the area thoroughly and then apply a covering to avoid irritation.

BODY ODOR

Perspiring is a normal bodily function — your body's response to physical exertion. When you perspire, your body is regulating its temperature and eliminating waste.

On average, your body secretes about a quart of water a day, in addition to mineral salts. Most of this moisture evaporates when it reaches the surface of your skin. The rest of the moisture, however, provides a great environment for bacteria to thrive in. And that's what causes the unpleasant odor.

Here are some natural ways to keep offensive odors at bay.

FENUGREEK The medicinal properties of fenugreek were discovered by the Egyptians. The plant has also been used by the Greeks, Romans and Chinese, all of whom ate it to eliminate body odor.

WITCH HAZEL Native Americans discovered the deodorizing applications of witch hazel extract, which they later passed on to European settlers.

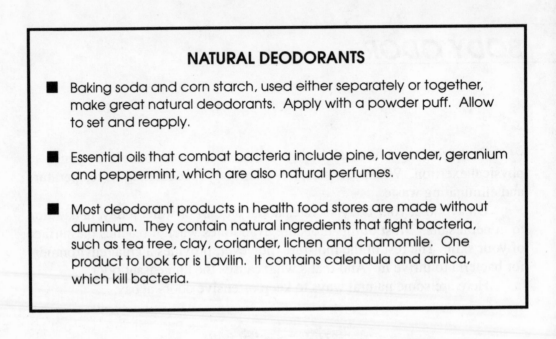

NATURAL DEODORANTS

■ Baking soda and corn starch, used either separately or together, make great natural deodorants. Apply with a powder puff. Allow to set and reapply.

■ Essential oils that combat bacteria include pine, lavender, geranium and peppermint, which are also natural perfumes.

■ Most deodorant products in health food stores are made without aluminum. They contain natural ingredients that fight bacteria, such as tea tree, clay, coriander, lichen and chamomile. One product to look for is Lavilin. It contains calendula and arnica, which kill bacteria.

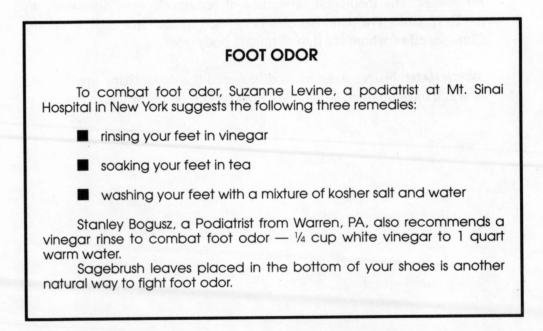

FOOT ODOR

To combat foot odor, Suzanne Levine, a podiatrist at Mt. Sinai Hospital in New York suggests the following three remedies:

■ rinsing your feet in vinegar

■ soaking your feet in tea

■ washing your feet with a mixture of kosher salt and water

Stanley Bogusz, a Podiatrist from Warren, PA, also recommends a vinegar rinse to combat foot odor — ¼ cup white vinegar to 1 quart warm water.

Sagebrush leaves placed in the bottom of your shoes is another natural way to fight foot odor.

BOILS

Boils, also called furuncles, are less common today than they were 100 years ago because of improvements in personal and public hygiene. They are still a concern, however, for travelers and inhabitants of undeveloped countries around the world.

Boils are usually caused by bacteria that find their way through breaks in the protective surface of the skin. In an open wound, these bacteria can cause infection. And if they attack hair follicles or oil-secreting glands, they can form a boil. Characterized by a localized infection, boils often resemble a common blister. The area becomes tender, red and filled with pus.

Most boils are not serious and disappear on their own. However, if a boil persists, have your doctor pierce it and apply a proper dressing. If you prefer to take care of it at home, try one of the following remedies. Remember, extreme care must be taken when treating boils in order to prevent bacteria from spreading to other parts of the body.

___**DANDELION**   In China, medical care is not centralized. So, in rural areas, local people are trained in first aid and minor procedures. They are called "barefoot doctors." To treat boils, these "doctors" simmer the leaves and tops of dandelions together to make a decoction. Or, they crush the plant and apply it to the boil as a poultice.

___**ECHINACEA**   Also called purple coneflower and Sampson root, Echinacea was used by Native American Indians to treat boils. A natural antiseptic, this plant has wound-healing properties when applied to the skin.

___**EGGS**   In England, a well-known cure for boils uses hard-boiled eggs. After the boiled egg has cooled, they carefully peel away the shell so that the thin inner membrane is left intact. Then they place this membrane over the boil and allow it to dry. The English say this relieves the soreness. Once the egg membrane has dried, they replace it with another.

FENUGREEK Fenugreek is well-known in the Mediterranean and the Middle East as a medicinal plant. It is a good source of vitamins and minerals, especially calcium. The seeds contain up to 30 percent mucilage (a plant gum) and make a good poultice. Fenugreek poultices have a healing effect and soothe boils.

HEAT This Irish treatment for boils uses wet heat: Fill a jar or bottle with hot water. Wait a few seconds — until the jar is thoroughly heated — and then pour out the water. Place the hot mouth of the jar over the boil. As the air in the jar cools and contracts, suction will draw out the core of the boil. Be careful not to squeeze the boil during this treatment, as you might spread the infection. Orientals use this same remedy. They call it "wet cupping."

KINO GUM The kino tree, one of the most widely cultivated trees in India, produces an oily gum, also called kino, that is prized for its astringent properties. Among other things, kino gum is used to treat all kinds of skin ulcers — including boils. The gum is harvested by piercing the tree bark. It is usually sold in cut or powdered form.

ONION The Cheyenne Indians used a poultice of onion bulbs and stems to treat boils. Onions, like garlic, contain large amounts of sulfur compounds (which are detoxifiers and antibiotics). Once the boil came to a head, the Indians washed out the pus with raw onion juice and water.

RADISHES An old English remedy is to place a slice of wild radish on the irritated area. Garden radishes contain sulphoraphine, a natural antibiotic, which may be why people in many European countries still use this treatment.

BRONCHITIS

Bronchitis is an inflammation or infection of the bronchial tubes — the airways that connect the windpipe with the lungs. Bronchitis can be caused by inhaling an irritant (such as dust or cigarette smoke) or by viral infection (such as the flu).

Acute bronchitis lasts for about 10 days and is best treated with bed rest, plenty of liquids, and protection from inclement weather. Chronic bronchitis is much more serious and is considered a chronic lung disease. It can last as long as four months or a lifetime and, if left untreated, can lead to pneumonia or severe lung damage.

Bronchitis is often indicated by the presence of excessive sputum (coughed up fluids and pus), either yellow, green or gray in color, and a persistent cough. Coughing during an attack of bronchitis should not be suppressed, as it is necessary to clear the lungs of excess mucus and trapped particles. Any cough remedy used should be an expectorant, not a suppressant. (See page 203 for natural cough remedies.)

Although chest pain is usually not a primary symptom of bronchitis, it may develop due to harsh or persistent coughing. A sore throat or tenderness around the "Adam's apple" is another typical complaint of bronchitis sufferers.

Serious cases of bronchitis require medical attention and possibly a prescription for antibiotics, such as ampicillin or tetracycline, to kill off the overgrowth of bacteria. Chest x-rays may also be ordered for serious cases of bronchitis. For a mild case, however, consider the following international remedies.

APPLE In Tudor times in England, bronchitis and severe coughs were treated with a well-liked remedy: an apple baked with honey and served mashed with butter. Canadian researchers have now determined that people who eat apples or drink apple juice on a daily basis tend to have a lower incidence of colds and upper respiratory ailments.

CHAMOMILE Prescribed by members of the medical community in France and Spain, hot chamomile tea is considered especially beneficial for children with bronchitis. Chamomile is high in calcium and magnesium, and also contains potassium, iron, manganese, zinc and vitamin A.

CHILI PEPPERS For bronchitis, the Swedes use hot chili peppers. When you bite into a hot pepper, your eyes water, and your nose runs. Your lungs and bronchial passages also produce watery secretions. The mucus in the lungs is thinned, and coughing is eased.

The compounds that give pepper its fiery effect are oily, and water can't dilute them. So, if you need to douse the fire after eating hot peppers, eat some cool yogurt or bread, or drink some milk. These substances will absorb the oils

EUCALYPTUS In Australia, boiling the leaves of the eucalyptus tree in water and inhaling the steam is a popular treatment for bronchitis. This softens mucus in obstructed airways and eases breathing.

IRISH MOSS For chronic bronchitis and other lung ailments, the high mucilage content in Irish moss is known to soothe the inflamed membranes of the respiratory tract. Irish moss's healing elements include iodine, calcium and sodium, as well as vitamins A, D, E and K. One recipe calls for 1 teaspoon of dried herb to 1 cup of water taken twice a day.

ONION A remedy for bronchitis popular throughout Europe may bring tears to your eyes — but it will also relieve your symptoms. In this treatment, a hot onion poultice is applied to the chest. Both the vapors and the heat ease breathing by clearing the airways.

PERU BALSAM The Indians of Peru, as well as many inhabitants of El Salvador, treat bronchitis the same way they treat asthma — by eating the thick sap of the balsam tree. The sap works especially well for bronchitis because it is an expectorant, which means it makes coughing easier. This clears out the lungs, thereby shortening the course of the illness. Peru balsam sap is available at most health food stores.

WARNING: Any cough that persists for more than a week, is accompanied by a fever, or shows signs of blood should be checked by a health care professional.

BRUISES

A bruise is the result of a blunt injury that doesn't break the skin. Tiny blood vessels rupture and show through the skin in varying shades of color. Mild bruises, the most common type, are slightly brown or gray. They fade after a few days. Bluish bruises, which are usually accompanied by pain and slight swelling, also disappear after a few days. Serious bruises are dark purple, nearly the color of a Concord grape. Often, the swelling accompanying this type of bruise stretches the skin so it looks shiny (which is where we get the term "shiner").

For the majority of healthy people, bruises heal over several days or weeks. Letting nature take its course is the logical resolve for healing black and blues (which change to reds before turning green and yellow as the blood is reabsorbed into the body.) Some bruises can be treated at home with the following natural remedies from around the world.

ADDER'S TONGUE Adder's tongue is used by American Indians as a remedy for bruises. The leaves and stem of the plant are mashed and made into an ointment which is applied to the affected area.

ARNICA Popular in Europe, Arnica tincture is effective in helping bruises heal. To make a tincture, refer to page 84.

BURDOCK The burdock plant is revered throughout Europe for its strong medicinal properties. The root of the plant is often used to treat bruises. To try it, break and mash the root until it produces a juice. Then rub the juice gently on the bruised area. The burdock plant grows wild in rubbish dumps and along roadsides, and is cultivated in gardens.

CHIVES The Chinese crush the leaves or roots of chives, a relative of the onion, and apply the juice to relieve the swelling and pain of bruises.

COMFREY English herbalists consider comfrey to be the most powerful healing agent in the plant world. They use it as a poultice for bruises, wounds, sores and insect bites. To make a poultice, use either fresh grated comfrey juice or boiled leaves and apply the liquid with a soft cloth.

HEAT A day or so after an injury, try putting heat on the bruise to speed blood flow and promote healing.

ICE Apply ice immediately after an injury to reduce the pain and swelling. And keep the afflicted area raised to decrease blood flow and minimize inflammation.

LAVENDER For centuries, lavender oil compresses have been used in France, Spain and other regions of Europe for soothing bruises. The oil has antibacterial properties.

LEMON The Germans treat bruises with a lemon-and-water preparation. A lemon is sliced in half and boiled. The resulting solution is cooled and given in doses of 1 cupful a day.

This treatment is especially effective if the patient is vitamin C deficient. The yellow outer skin and the white inner skin of the lemon peel contain healing agents (bioflavonoids). These agents combine with the vitamin C of the lemon pulp to help strengthen the small capillaries throughout the body and accelerate the healing of bruises. (This treatment can also be used to help prevent deficiency-related bruises.)

POTATO American folklore mentions many uses for the potato. Raw potato juice or hot potato water is said to relieve bruises and sprains. This probably works because potatoes contain many minerals that help with healing.

WITCH HAZEL You can bet that the Mohawk Indians, mighty hunters and warriors, suffered their share of bruises. The Mohawk treatment used the bark and leaves of the witch hazel tree which they boiled and applied to the skin — after the preparation had cooled, of course.

WARNING: If you bruise with overwhelming ease or frequency, you should consult a physician. You could have a vitamin C deficiency, a blood disorder, or a reaction to cortisone medication.

BURNS

It doesn't take much. A quick brush with a hot iron, a tiny drop of hot oil from a sizzling skillet — or too many minutes under the hot sun. Burns, even minor ones, can be extremely painful.

Burns are measured in degrees, according to the extent of the tissue damage. First-degree burns are red and tender and sometimes cause swelling. They injure only the first layer of skin, the epidermis. A mild sunburn is a first-degree burn. (See page 477 for natural sunburn remedies.)

With a second-degree burn, there is blistering, which indicates that tissue damage has extended past the epidermis and into the dermis, the second layer of skin. Second-degree burns that cover only a small area should be rinsed gently with soap and water to remove any loose skin. A second-degree burn that covers a large area of the body is serious and requires medical attention. This type of burn may take two weeks or longer to heal.

Third-degree burns are the most severe and require immediate medical attention — possibly even hospitalization. A third-degree burn causes complete destruction of the full thickness of skin and maybe even the tissue underneath.

Get professional help immediately for any serious burn. Minor burns, however, can be treated effectively at home using one of the following remedies.

ALOE Aloe has been prized for centuries as a burn remedy. Its clear gel, which oozes out of the broken stems and leaves, can be directly applied to burns. The mucilaginous fluid in the leaf relieves pain and has a soothing effect on the injured skin.

The Greeks used aloe as a healing herb as far back as 2,000 years ago. And its reputation was so widespread in 333 B.C. that Alexander the Great sent a special emissary to the Island of Socotra to retrieve some.

BURDOCK The root of the burdock plant is effective in the treatment of minor burns. This plant, considered a weed, grows wild. But because Europeans find it so helpful to treat various ailments, they often cultivate it in their gardens.

CUCUMBER The Chinese rub cucumber juice into the skin to treat burns.

GINGER The healing magic of ginger stops the pain of superficial burns instantly, reduces swelling and helps to eliminate blistering. Whatever the source of the burn, it can be treated by crushing fresh ginger, squeezing out the juice and applying with a cotton ball.

GOTU KOLA In the Fiji islands, healers treat burns with the gotu kola plant, a weed that is commonly found in mountainous tropical regions. Fiji healers claim that the plant accelerates the healing of burned tissue.

HONEY Descendants of the Norse people still mix honey and cod liver oil into a preparation that they use to treat minor burns. Nutrients in the oil (vitamins A and D) and honey accelerate healing by nourishing surrounding areas of healthy skin. It decreases bacterial growth, but does make a sticky mess.

LAVENDER Lavender oil compresses are commonly used in Europe for soothing burns.

LEEKS For minor burns, the Romans used leek juice. Like the onion, it is a natural antiseptic. The juice was extracted from a whole plant and applied as a salve to the burnt area. The Egyptians, too, used leek juice as a burn treatment to soothe and heal damaged skin.

ONION On the Ivory Coast of Africa, onion juice is used to treat burns. The juice does not necessarily relieve pain, but it does act as an antiseptic.

ST. JOHN'S WORT For minor burns, many people use the oil form of St. John's wort, which can be gently dabbed on the injury to promote healing.

SLIPPERY ELM Slippery elm is a food and a medicine that American Indians used for a variety of ailments. Today, slippery elm powder is made from either the inner or outer bark of the red elm tree. Mix the powder with water to make a poultice and apply. The soothing, healing properties come, in part, from the high mucilage content.

VITAMIN A Vitamin A is an antioxidant, which can speed healing. Good food sources of vitamin A include green fruits and vegetables.

VITAMIN C Vitamin C is another antioxidant. Good food sources of vitamin C include citrus fruits, potatoes and broccoli.

VITAMIN E Vitamin E soothes burns and may also help prevent scarring. Apply it by splitting open a capsule and applying it directly.

Turn to page 50 for a chart listing food sources for vitamins and minerals.

CANCER

Cancer is still one of the most feared and misunderstood diseases in the world, despite the fact that we are learning more about it every day. The good news is, we now have successful treatments for many cancers. More important, we have learned how to take positive preventive steps — by making simple lifestyle changes — to help lower the risk of developing this disease in the first place.

All cancers, and there are many types, have one thing in common — they are characterized by rapid, excessive and uncontrolled cell growth. This is why early detection is so critical, and why knowing what to look for gives you the upper hand when dealing with this disease. Some of the early warning signs of cancer include:

- Unusual bleeding or discharge
- Sores that fail to heal
- Lumps that grow on or under the skin
- Chronic fever
- Unusual bruising
- Unusual changes in bowel habits
- Persistent difficulty in swallowing
- Recurring indigestion
- Obvious change in wort or mole
- Nagging cough or hoarseness

Because these symptoms can be a sign of less serious ailments, many people tend to ignore them. But it is vital for you to recognize that these symptoms are also consistent with cancer, and must be looked at by a doctor — as soon as possible — if you have any doubts whatsoever.

Cancer doesn't just happen overnight. It takes a long time, and a combination of factors, to develop. We get cancer cells in our bodies all the time when normal cells go haywire. Out of control, these cells can keep growing until a cancer is established. If our immune systems are working properly, those first few cells are destroyed. If, however the

Eat to Beat Cancer

Many physicians believe that anywhere from 10 to 70 percent of all cancers can be traced to poor dietary habits. The National Cancer Institute agrees that the risk of cancer can be diminished by what we eat and has developed these general guidelines to improve your chances:

- ■ Reduce your intake of saturated fat.
- ■ Avoid salt-cured, smoked and nitrate-cured foods such as bacon, cheese and luncheon meats. (It's interesting to note that while the Japanese have a low incidence of cancer, those that do get the disease seem to favor a diet high in smoked, pickled and salt-cured foods.)
- ■ Eat plenty of high-fiber foods like whole grains, fruits and vegetables.
- ■ Adults should eat at least 5 servings of fruits and/or vegetables a day, especially those rich in the antioxidant vitamins beta-carotene (which becomes vitamin A in the body) and vitamin C.

It is also recommended that you avoid alcoholic beverages, reject tobacco, and reduce refined sugar and sodium.

immune system malfunctions — perhaps weakened by repeated exposure to toxic substances, poor nutrition or continual mental stress — it can't protect us. That's why our first line of defense against cancer is to take preventive measures to keep the immune system strong.

AGRIMONY The Chinese prevent colon cancer by mixing an extract of the hairyvein agrimonia (agrimony) plant with ethyl alcohol (drinking alcohol). Agrimony is available at most health food stores.

ANTIOXIDANTS These vitamins — especially beta-carotene and vitamin C — may halt the processes that lead to cancer.

The best food sources of beta-carotene are cantaloupes, carrots, apricots, mangos, oranges, nectarines, tangerines, peaches, papayas, broccoli, prunes and pumpkins. Though all orange and deep yellow fruits and vegetables are rich in beta-carotene, Polish researchers discovered that the seeds and pulp of deep orange pumpkins and winter squash, in particular, contain substances that may inhibit cancer.

The best food sources of vitamin C are citrus fruit, Brussels sprouts,

Preventing Breast Cancer

More than half of all women will detect breast lumps during their lifetimes — and about 10 percent of these lumps will be cancerous. That's why it's so important for all women to learn how to do self exams, in addition to scheduling regular clinical exams and mammograms. If you are not yet familiar with the technique of self-examination, check with your doctor. There are also many pamphlets available at your local library that clearly illustrate the various steps. And if you find a lump, see your doctor immediately. Remember, if detected early, breast cancer is highly treatable.

Diet. Recent scientific findings suggest that diet is especially important in breast cancer prevention. For example, in one very recent study, researchers from the New York University Medical Center and the Strang Cancer Prevention Center in New York discovered that the level of bile acids (which can be carcinogenic) found in breast cyst fluid is 100 times greater than in the blood. They also discovered that the origin of this high concentration of bile acids came from food being digested in the intestines — indicating a strong link between diet and the risk of breast cancer.

And additional studies done at the Strang-Cornell Cancer Research Laboratory in New York suggest that compounds called "indoles" — which are found in cruciferous vegetables — may protect against breast cancer by preventing the body from producing a kind of estrogen that is often found in women who have breast cancer. Instead of producing this highly reactive, cancer-stimulating kind of sex hormone, it appears that indoles encourage the production of a hormone that is relatively inert.

Exercise. According to a recent study published in the *Journal of the National Cancer Institute*, regular, moderate physical activity may help premenopausal women (women ages 40 and under) reduce their risk of developing breast cancer. And because professional athletes (and other women who exercise strenuously) typically have a low risk of breast cancer, the researchers are currently studying post-menopausal women to see if vigorous physical exercise has the same beneficial effect as moderate exercise.

broccoli, cauliflower, strawberries, potatoes, tomatoes, sweet potatoes, spinach, leafy greens, honeydew melons, papayas and sweet peppers.

All of these fruits and vegetables are also chock-full of phytochemicals, which have been shown to stunt the growth of cancer cells in test-tube studies.

APRICOT This fruit is an excellent source of beta-carotene, a form of vitamin A that has proven to be especially helpful in thwarting lung and skin cancer. (Dried apricots contain more beta-carotene than the raw fruit.)

BEANS This nutritious vegetable, which is readily available in many varieties, has a multitude of effective preventive properties.

Beans are high in fiber, which has been widely credited with helping to prevent both cancer and heart disease. They are also a source of saponins, which help to slow down the runaway cell division associated with cancer and protease inhibitors, which suppress certain enzymes in cancer cells to slow the rate of growth.

Specifically, beans provide a defense against colon cancer by inhibiting the over-production of cells in the large intestine. And the isoflavens in this vegetable help prevent breast and ovarian cancers by reducing the possibly carcinogenic estrogens from increasing.

BROCCOLI This highly nutritious veggie belongs to the group of vegetables called "crucifers," which have been linked with lower development rates of some cancers. Broccoli contains dithiolthiones,

---

Herbs and Spices May Help

Preliminary research suggests that some herbs and spices, particularly rosemary, tumeric and cumin, may have anti-cancer properties. Curcamin, which gives curry its yellow color, may also ward off cancer. Researchers at Rutgers University hypothesize that these substances may act like antioxidants, gobbling up free radicals before they can damage cellular DNA.

which stimulate your body's immune system to fight cancer on its own. In addition, broccoli (along with the other crucifers) contains indoles which have been linked to lowering the risk of breast cancer.

Other crucifers include cauliflower, cabbage, Brussels sprouts, collard greens, kale, mustard greens and turnips. For the greatest health benefits, eat these vegetables raw or lightly cooked.

BURDOCK A common vegetable side dish in Europe is burdock. This veggie reputedly neutralizes poisons — and preliminary research suggests that it may also be valuable as a tumor preventive.

BRUSSELS SPROUTS Brussels sprouts are loaded with beta carotene and chlorophyll, and eating them has been linked to lower rates of colon and stomach cancer. Scientists suspect that chemicals called glucosinolates, which are found in high levels in the vegetable, are why they are so potent.

CARROTS Carrots are loaded with beta-carotene, which has been tied to a variety of lowered cancer rates. One study in Edinburgh, Scotland specifically tied carrots to a lowered risk of colon cancer.

CITRUS Rich in fiber and vitamins A and C, oranges, grapefruits, lemons and limes also contain a substance called limonene that may work by

---

NATURE'S MEDICINE CABINET

The people of Hunza who live in the Himalayas of West Pakistan live long and healthy lives — past the age of 100 in some cases. And they are virtually free of cancer. This may be due to the Hunza diet, which includes large amounts of buckwheat, peas, broadbeans, lucern, apricots and apricot seeds, cherries and cherry seeds, and sprouting legumes — all of which contain vitamin B17, which is also known as laetrile.

At one time, laetrile was used as a cancer drug in the United States, but there was a lot of controversy over it because it contains cyanide. The laetrile is present in very small amounts in the foods in the Hunza diet (except for the cherry and apricot pits), and so is considered not harmful.

stimulating the body to produce cancer-inhibiting enzymes.

In animal studies, when rats were given a drug known to cause breast cancer, orange peel oil reduced the incidence of the disease. In Japanese studies, grapefruit extract has been shown to stop tumor growth. And Dutch and Swedish research indicates that people who eat citrus fruit have less risk of getting cancer of the pancreas and stomach.

FENUGREEK Dr. Max Gerson, author of *A Cancer Therapy*, reports that he witnessed the disappearance of two breast cancers after the use of large

---

Preventing Colon Cancer

Colon cancer is the second most common lethal cancer in the United States, killing about 60,000 people every year — which is the reason so much research is focused on eradicating this form of the disease. Though colon cancer is a major killer of both men and women, it is found most often in men over the age of 40. Though we are learning more and more about how to prevent colon cancer, early detection is still the key to successful treatment — and the reason you should see your doctor at the first sign of rectal bleeding or changes in your bowel habits.

Diet. It is becoming increasingly evident that a high-fiber, low-fat diet is the primary factor in preventing colon cancer. Research has shown that a high-fat diet has a direct effect on carcinogenic changes in the colon. That's why the National Cancer Institute recommends you reduce your fat intake to less than 30 percent of calories. And while the average American gets about 10 grams of fiber a day, cancer experts recommend you increase your fiber intake to 20 to 30 grams daily.

You can easily get more fiber in your diet by eating high-fiber cereals, whole-grain breads and muffins, and plenty of fresh fruits and vegetables. Cruciferous vegetables are especially good. Research in Greece, Japan and the United States indicates that eating raw or cooked broccoli or cabbage once a week can significantly decrease your chances of getting colon cancer. And Norwegians, who typically include a lot of crucifers in their diets, have fewer and smaller pre-cancerous polyps of the colon.

Exercise. Daily exercise — along with a high-fiber diet — can help you have regular bowel movements. And that, in itself, will lower your risk of getting colon cancer.

amounts of fenugreek seed tea in combination with a salt-free vegetarian diet. This may be because fenugreek contains plant hormones, and some breast cancers respond to hormones that counteract estrogen.

FIGS Figs and fig extracts contain the compound benzaldehyde. In her book *Food — Your Miracle Medicine* (Harper-Collins), Jean Carper reports that Japanese researchers have used this compound to successfully shrink tumors in human beings.

> ## EXERCISE!
> Studies have shown that regular exercise can lower your risk of certain cancers, especially cancers of the colon and breast. Try to exercise at least 4 hours a week. Walk, bike, swim, jog, hike, dance — anything you like. The important thing is to pick an activity you enjoy. Then you'll be more likely to stick with it.

GARLIC Dr. Gerson also says that in countries like Italy, Greece and Yugoslavia, where a lot of garlic is used, the cancer rate is low. He notes that in China, people who routinely eat garlic and onions have a lower incidence of stomach cancers. This may be because these vegetables contain allyl sulfides, which help the body excrete carcinogens before they can do any damage.

GRAINS Grains such as rice, wheat and barley have earned a good nutritional reputation because of the many health benefits they offer. And now we have indications that the phytic acid found in all grains may provide an additional cancer-preventing benefit. It appears that phytic acid binds to the mineral iron and may prevent it from causing free-radical damage that could lead to cancer.

GREEN TEA For many years, green tea has been the beverage of choice for millions of Asians. Now research is finding that this ancient brew may help lower your risk of cancer of the esophagus.

According to a study in the *Journal of the National Cancer Institute*, the risk of esophageal cancer in a group of people who regularly drank green tea and were non-smokers and non-alcohol drinkers was reduced by 57 percent for men and 60 percent for women. The researchers speculate that this has something to do with the polyphenols found in green tea. In animals, these compounds have been shown to protect against cancer by stopping the production of enzymes that produce cancer-causing substances.

JOB'S TEARS The Chinese believe that this herb may inhibit the growth of cancer cells. Taken as a tea, Job's tears has a sweet, light flavor. It is available in health food stores.

KALE All dark green, leafy vegetables are excellent sources of vitamins and minerals that boost the immune system. Researchers have found that Hawaiians (whose diet is especially rich in these vegetables) have lower rates of lung cancer. And in Singapore, people specifically eat raw or cooked kale to prevent this disease.

SEAWEED One culture that has a particularly low incidence of cancer is the Japanese. Traditional Japanese cooking uses a lot of seaweed. Nori, a particular kind of seaweed favored in sushi dishes, actually may contain anti-tumor compounds that prevent cancers of the digestive tract.
Another type of seaweed, kelp, is a Japanese diet staple. It is added

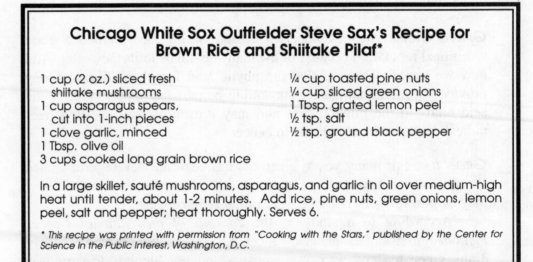

Chicago White Sox Outfielder Steve Sax's Recipe for Brown Rice and Shiitake Pilaf*

1 cup (2 oz.) sliced fresh
   shiitake mushrooms
1 cup asparagus spears,
   cut into 1-inch pieces
1 clove garlic, minced
1 Tbsp. olive oil
3 cups cooked long grain brown rice

¼ cup toasted pine nuts
¼ cup sliced green onions
1 Tbsp. grated lemon peel
½ tsp. salt
½ tsp. ground black pepper

In a large skillet, sauté mushrooms, asparagus, and garlic in oil over medium-high heat until tender, about 1-2 minutes. Add rice, pine nuts, green onions, lemon peel, salt and pepper; heat thoroughly. Serves 6.

This recipe was printed with permission from "Cooking with the Stars," published by the Center for Science in the Public Interest, Washington, D.C.

to salads and entrees, eaten as a vegetable, and is used as a seasoning in soup. And the Egyptians and Chinese have been eating brown kelp (laminar) for centuries. This type of seaweed is said to be one of nature's pharmaceutical miracles — and a possible cancer preventive.

SHIITAKE MUSHROOM Lentinan, an extract made from the shiitake mushroom (a common ingredient in Japanese cooking) is now being studied for its effectiveness in the treatment of cancer. In particular, the shiitake is believed to work on stomach and cervical cancer.

SOY Research indicates that the low incidence of breast cancer in East Asian women could be due to the high level of soy protein in their diets. Good food sources of soy protein include tofu, tempeh, soy flour and soybeans.

SPINACH In the U.S. and the rest of the world, people are finding out just how healthy spinach can be. Dr. Richard Sekelle, a scientist at the University of Texas, found that people who ate spinach (and other foods high in beta-carotene) had 8 times less of a chance of developing lung cancer than people who didn't eat these foods. Italian researchers proved that spinach can block the formation of nitrosamines — some of the most potent cancer-causing chemicals.

STRAWBERRIES Strawberries — and grapes — are especially good sources of two phytochemicals (ellagic acid and phenethyle isothiocyanate) which have been found effective in preventing and treating cancer of the esophagus by prohibiting cells from becoming cancerous when exposed to a cancer-causing chemical.

TOMATO Nitrosamines are by-products of our digestive process that have been proven to cause cancer. But two phytochemicals found in tomatoes (p-coumaric and chlorogenic acid) can prevent the formation of nitrosamines. (Strawberries, grapes, carrots and green peppers, as well as other fruits and vegetables, also contain p-coumaric acid and chlorogenic acid.)

In addition, tomatoes contain another cancer-fighting substance — lycophene, an antioxidant that may reduce your risk of cancers of the mouth, esophagus, stomach, colon and rectum. Some researchers suggest that you eat 7 or more tomatoes a week.

TUMERIC Tumeric may not find its way into many American dishes, but it is an extremely popular flavoring in India, especially in the eastern part of the country. And now there is evidence — demonstrated by the lower rate of cancers in this part of India — that this spice may have cancer-preventing properties.

WHEATGRASS A rich, nutritional food called wheatgrass was discovered by Dr. Ann Wigmore. Dr. Wigmore believes that its extremely high vitamin and mineral content is helpful in the prevention of cancer and other disorders. In many juice "bars," wheatgrass is added to mixtures of fruit and vegetable juices.

CANKER SORES

Canker sores are small, painful ulcers that can occur anywhere inside the mouth. The most common sites for these small, white and red ulcers are on the tongue, gums or inside the cheeks. The sores can appear singly or in groups. Most of them clear up within two weeks, though some can last months.

Canker sores are more common in women than men, and although doctors aren't really sure what causes them, people at higher risk tend to have low levels of iron, vitamin B12 and folic acid. That's why, if you are prone to canker sores, you might want to add these foods to your diet:

- Steamed clams, oysters and mussels (for vitamin B12)
- Peas, beans, wheat germ and lentils (for folic acid)
- Fortified cereals, lean cuts of beef and tofu (for iron)

A vitamin B-complex supplement (providing 100 milligrams of each of the B vitamins) may also help. And to treat canker sores once they've developed, try some of the following tried-and-true natural remedies.

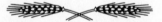

BURNET Some herbalists recommend burnet to help heal mouth ulcers. Crush a teaspoon of fresh leaves and place inside your mouth on the sore. Leave it there for 20 minutes. Repeat this procedure 2 or more times a day until the pain subsides.

GOLDENSEAL This small woodland plant is important in Native American medicine. To use it to treat canker sores, make a mouth rinse composed of 1 cup of warm water, ¼ teaspoon of salt, and ½ teaspoon of goldenseal (or the contents of one capsule of goldenseal powder). Goldenseal is available in health food stores.

SAGE North American Indian tribes believed that sage offered many benefits, including spiritual salvation. And at the other end of the globe, Chinese and Arabic herbalists shared these beliefs. Modern herbalists recommend sage as a treatment for canker sores. This herb contains camphor and other volatile oils which have antiseptic and astringent properties to help clean and shrink the sores.

To make a sage mouthwash, steep 1 teaspoon of fresh sage (or ¼ teaspoon dried) in 1 cup of hot water, covered, for 4 minutes. Then swirl in ¼ teaspoon of salt and 1 teaspoon of cider vinegar. Swish the mixture around in your mouth while it's still hot.

TEA A popular home remedy for canker sores is to apply a wet tea bag to the area. Black tea is said to work best, due to its high tannin content, which acts as a pain-relieving astringent.

VITAMIN C Vitamin C can be very helpful in preventing and treating canker sores — especially those caused by stress or trauma to the mouth. Good food sources of vitamin C include red, yellow, and orange vegetables, and citrus fruits.

VITAMIN E Some people find relief by squeezing a capsule of vitamin E oil directly onto the sore.

Helpful Hint

To create a harsh environment for canker sores, gargle with a mixture of three parts water to one part hydrogen peroxide.

CARPAL TUNNEL SYNDROME

If you spend much of your day doing repetitive arm and wrist motions — for example, if you're a computer operator, a hair stylist, or a seamstress — you are putting continuous stress on your hands, wrists and arms. This kind of stress can lead to numbness and tingling in the fingers, accompanied by pain, stiffness and swelling. These symptoms can become severe, even spreading to the elbows and shoulders. In extreme cases, the entire arm becomes so weak that weight cannot be supported.

If these symptoms sound familiar to you, you may be experiencing carpal tunnel syndrome (CTS) — along with about 23,000 other people who suffer from it each year. CTS affects the carpel tunnel at the base of the hand that is formed by your wrist bones and ligaments. Repeated extension and flexing causes these ligaments to become inflamed, putting pressure on the median nerve.

Fortunately, there are several easy things you can do to reduce the pain, prevent it from getting worse, and even lower your risk of getting carpal tunnel syndrome in the first place.

REST Take periodic 2-minute breaks during long work sessions to give your hands a rest.

VITAMIN B6 There is scientific evidence that this nutrient can not only successfully treat mild to moderate cases of carpal tunnel syndrome, it can act as a preventive. For example, researchers from the Kaiser Pernanente Medical Center in Hayward, California had success with a vitamin B6 dosage of 200 milligrams per day administered over a period of three months. How does it work? Carpal tunnel syndrome causes a reduction in the rate at which nerve impulses travel, and vitamin B6 therapy seems to speed up the nerve impulses to the hand, reducing the pressure and pain.

If your daily work puts you at risk of developing CTS, take 50 to 100 milligrams of B6 daily. And add some good food sources of this vitamin — whole grain cereals, fish (especially salmon), chicken, liver and egg yolks — to your diet.

WATCH YOUR POSTURE It may seem a bit awkward at first, but this can help ease the pressure and pain of CTS: Simply keep your hands and wrists as straight as possible while you work. Once you get into the habit of working this way, your symptoms should subside.

WEAR A SPLINT The goal here is to relieve the pressure on the median nerve in your wrist. By wearing a splint at night, you'll be able to accomplish this and still be able to handle your daily work activities. You can obtain a splint through an occupational therapist or at your local drug store.

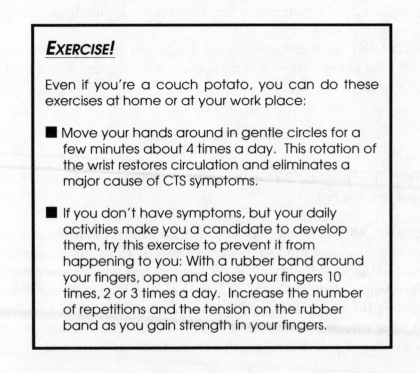

EXERCISE!

Even if you're a couch potato, you can do these exercises at home or at your work place:

■ Move your hands around in gentle circles for a few minutes about 4 times a day. This rotation of the wrist restores circulation and eliminates a major cause of CTS symptoms.

■ If you don't have symptoms, but your daily activities make you a candidate to develop them, try this exercise to prevent it from happening to you: With a rubber band around your fingers, open and close your fingers 10 times, 2 or 3 times a day. Increase the number of repetitions and the tension on the rubber band as you gain strength in your fingers.

CELLULITE

Cellulite is the term used to describe the dimpled, lumpy fat deposits that form on the thighs, buttocks and upper arms. These deposits tend to be worse in women who retain fluid — however, the main cause is too much fat in the diet, combined with not enough exercise. So, to help you win your battle with these unsightly bulges, here are our diet and exercise tips.

CALCIUM Calcium is one of the common minerals that helps keep skin healthy. Magnesium, zinc and potassium also are recommended for eliminating cellulite. Turn to page 50 for natural sources of these minerals.

DIET Aim for a low-fat, high-fiber, low-sodium diet that's about 25 percent calories from fat. Eat plenty of fruits, vegetables and whole grains. (Naturalists specifically recommend millet to combat cellulite.) Keep meats to a minimum and read the labels on prepared foods. For more information on weight loss, refer to page 509.

EXERCISE Pick an aerobic activity you enjoy and stick with it for at least 20 minutes 3 times a week. Walking, hiking, dancing and running are all excellent ways to get rid of cellulite — and improve your general health at the same time. Try lifting weights to firm up flabby arms and thighs. Start with a book that has weightlifting exercises specifically designed for women. Then consult with a fitness professional before you join a gym or set up a workout space at home.

EXFOLIATION The better your circulation, the less likely you are to develop cellulite. Use a loofah with a natural abrasive such as sea salt or an almond scrub to stimulate blood flow in the tissues.

MASSAGE A daily massage with vitamin E oil or vegetable oils such as safflower or rice oil also improves circulation.

MOISTURIZE Keeping the skin's surface hydrated helps in the battle against cellulite. Lotions that include vitamin E and aloe are your best bets.

WATER Diet, exercise and drinking plenty of water are the 3 keys to getting rid of cellulite. Eight glasses of water every day is the suggested amount.

WARNING: Stay Away From Those "Miracle" Creams!

American women spend millions trying to get rid of cellulite with creams, gels and other pricey preparations. But, according to an independent research team at Johns Hopkins University in Baltimore, none of the cellulite-reducing products they tested worked. The Food and Drug Administration is now monitoring claims made by the manufacturers of these products, many of which are imported from other countries.

Helpful Hint

You can use anything — even fighting cellulite — as an excuse to treat yourself to an herbal bath. Cal-a-Vie's Spa recommends perfuming the water with sage, cypress and/or juniper oils.

CHICKEN POX

Chicken pox is a contagious disease which is most common in children between two and six years old, although it can affect people of any age. Although the itching that accompanies chicken pox is extremely uncomfortable, additional side effects are rare — and immunity is usually permanent.

There's very little advance warning before the onset of chicken pox, except for the possibility of a slight fever before blisters begin to appear on the body. The blisters usually dry up and disappear by the fourth day — without scarring — as long as the patient is prevented from scratching them. This is easier said than done, especially when you are dealing with very young children. However, to that end, we offer some effective ways from around the world to cut down on the intensity of the itching and keep your little patient comfortable.

BORAGE As a topical remedy, borage tea helps to clear up the blisters caused by chicken pox. Simply apply the cooled liquid to the blisters with a cotton swab.

CHICKWEED This herb can be used in two ways to relieve inflammation and itching — as an additive to the bath, and as an after-bath salve.

To use in the bath, add the chickweed to about 2 pints of water. Bring it to a boil, then remove from the heat and let it cool for about 15 minutes. Then strain the mixture and add it to the bath water.

To make chickweed salve, mix about 8 ounces of chopped chickweed with 6 ounces of petroleum jelly and 1 ounce of beeswax in a warmed ovenproof bowl. Then cover the bowl and keep it in a low oven for 4 hours. Strain through muslin or nylon cloth, cover and keep cool.

COMFREY Native Americans mix powdered comfrey, powdered Oregon grape root and green clay to make a salve that is both healing and soothing.

LANTANA In the Bahamas, the leaves of this plant are applied to the blisters to ease the itch.

OATMEAL One of the oldest remedies in the book for relieving the chicken pox itch is a tepid bath with oatmeal. After the bath, don't towel-dry — let the skin dry naturally to retain some of that soothing oatmeal residue.
CAUTION: *The bottom of the bathtub can become very slippery when oatmeal is mixed with the water.*

TEA The Chinese grind tea leaves into a powder and dissolve them in boiling water to make a strong tea that they apply to the blisters 2 to 3 times a day.

ZINC OXIDE Australians make a soothing powder of equal parts of zinc oxide, boric acid and cornstarch to help relieve the itch of chicken pox.

CHRONIC FATIGUE SYNDROME

Chronic Fatigue Syndrome (CFS) has been identified only in the recent past, primarily because its many symptoms are common to a vast number of other illnesses. CFS is sometimes mistakenly confused with the Epstein-Barr virus which causes infectious mononucleosis (though no evidence exists which links the two). To make diagnosis even more difficult, standard medical testing doesn't help. And some physicians still maintain that CFS does not exist.

CFS is also known as Chronic Fatigue Immune Dysfunction Syndrome (CFIDS), Post Viral Syndrome and "yuppie flu." Most people who are stricken are between the ages of 20 and 40. And, statistically, women have twice as much chance of getting it as men.

Symptoms of CFS fall into three categories:

Physical symptoms. Flu-like symptoms are most common, including fatigue, sore throat, low-grade fever, and aches and pains. In addition, CFS may cause weakness, clumsiness, "pins and needles," twitching muscles, headache, sensitivity to light and noise, palpitations, giddiness, gastrointestinal upset, nausea, swelling of the lymph glands, cough, rashes, loss of appetite, weight loss or gain, and swelling of the fingers.

Mental or cognitive symptoms. Memory loss, confusion, and the inability to concentrate or think clearly.

Emotional symptoms. Depression, anxiety, panic attacks, weepiness, irritability and an inability to handle stress.

The presence of some of the above symptoms are not sufficient to diagnose CFS. They must also be accompanied by fatigue — sometimes disabling fatigue that makes it almost impossible for the patient to function.

At this time the scientific community has been unable to determine a specific cause for CFS, nor have they found a cure. However, we do know that it's important for you to maintain a diet which is low in protein, low in fat and high in carbohydrates. Plus, you can take these additional steps to help you feel better and function more normally.

ANTIOXIDANTS Some symptoms of CFS may be relieved by taking an antioxidant vitamin formula plus a B-complex supplement.

ECHINACEA Once used by Native Americans as an antiseptic and analgesic, echinacea may also help provide a significant immune-stimulating effect which is helpful for people suffering from CFS. Echinacea is available in capsule form in health food stores.

GERMANIUM A biologically active trace mineral called germanium has good immune-enhancing effects which may help overcome some symptoms of Chronic Fatigue Syndrome. Organic germanium is available in health food stores as Ge-132.

MAGNESIUM Researchers have found that many CFS patients have low magnesium levels. So eat plenty of magnesium-rich foods like dark green, leafy vegetables, peas, nuts, whole grains, mustard seeds, brown rice and soybeans.

Helpful Hints

■ It's been proven that CFS is tied to stress. That's why it is especially important for people with CFS to learn how to reduce stress in their daily lives. Turn to page 467 for more information about lowering stress.

■ Though you might not think that people who are fatigued would have trouble sleeping, restful sleep is even more essential for CFS sufferers than most other people. Refer to the insomnia section of this book on pages 331 to 336 to learn how to improve the quality of your sleep.

COLD SORES

Cold sores are small lesions (caused by the herpes simplex virus) that appear on the lips and face. Also known as fever blisters, they have the bad habit of returning to the same spots over and over again.

You may not notice any symptoms before a cold sore becomes active. Or, you may have some flu symptoms before you develop a burning sensation that turns into a blister. Once the sores subside, many factors can reactivate them, including high fevers, colds, stress, hot weather, anxiety or nutritional deficiencies (which is the reason adding higher amounts of raw vegetables and cultured products such as yogurt and sauerkraut may have a positive effect on preventing cold sores from developing).

While cold sores can't be "cured," they can be treated and controlled. Here, then, are some steps you can take to ease your discomfort and encourage healing.

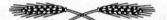

CALENDULA Calendula is used throughout the world for soothing skin ailments. Aromatherapists treat cold sores with a mixture of calendula oil, geranium oil, eucalyptus oil and lemon oil that is applied topically.

ECHINACEA This Native American herb boosts the immune system when taken internally, and has natural antibiotic healing properties when applied topically.

EUCALYPTUS Dilute two drops of eucalyptus oil in approximately ⅓ ounce of sunflower oil to make a natural antiseptic treatment for cold sores.

GOLDENSEAL This Native American Indian favorite is a very strong

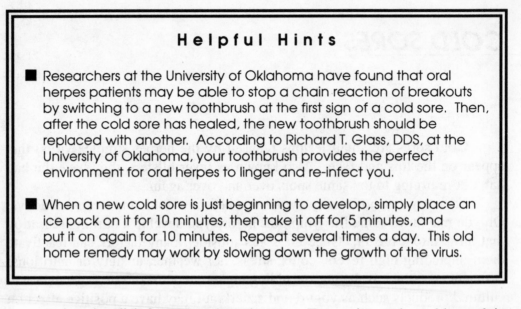

Helpful Hints

■ Researchers at the University of Oklahoma have found that oral herpes patients may be able to stop a chain reaction of breakouts by switching to a new toothbrush at the first sign of a cold sore. Then, after the cold sore has healed, the new toothbrush should be replaced with another. According to Richard T. Glass, DDS, at the University of Oklahoma, your toothbrush provides the perfect environment for oral herpes to linger and re-infect you.

■ When a new cold sore is just beginning to develop, simply place an ice pack on it for 10 minutes, then take it off for 5 minutes, and put it on again for 10 minutes. Repeat several times a day. This old home remedy may work by slowing down the growth of the virus.

antiseptic, disinfectant and astringent. To try it, apply goldenseal in powdered form directly to the cold sore — or make a rinse by mixing the powder with warm water and salt.
CAUTION: *Goldenseal should not be used during pregnancy. It stimulates the uterus to contract.*

LAVENDER Mix 10 drops of lavender oil in about 1 ounce of sunflower oil. Apply directly to the sores for soothing, healing relief.

LEMON BALM The Greeks make a salve from the lemon balm plant (which has natural antiviral properties) to treat cold sores. And aromatherapists suggest mixing the essential oil of lemon balm with rose oil to make a topical treatment.

LYSINE Introducing more of the amino acid lysine into your system can help overcome the effects of arginine, which works in your body to induce the growth and reproduction of the herpes simplex virus. Food sources of lysine include dairy products, potatoes and brewer's yeast. It can also be purchased in capsule or cream form.
CAUTION: *Avoid foods high in arginine, like chocolate, peanuts and most cereal grains.*

SAGE Sage contains camphor, volatile oils and tannin, which work as healing agents. To make a sage mouthwash, steep 1 teaspoon of fresh sage (or ½ teaspoon of dried sage) in 1 cup of hot water. Cover and add ¼ teaspoon of salt and 1 teaspoon of cider vinegar. Swish this mixture around in your mouth while it's hot, then spit it out.

TEA Because the tannins in tea are antibacterial and antiviral, Indian scientists believe that tea can help heal cold sores. Hold a hot, wet tea bag on the sore several times a day.

TEA TREE OIL Tea tree oil has been used in Australia since the 1700s for external wounds of all types, including cold sores. It works as an antibiotic and stimulates the immune system.

VITAMIN E Vitamin E contains many healing properties that promote tissue regrowth. To apply to a cold sore, break open a capsule and rub the liquid directly on the sore — or saturate a gauze pad with vitamin E oil and place it on the affected area.

WINE CONCENTRATE A Canadian researcher tested freeze-dried wine concentrate on a cold sore. The researcher suspected that the concentrate might help heal cold sores because the sticky residue left after wine evaporates contains tannins. And, yes, the lesion was healed with no scar.

ZINC Zinc sulfate, applied topically, has been found to be effective in slowing the outbreak of cold sores and helping to induce healing.

COLIC

Many very young infants (more who are bottle-fed than breast-fed) suffer from a very painful condition called "colic." The muscular walls of the abdomen contract, creating acute spasms that last for hours. The infant becomes fretful and inconsolable, crying almost continuously and drawing up his or her legs when the spasms occur.

Given a few months, babies always outgrow colic. Still, there's no need for them to suffer through that time. To ease your baby's pain — and your frustration — we offer these remedies from around the world.

___**CATNIP** The Pennsylvania Dutch are well-known for their unique traditions, many of which can be traced to their European roots. One such tradition is to use very weak catnip tea to treat infants suffering

---

Helpful Hints

■ Because the following foods are difficult to digest (for you and baby), avoid them if you are nursing: Coffee, green peppers, beans, cucumbers, chocolate, eggs, alcohol, onions, leeks, garlic, eggplant, lentils, zucchini, tomatoes, sugar, and too much fruit.

■ Try gently rubbing baby's belly with a warm cloth. This can have a soothing effect.

from colic. This treatment is also popular in other parts of the world.

DILL Dill is one of the oldest remedies known for calming colic. In addition to being an antispasmodic, it has gentle tranquilizing properties which soothe an upset infant. Europeans give their babies 1 teaspoon of very weak dill tea when colic flares up.

FENNEL In Italy, the water from boiled fennel seeds is given to babies to stop colic. Fennel is very gentle and is a common remedy for all types of digestive disorders.

PEPPERMINT Herbalists suggest a teaspoon of warm peppermint tea for babies suffering from colic. Peppermint has antispasmodic properties that gently soothe the baby's irritated digestive tract.

SLIPPERY ELM If you're a nursing mother, try drinking warm water mixed with slippery elm powder to calm your colicky baby. The soothing properties of the herb will be passed on to the baby through your breast milk.

COLITIS

Colitis is a chronic digestive disease that causes abdominal pain, diarrhea, fever, rectal bleeding and an almost continual need to eliminate. It occurs when the lining of the colon (mucosa) becomes inflamed. Ulcerative colitis — which almost always produces bloody stools — occurs when the inflamed colon is also lined with ulcers. Ulcerative colitis is an uncommon disease, which requires a physician to diagnose and treat. More common and less serious forms of colitis may be related to diet and elimination habits.

While the causes of colitis are still being studied, the leading theory suggests that it has something to do with a microbe interacting with the body's immune system. Repeated use of antibiotics over a long period of time may kill off protective bacteria living in the intestine. As a result, the bad bacteria are allowed to grow and produce an irritating toxin which inflames the lining of the colon. And another form of colitis, ischemia — which affects elderly people who have atherosclerosis (narrowing of the blood vessels) — is apparently caused when the blood supply to the intestinal wall is impaired.

If you suffer from colitis, here are some effective ways to find relief.

ALFALFA Research has shown vitamin K to be helpful in aiding colitis — and alfalfa is an excellent source of this nutrient. Alfalfa capsules can be purchased in health food stores.

CAYENNE This spice from Central and South America helps relieve diarrhea and cramps and allows the colon to heal itself. One recipe that's suggested for colitis is to mix ¼ teaspoon of cayenne with ½ cup of distilled water, 1 tablespoon of cider vinegar and 1 teaspoon of honey. Drink morning and night.

Eat to Beat Colitis

■ **There's no question that your appetite will be affected when colitis strikes.** Therefore, it's especially important for you to provide yourself with proper nourishment between attacks.

■ **Stay away from fiber during a flare-up.** Fiber helps you have more bowel movements — and this will simply irritate your condition. When you're feeling better, though, gradually reintroduce high-quality foods containing fiber — such as oat bran, brown rice, whole grains and lentils — into your diet.

■ **Avoid fats and oils.** They can encourage the onset of diarrhea. (Sorry, no fried foods.)

■ **If you have colitis, you may also be borderline lactose intolerant.** If so, stay away from dairy products. Many high-quality dairy substitutes are available today which will allow you to enjoy "cheese," "ice cream," etc. without paying for it later.

■ **Eat your vegetables, but don't eat them raw.** It's better to steam them.

■ **Peel all fruits** — even grapes — and avoid eating them on an empty stomach.

■ **Try eating baby food to supplement your diet.** It's easy on your system and easy to digest.

_____ **FENUGREEK** It is believed in some cultures that fenugreek can lubricate the colon and help the body rid itself of excess mucus. Health food stores sell fenugreek in pill and tea form.

_____ **PECTIN** Add this gentle, soluble fiber to your diet. It is found in vegetables and fruits such as apples. You can also get pectin by drinking diluted fruit juice.

_____ **YOGURT** Acidophilus, an ingredient found in yogurt, can normalize your intestinal bacteria. And this will help relieve your symptoms. It's best to have some yogurt twice a day on an empty stomach.

Helpful Hint

Everyone's digestive system reacts somewhat differently to various foods. So it's a good idea to keep track of which foods cause your flare-ups, and which seem to improve your condition. A diary will help you pinpoint the troublemakers. Chances are, you'll discover you might have food allergies you were not aware of.

And since stress has also been implicated with colitis, your diary should keep track of your emotional ups and downs. Some diseases require a major commitment to lifestyle changes — and colitis is one of them. So if stress is a major trigger for you, take steps to correct the situation by trying some of the remedies for stress on page 467.

COMMON COLD

Sneezing, coughing, congestion, runny nose, sore throat, watery eyes — all are familiar symptoms of the common cold. Few people escape it — probably because there are more than 100 microorganisms (called rhinoviruses) that can cause a cold. And all of these viruses are easily transmitted from person to person.

Contrary to popular belief, the common cold is not caused by wet feet, wet hair or cold weather. Rather, the viruses infect you when your resistance is low — for example, when you are under some type of emotional or physical stress as a result of poor diet, overwork or lack of sleep.

While the cure for the common cold continues to elude doctors and scientists, treatments for its symptoms abound. Sniffle or cough within earshot of friends, and you are certain to be bombarded by a barrage of home remedies — like those that follow — to help make your cold more bearable.

ACEROLA CHERRIES If there is still any controversy surrounding the effectiveness of vitamin C in preventing colds, the Indians of Ecuador have no part of it. For centuries, they have prevented colds by eating acerola cherries, which are so rich in vitamin C that some of the annual crop is exported to the United States to provide a supplement for baby foods.

ANGELICA Native Americans have long known the medicinal value of angelica. To combat a cold, they boil or steep 1 teaspoon of the dried root or seeds in 1 cup of water and drink as needed. The plant contains pinene, which is an expectorant with antimicrobial properties.

CITRUS When European explorers found their way to the islands of the

Caribbean, they discovered that the natives of these islands had a much higher resistance to colds than they did. Observation also revealed that these natives ate large quantities of grapefruits and pineapples. The natives of the Caribbean Islands were not the only ones to make this connection early on. The Seminole Indians of Florida traditionally gargled grapefruit juice to prevent colds and to alleviate sore throats.

The early explorers knew no more about vitamin C than did the natives. But they all made the connection between citrus fruits and warding off colds.

ECHINACEA Many herbalists believe echinacea (or purple coneflower) stimulates the immune system by increasing the body's ability to produce white blood cells (which destroy viruses and bacteria). Echinacea is available in tea and capsule form in most drug stores and natural products stores.

GARLIC The Egyptian pharaohs ate garlic to fight infections. And today, the Irish (who live in a damp, cold climate that makes them prone to lung infections), along with many other European and Asian people, make garlic syrups to ease coughs. Because of its strong immune-enhancing properties, garlic really is a good preventive and treatment for the common cold.

To keep your immune system strong, chew about 3 raw cloves a day and add as much garlic as possible to your cooking. If you're concerned about keeping your breath kissing sweet, or if you can't tolerate the strong taste, try odor-free garlic tablets. They work almost as well as the fresh cloves.

GINGER To treat a cold the Asian way, boil fresh gingerroot in milk and inhale the vapors. To prevent future colds, follow the Asian example again and chew a small piece of gingerroot before meals.

The English prefer to take their ginger in the form of ginger tea that they sweeten with honey to break up a cold. According to most British, the best time for this treatment is just before bedtime. To make it, grate a handful of fresh ginger and squeeze about 2 teaspoons of the juice into a teacup. Cover with boiling water and sweeten to taste. No need to stir.

LEMON Before bedtime, Europeans who are fighting a cold sip one or more glasses of hot water with lemon juice. Any hot drink is relaxing, reduces congestion and encourages perspiration that may break a fever. In addition, the lemon contains vitamin C to fight the cold, and the juice helps to ease sore throat pain.

NASTURTIUM This flower has been used for centuries by Peruvian Indians as a remedy for colds, cough and the flu. They make a tea from 2 teaspoons of bruised fresh leaves steeped in a cup of hot water for 10 minutes.

Modern research supports this use of nasturtium as a cold and flu treatment. Many herbalists believe fresh nasturtium has antibiotic properties.

POMEGRANATE The pomegranate, a tree fruit that is common to regions in the Middle East, is a popular treatment for the common cold. Its bright-red juice is equally effective against all the usual symptoms, including sore throat, cough, congestion and fever. Pomegranates, which are loaded with vitamin C, can be found seasonably in most grocery stores.

SASSAFRAS The Seminole, Mohawk and Iroquois Indians all used sassafras roots to treat a number of ailments, including the common cold.

The Truth About Chicken Soup

The first thing my Grandma (and maybe yours) did when someone in the family came down with a cold was serve up a bowl of hot chicken soup. And it turns out that Grandma may have been on to something. Studies at Harvard Medical School and Mount Sinai Hospital in Miami, Florida show that chicken soup is as effective against a cold as any over-the-counter remedy — although researchers are just beginning to understand why it works.

Here's one good recipe for chicken soup: Cover a stewing chicken with water and bring to a boil. Add celery, onions, carrots and a garlic clove or two. Simmer until the chicken falls off the bone. Cool and strain the broth, discarding any fat. Put thin slices of lemon on top and enjoy.

Not only does sassafras tea shorten the length of the illness, but those who drink the tea on a regular basis develop a much higher resistance to future colds. It has antiseptic properties, and an infusion of the roots can bring down fever.

VINEGAR A cold remedy that dates back to colonial times is to drink 2 teaspoons each of apple cider vinegar and honey in a large glass of water 3 times a day. Today, herbalists believe this mixture creates an unfavorable environment for cold viruses.

For more remedies for cold symptoms, read the congestion section which follows and the cough section on page 203.

CONGESTION

Congestion that accompanies a cold, flu or allergy attack is caused when the mucous membranes in the respiratory system become irritated and inflamed. Your head aches, you have difficulty breathing — and you feel miserable. Drink plenty of fluids to help loosen the stuffiness, and take advantage of the following herbal remedies to ease your discomfort.

BASIL In the 16th century, Europeans made a tea to treat the stuffiness caused by inflamed mucous membranes by steeping 5 grams of fresh basil in a cupful of water. The Japanese use basil tea for this same purpose. Pungent oils such as thymol and camphor in the plant help open clogged passages.

FENUGREEK When someone in Greece comes down with a bad cold, he or she promptly boils the seeds of the fenugreek plant into a tea. Despite its name, this medicinal plant was discovered by the Egyptians. Today, its therapeutic powers are recognized in many parts of the world, including Greece and China. When taken as a tea, fenugreek eases congestion. As residents of Athens can tell you, this treatment is especially useful in highly polluted areas.

HYSSOP Greek master herbalists boiled the leaves and flowers of hyssop (a shrub plant in the same family as mint, sage and balm) in water and mixed it with honey to ease persistent coughs. And the Cherokee Indians used hyssop to relieve congestion. Modern research indicates that the volatile oils in hyssop may relieve mild respiratory symptoms, especially those related to colds. Hyssop also contains the compound marrubin, which acts as an expectorant.

To prepare hyssop tea, steep 1 teaspoon of fresh hyssop (½ teaspoon if you use dried hyssop) in ¾ cup of hot water for 4 minutes. Drink hot to relieve congestion. Some herbalists believe that adding an equal amount of sage when steeping hyssop will boost its decongestant properties. And, of course, honey can be added for flavor.

MORMON TEA Mormon Tea — which was used by early Mormon settlers in the United States as a substitute for coffee and tea — is commonly used in Europe as a cold remedy. It is made by steeping 1½ ounces of dried ephedra branches in 1 pint of boiling water for no more than 20 minutes. This treatment works because the ephedra plant contains the substance ephedrine, a natural decongestant.
CAUTION: *This remedy should not be used by people with hypertension.*

MUSTARD Because the Chinese believe that leaf mustard provides a warm energy, and that the pungent taste promotes circulation in the lungs to relieve mucus discharge, they make a tea by boiling 5 grams of fried leaf mustard seeds with 10 grams of fried radish seeds, 5 grams of dried orange peels, and 5 grams of licorice — and drink as needed.

In other parts of the world, people prefer a topically applied mustard paste. To try this, make mustard powder into a paste by adding water. Heat the paste, spread it on a cloth, and apply the cloth to the chest. This will draw the blood to the surface, and decrease congestion.
CAUTION: *This remedy can be irritating to the skin of sensitive people. But the irritation can be reduced if the mustard powder is mixed with rye flour.*

PEPPERMINT The menthol in peppermint clears head congestion in some people. Peppermint tea, a popular Native American herbal remedy for the common cold, is made by combining 2 teaspoons each of dried peppermint leaf and dried elderflower, and steeping, covered, in 1 cup of hot water for 10 minutes.

PERU BALSAM In South America, the thick, syrupy sap of the balsam tree is used as an expectorant. Because this sap makes coughs more productive, it also helps shorten the length of illness. The medicinal qualities of balsam sap were first discovered by the Indians of El Salvador. It was later introduced to Peru, where it remains in use today. Peru balsam sap is available in health food stores and through mail order.

H e l p f u l   H i n t

A foot bath feels great when you're not feeling 100 percent. Simply soak your feet and ankles in water that has been heated to about 100° F to increase blood flow throughout your entire body — and help relieve head congestion.

CONSTIPATION

Constipation, though uncomfortable, is not very serious — except in rare cases when it is caused by a tumor or intestinal obstruction. You can get constipated when your fluid or fiber intake is too low, when you are inactive, when you resist your body's signal to visit the bathroom, or as a reaction to stress or to certain drugs.

The term comes from the Latin phrase *con stipati*, which means "crammed together" — and that's exactly what happens to the waste materials in your intestines to cause this problem. Waste materials surrender a significant amount of water before being expelled, but if too much water is removed, they dry up and pack tightly into the large intestine.

Basically, keeping your bowels working normally is a function of eating a balanced diet on a regular basis. If you are often constipated (and there is no obstruction, disease or infection), you are either not getting enough fluid, or you are not getting enough roughage. Though there are many over-the-counter laxatives on the market, you're better off staying away from them. Your body can become dependent upon these products, and you may not be able to stop taking them without becoming constipated again. Instead, try some of the natural remedies we have scouted out for you.

ALOE Naturalists suggest mixing 6 ounces of aloe vera juice or gel in water or juice to relieve constipation.

APPLE Canadians eat 1 or 2 apples without other food or beverages each morning before breakfast to avoid constipation. To aid digestion, chew the peel thoroughly. Baked apples will also help overcome sluggish stools.

BANANA The Chinese try for the same effect by eating a ripe banana or ripe figs first thing in the morning on an empty stomach.

BARLEY To clear up constipation, Israelis eat 3 or 4 muffins or biscuits made with barley flour each day. The French prefer muffins and biscuits made with oat bran meal.

BRAN A daily dose of bran may be all you need to prevent constipation. A group of Swedish researchers discovered that eating 3 to 6 pieces of fiber-rich crisp bread made from whole rye meal and wheat bran does the trick. Other good sources of bran include hot and cold breakfast cereals, whole-wheat bread, multi-grain bread and bran muffins.

CABBAGE This leafy veggie, uncooked and well chewed, can have a

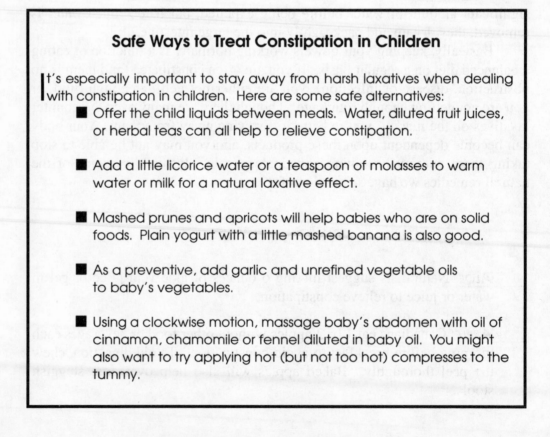

Safe Ways to Treat Constipation in Children

It's especially important to stay away from harsh laxatives when dealing with constipation in children. Here are some safe alternatives:

- Offer the child liquids between meals. Water, diluted fruit juices, or herbal teas can all help to relieve constipation.

- Add a little licorice water or a teaspoon of molasses to warm water or milk for a natural laxative effect.

- Mashed prunes and apricots will help babies who are on solid foods. Plain yogurt with a little mashed banana is also good.

- As a preventive, add garlic and unrefined vegetable oils to baby's vegetables.

- Using a clockwise motion, massage baby's abdomen with oil of cinnamon, chamomile or fennel diluted in baby oil. You might also want to try applying hot (but not too hot) compresses to the tummy.

positive laxative effect on your system.

COCONUT To cure constipation, the Chinese eat fresh coconut meat in the morning and evening. This probably works because coconut is rich in natural oils.

> **EXERCISE!**
>
> Any aerobic exercise helps keep your body in tune, and that includes preventing constipation. Exercises such as walking, jogging, or running increase blood flow to the intestines, which can help improve bowel regularity.

COFFEE Dr. Andrew Weil, from the University of Arizona College of Medicine, recommends a cup of strong coffee on an empty stomach, first thing in the morning, as a quick treatment for occasional constipation. (Decaffeinated coffee works as well as regular.)

DANDELION A German remedy for mild constipation is dandelion tea. Prepackaged tea bags are available in health food stores.

DATES Dates dipped in ghee (clarified butter) are a great tasting natural laxative. Ghee is made by melting butter and straining out the milk solids that form on top.

GINGER Because ginger helps normalize intestinal movement, it can be helpful for constipation when taken in combination with cascara sagrada or rhubarb root (two natural laxatives).

HONEY The Chinese mix honey in warm water to treat constipation. The Egyptians and Indians add honey to tea made with fresh or powdered ginger, tumeric or cumin.

LEMON An old folk remedy for constipation is to drink lemon juice in a cup of warm water (without sweetener) 30 minutes before eating breakfast. In China, they like to use grapefruit juice instead.

LICORICE Licorice, which you probably recognize as a flavoring agent in various confections and liqueurs, comes from a tall, spiky plant that has small blue flowers. This plant, whose name means "sweet root" in Greek, was used by the ancient Greeks as a laxative. Known as "the grandfather of herbs," licorice has been used medicinally since the days of Caesar.

MUSTARD SEEDS The French eat whole mustard seeds to treat indigestion and nausea. The seeds are also an effective laxative.

PSYLLIUM Another natural laxative calls for psyllium husks or seeds. Mix 1 to 2 teaspoons of powdered husks in a large glass of water and drink after meals. Psyllium powder is available in most drug stores.

PUMPKIN SEEDS Ethiopians may not know the nursery rhyme about Peter, the pumpkin eater, but they do chew pumpkin seeds (which contain fiber) as a natural laxative.

RHUBARB Since American settlers trekked westward, rhubarb has been used as a laxative. One tasty laxative remedy is made by pureeing cooked rhubarb stems and adding apple juice and honey to taste. The ancient Chinese variety of rhubarb (tahuang) has the strongest laxative properties. Tahuang is dried, cut and pulverized into a yellow powder before being used.
CAUTION: *Rhubarb can produce a laxative action. But because rhubarb contains oxalic acid, those who suffer from arthritis, rheumatism and gout should avoid this treatment.*

SENNA Senna is one of the world's safest and most thorough laxatives. Senna not only cleanses the bowel, it also tones it. The senna pods are more effective than the leaves. A tea cup of senna infusion at night on an empty stomach will make the bowels work by morning. Use 6 to 10 pods to make an infusion for adults. Use 3 to 5 pods for children.

SUNFLOWER SEEDS The Chinese prefer sunflower seeds as a laxative. They shell approximately 30 grams, crush them, add 1 cup of boiling water, and stir in some honey. They drink this combination in the morning and evening.

_____**SWEET POTATO** The Chinese eat sweet potatoes seasoned with salt or sugar before bedtime to cure chronic constipation.

_____**WALNUTS** In China, a common treatment for constipation is to slowly chew about 3 ounces of walnuts.

_____**WATER** Drink at least 8 to 10 glasses of water a day to soften stools. This is especially helpful if you are over 60 years of age, when stools can become harder and more difficult to pass. An easy way to do this is to fill a thermos with water and sip it every half hour or hour all day long.

The Chinese depend on only one cup of water — salt water — taken before breakfast. And they sometimes boil pork, skim off the excess fat, and then drink the soup for relief.

Helpful Hints

■ **Avoid dairy products.** Cut down on milk, cheese and yogurt. These products can bind up your system and be difficult to digest. If you're concerned about your calcium intake, refer to the osteoporosis section on page 395.

■ **Bulk up on natural laxatives.** Foods that are excellent sources of soluble fiber include pearled barley, black-eyed peas, blackberries, chick peas, lentils, lima beans, black beans, figs, raspberries and kidney beans.

■ **Cook your vegetables.** All vegetables are good for you, but they should be cooked if you're suffering from constipation. Eaten raw, they are harder to digest, which is something you don't need if your digestive system has slowed down.

CORNS AND CALLUSES

Corns and calluses are nothing but hardened patches of skin, caused by continuous friction or pressure, that are painful only if pressed against the soft tissue underneath. To avoid corns and calluses on your feet, never wear shoes that don't fit — no matter how great they look. Unfortunately, calluses on other parts of the body are not so easily prevented. Most people who do physical labor have them. And musicians who play stringed instruments purposely build up calluses on their fingers. In these cases, the calluses actually help protect the skin from serious injury or infection.

Protective or not, both corns and calluses can be unsightly — and a problem for the average person whose physical labor is limited to activities like gardening, jogging, golf or tennis. There is, however, no need to seek professional treatment to get rid of them. Here are some safe, easy ways to take care of them yourself.

___**BREWER'S YEAST** The Bavarians of Germany spread brewer's yeast on a cloth, and bind the cloth to their corns and calluses. They repeat this process daily until the callus disappears — usually within three to four weeks.

___**CHAMOMILE** Try soaking your callused hands or feet in a very weak solution of chamomile tea and warm water to soften the hardened skin. (Wash with soap and water afterwards to remove any staining.)

___**DANDELION** This corn remedy is popular among the shepherds of Australia: They simply break a dandelion stem in half and drip the milky white sap on the corn. They repeat the sap application for several days. Then, in a week or two, they say that the corn turns dark and falls off.

GARLIC The Brahman physicians of India treat corns with a combination of castor oil and garlic. Castor oil is loaded with vitamin A, which is known to be effective in treating skin ailments in general. And raw garlic irritates the skin just enough to attract the defenses of the body's immune system to the area.

IVY The Osage Indians bound their corns and calluses with bruised ivy leaves, a practice that was said to bring results in 2-3 weeks.

LEMON In Sicily, people bind a lemon slice to the painful area, and leave it there overnight. They continue this treatment until the irritation disappears.

ONION A home remedy is to tape a slice of raw onion to the corn. Try this every night for 3 to 4 weeks, until the corn disappears.

PAPAYA Hawaiian medicine men applied pure papaya juice or a piece of fresh papaya pulp directly on a corn. The area was then bound and the bandage left on overnight.

PUMICE This treatment has been used for years — and it still works. Soak your callus in warm water, then use a pumice stone or callus file to remove the hardened skin. For a corn, moisten the stone with warm water, and gently rub the corn to help reduce its size. Follow with an application of a soothing, moisturizing lotion.

Helpful Hint

Here's a remedy you may want to continue long after your corns and calluses have disappeared because it feels so-o-o good! Soak your feet several times a day in a warm water bath with baking soda added.

COUGH

Whether it's a dry, hacking cough caused by irritants in the air, or the phlegmy, loose cough usually associated with an allergy or virus, a cough should never be ignored. Because it is often a symptom of a serious underlying condition, you should always seek medical attention if a cough persists for more than a few weeks. In most cases, however, the following self-care treatments should suffice.

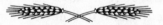

ANISE Anise oil, extracted from the seed of the anise plant, is a popular ingredient in German cakes. It is also used in Spain, Italy, France and South America as a flavoring for liqueurs. And the people of these countries have discovered that anise oil has another use as well — it's an excellent remedy for dry coughs.

In England, too, during the 17th century, a natural cough medicine was made from aniseed mixed with sugar candy or sugar, powdered licorice and coriander seeds. Anise is an expectorant, and licorice (which is common in many modern commercial cough syrups) is not only an expectorant, it also reduces throat irritation, acting like codeine. It is also antibacterial and can neutralize many toxins produced by bacteria.

BERRIES In Finland, lingonberries, which are like miniature cranberries, are considered an excellent cough remedy — and they taste a whole lot better than any cough syrup. (Look for lingonberry jam in gourmet specialty shops.)

And here are recipes for three more especially tasty, berry-based cough treatments: (1) Simmer elderflower and/or black currants in a little water, sweeten with honey, pour in a wineglass and drink while still hot. Ginger and cloves can be simmered along with the berries to add warmth and antiseptic properties to the mixture. (2) Mix the juice of black currants with honey to make a syrup. Then take it, as needed, by the teaspoon. (3) Mix raspberry juice with honey, and take 2 teaspoons as needed.

CABBAGE In England, people with coughs and hoarseness get out their blenders and make a healthy, if not particularly appetizing, home remedy. Cabbage syrup is made by liquefying a red cabbage. The juice is strained and weighed, and half its weight in honey is added. The mixture is then simmered over a low heat until it becomes syrupy. Several doses of 2 teaspoonfuls each can be taken in quick succession. (Cabbage is an excellent source of vitamin C, and the honey soothes the throat.)

COMFREY A home remedy that's said to quell a cough is to put ½ ounce of crushed, dried comfrey root into a saucepan with ½ pint each of milk and water. Bring the mixture to boil and simmer for 20 minutes. Strain and cool. Then take by the spoonful whenever needed.

EUCALYPTUS To relieve coughs, put a few drops of essential oil of eucalyptus into a large pot of boiling water. Cover your head with a towel and inhale the vapors.
CAUTION: *Be careful not to burn your face.*

FIG Figs contain demulcents, which are substances that soothe irritated mucous membranes in the mouth, throat and respiratory system. Whether or not the Greeks and Romans knew this, they did use figs in many medicinal recipes. For example, one cough remedy called for 6 figs to be boiled in milk for 10 minutes. A cupful of this liquid was taken several times a day. Another remedy was to roast 6 figs until dry and grind to a powder. The powder could then be made into a drink like coffee or tea and taken when required. Following this ancient example, grain beverages containing figs can be found in health food stores today.

GRAPEFRUIT In China, they still make a mixture of steamed, peeled grapefruit, half a cup of rice wine and 1 cup of honey, and keep it on hand to drink throughout the day to relieve a cough.

An Ancient Chinese Secret That You Can Find in the Veggie Bin at Your Local Supermarket

Chinese health secrets have been passed down through the centuries and across the generations on illustrated scrolls and via the teachings of masters to their pupils. One of these secrets is a vegetable known as t'ien men tung that is made into a soup used to treat dry coughs. Fortunately, you don't have to make a pilgrimage to Inner Mongolia or Guangdong to take advantage of the healing benefits of t'ien men tung. Just pick up some asparagus at your grocery store. By any name, this remedy is an effective one.

HORSERADISH A cough syrup made by herbalists in Old England used horseradish as the main ingredient. Since horseradish can be an eye, nose, and throat irritant, open the windows when preparing the following remedy: Scrape some fresh horseradish root into a clean bowl. Cover the grated root with sugar and turn frequently for a day until there is a layer of syrup at the bottom of the bowl. Drain the syrup off into a clean bottle. Take 3 times a day, 1 tablespoon at a time.

LEEKS A home remedy for coughs is to cook 2 sliced leeks in very little water or milk, then squeeze the juice through a coarse cloth or press it through a fine strainer to make a puree. Stir in enough honey to make a syrup and eat a spoonful to two as needed.

LEMON Another way to use lemons — a favorite old Italian remedy that is also good for coughs — is to take 3 whole lemons cut in half and simmer them in a cup of water with honey until the liquid reduces to a about a third of a cup. Take 2 tablespoons every 2 hours. (The simmering gets the bioflavonoids in the lemons out and into the liquid.)

ONION The French treat coughs with a homemade syrup made by sprinkling sugar on sliced onions, and then letting the sugared onions sit overnight in a covered dish. A syrup results, which they take as needed.

PAPAYA Fresh papayas (and mangos), including the peel, are a good source of vitamins C and A, and are eaten in China to help ease chronic coughs.

POTATO WATER The Irish make a cough remedy from potato water. After boiling potatoes, they keep some of the water and sweeten it with sugar or honey. Then they take a teaspoonful as needed.

SUGAR In China, rock sugar, steamed with 5 fresh pitted olives for half an hour, is eaten to control coughing.

SUNFLOWER SEED The French make a decoction of sunflower seeds mixed with honey to treat a cough. One recipe calls for 1 ounce of seeds to 2½ cups of water, with honey added to taste. For more detailed instructions on how to make a decoction, turn to page 82.

THYME Thyme tea can be an effective cough treatment for both adults and children. To prepare thyme tea, steep 2 tablespoons of fresh thyme (1 tablespoon if you use dried thyme) in a cup of hot water. Herbalists also recommend brewing a tea using half thyme and half plantago, especially when a stuffy nose accompanies the cough.

CRADLE CAP

Cradle cap commonly occurs in infants. In most babies, these greasy, yellowish scales on the scalp are caused by overactive oil glands. But cradle cap can also be caused by food allergies — and it was recently linked by researchers to an overgrowth of yeast.

Here are several tips to help clear up the condition.

BABY OIL Use a soft toothbrush to gently rub the scalp with baby oil. (Instead of baby oil, you can use an opened biotin capsule.)

DON'T WASH Don't wash baby's hair too frequently. Your first reaction may be to scrub away at the scales with shampoo or soap. But cradle cap has nothing to do with cleanliness or hygiene — and too much shampooing can aggravate the condition by increasing sebum secretion.

ESSENTIAL OILS Mix olive oil with a few drops of essential oil of lavender, rosemary or lemon, and regularly rub it gently into the scalp. Leave the scented oil on overnight, and wash off the loosened crust with shampoo the next day.

HERBS Try herbal rinses. Meadowsweet, burdock infusion or ordinary tea can help loosen crust after a shampoo. Remove flakes with a hairbrush or clean fingernail, but never pick off crusts that are not loose. This can cause bleeding, inflammation or infection of the scalp.

VITAMIN B If you're a nursing mother, increase your intake of vitamin B. In some instances, cradle cap in nursing babies was linked to mothers who had a biotin deficiency — a condition that cleared up when these women took extra B vitamins.

CROHN'S DISEASE

Crohn's Disease is a chronic inflammatory disease which can affect any part of the gastrointestinal tract, but most commonly strikes the terminal ileum (the point where the small intestine joins the large intestine). The disease causes the inflammation to progress through all layers of the intestine, which becomes very thick, sometimes forming patches of ulcers and abscesses. It strikes both men and women, usually before age 30, with the peak age being between 14 and 24. The severity of the disease varies widely, and surgery is sometimes necessary to remove the ulcers. Typical symptoms include chronic diarrhea with abdominal pain, fever, weight loss, and a feeling of fullness in the lower abdomen.

Although doctors are not sure what causes Crohn's Disease — and, so far, there is no cure — it seems that (as with other gastrointestinal problems) it may be linked to a food intolerance in some people. And, in fact, doctors at Addenbrookes Hospital in Cambridge, England, have been successfully treating Crohn's patients by changing their diet.

Here are some tips to help you relieve your symptoms.

■ Keep a diary. By keeping a diary of the foods you eat you will be able to determine the types of foods which trigger flare-ups and adjust your diet accordingly.

■ Pay particular attention to your reaction to common trigger foods. These include wheat, dairy products, cruciferous vegetables (cabbage, broccoli, cauliflower, Brussels sprouts), yeast, tomatoes, citrus fruits and eggs. A high sugar intake has been linked to Crohn's. And some people react unfavorably to dairy products. In addition, researchers at Ninewells Medical School in Scotland discovered that yeast caused flare-ups in some patients — and that the symptoms subsided when yeast was eliminated from their diets.

■ Add the "right" foods to your diet. These foods are different for different people, but some researchers recommend eating more anti-inflammatory fatty fishes, while avoiding inflammatory animal fats and omega-6 vegetable oil.

CROUP

This respiratory illness, usually occurring in children between two and five years of age, is caused by a virus which inflames the larynx (voice box). The result may be a brassy, barking cough along with fatigue, fever, runny nose, hoarseness, sore throat and difficult, "noisy" breathing. In its most severe form, irritation to the larynx can establish spasms which can close off the airways and even become life threatening.

Because croup can strike suddenly, usually at night, it is vital for parents to react quickly, and to know what to do to reopen the larynx and induce normal breathing.

_____ **EUCALYPTUS** The Australian Aborigines were the first to discover that eucalyptus has strong decongestant powers. Put a handful of eucalyptus leaves or a few drops of eucalyptus oil into a pot of boiling water and have the child inhale the vapors for 5 to 15 minutes. A few drops of the oil may also be used in a room humidifier.

_____ **HYSSOP** This member of the mint family is effective in treating irritations of the respiratory tract and is a good expectorant. To treat croup, prepare a tea by steeping 2 teaspoons of fresh or dried hyssop in 1 cup of boiling water. Because this herb has a bitter taste, add honey or sugar to taste.

_____ **MULLEIN** This European remedy heals and soothes irritations of the respiratory tract. Use it as a tea by steeping 1 or 2 teaspoons of the dried leaves in 1 cup of boiling water. Add honey and lemon to overcome mullein's bitter taste.

_____ **THYME** This old favorite can be used to make a tea which loosens and removes mucus from the respiratory tract and relaxes the muscles to make breathing easier. It can also be used as an inhalant.

Prepare thyme tea with 2 teaspoons of dried herbs per cup of boiling water. Steep for 10 minutes.

First Aid for Croup

If your child is having difficulty breathing, the quickest remedy is steam — and plenty of it. Bring the child into the bathroom, have him or her sit on the toilet and turn the shower on as hot as you can make it. Your wallpaper may come loose, but you won't care, because the steam will correct the breathing trouble and the coughing will subside quickly.

Another way to get moisture into the child's larynx is with a good hot (but not too hot) bath. After the bath, prepare a hot compress to place on the throat. This moist heat will increase the blood flow through the congested area. When the child is comfortable, remove the compress, quickly bathe the neck and chest with cold water, dry the area and massage it with olive oil.

CUTS

The fact that a cut can heal in just a few days is an excellent example of the power of the body's natural immune system. The damaged blood vessels slowly contract, slowing or stopping the flow of blood. A clot forms to plug the wound. As the skin around the cut regenerates, the scab gets smaller and smaller — until the cut disappears.

However, even the smallest cuts can benefit from a little external attention. So be sure to keep your cuts clean and protected from infection so the natural healing process can continue, unhindered. And check out the following healing aids used by people all over the world.

ACACIA The acacia tree, found in upper Egypt and Senegal, is a prickly tree that flourishes in the desert. The tar that exudes from its bark has several medicinal applications. When dried and powdered, for example, acacia gum can be used to stop bleeding caused by superficial lacerations.

BETONY To the Egyptians, Spanish and Romans, betony has been known as a useful medicinal herb, valued mainly for its astringent quality. The juice is used to heal cuts, skin ulcers and sores.

CALENDULA Modern science recognizes that the essential oil compounds found in calendula can soothe inflamed cuts and help form new tissue. Herbalists recommend using the leaves (steeped in boiling water) as a poultice.

COMFREY The wound-healing powers of comfrey have been known since Greek and Roman times. Potions and poultices made from the leaves, stem and flowering parts of the plant are applied to injured skin. The allantoin in the comfrey promotes multiplication of cells and, thus, tissue growth. The plant also contains anti-inflammatory agents and seems to regenerate aging skin. Comfrey also breaks down damaged red blood cells and so makes bruises heal more quickly. (Another name for comfrey is bruisewort.) Tannin in the leaves is also very astringent.

ECHINACEA The healing properties of echinacea are well documented, so it's no surprise that one effective remedy for treating cuts is a tincture of echinacea. For directions on how to make a tincture, turn to page 84.

NATURE'S MEDICINE CABINET

The Egyptians and Chinese independently discovered that moldy bread can be used to heal boils, and over the centuries other cultures have discovered that moldy bread also can be used to treat cuts and severe wounds. For example, both North American Indians and the Mayas used moldy bread to treat battle wounds. And it has been documented that knights during the time of King Arthur treated their battle wounds with yeast and moldy bread.

What all these cultures inadvertently discovered was the drug that would later be named penicillin — a drug that changed the face of history. The man credited with the discovery of penicillin, Englishman Alexander Fleming, also discovered it unintentionally. While searching for a drug to treat infectious diseases, he accidentally left one of his petri dish samples uncovered. It started to grow mold. At first, Fleming thought the sample would have to be thrown away. But then he noticed that the infectious bacteria around the mold had been destroyed. Further tests showed that the normal cells had not been affected. Fleming isolated the mold, penicillin was born — and Fleming was knighted for his discovery.

GARLIC During World War II, the Russians discovered this remedy for cuts and wounds that is still used in parts of Russia today: They put raw cloves of garlic on the edges of a wound to promote healing. Although this treatment may sound like the product of superstition, it has a scientific basis — natural chemicals in garlic are known to act as antiseptics.

GOTU KOLA In the Fiji islands, healers treat cuts with the gotu kola plant, a weed that is commonly found in mountainous tropical regions. Fiji healers claim that the plant is an effective antiseptic.

HONEY South American Indians had a really sweet treatment for cuts and other skin injuries. Before dressing a wound, they doused the bandages with honey. Scandinavians also use honey, which they mix with cod liver oil and apply to wounds.

In fact, many cultures throughout the ages have used honey as a healing agent — from the ancient Egyptians to the Aztecs of Central America to the medieval Europeans. Though they all learned from experience that honey dressings help heal wounds, they had no way of knowing that high organisms such as bacteria.

Curiosity Box

Residents of the Fiji islands routinely use papaya to treat wounds. But they don't use the leaf or the fruit. Instead, they take the raw milky-white sap from beneath the bark of the tree and apply it directly to the wound. And a staff member at a large London hospital recalls an incident in which this papaya treatment saved a life:

A patient had an infected wound following a kidney transplant. Antibiotics were not working, and the wound would not heal. The doctors were desperate for another solution. Then someone remembered hearing about the use of papayas in Africa. A papaya was purchased from a local market, and strips of the fruit were placed over the wound. It healed within a week.

Papase, from papaya, is readily available as an enzyme in extract form.

Today, in South Africa and other developing countries, physicians routinely smear wounds and sores with honey as a disinfectant ointment. And in Europe, honey ointments are often made by mixing a little flour and honey.

Make your own healing ointment by combining a teaspoon each of wheat germ oil, comfrey root, tea and honey. Heat this in the top of a double boiler until blended well. The wheat germ oil contains vitamin E, which promotes healing of the skin. And, as we said earlier, comfrey contains allantoin, which promotes the growth of connective tissue — and is easily absorbed through the skin.

LAVENDER Herbalists believe lavender possesses antiseptic and other healing properties. So, they recommend dotting pure essential oil of lavender on cuts and scratches.

LEMON A Greek home remedy is to rub lemon directly on a cut. (Ouch!)

MARIGOLD Tincture of marigold is in the same family as arnica, and has many of the same wound-healing properties. It is antiseptic and antibacterial, and is also effective against fungal infections. In fact, British physicians used marigold during World War I to dress wounds.

To make a healing dressing, soak bandages in a cup or more of boiled water to which a few drops of tincture of marigold have been added. Keep the dressing wet.

ST. JOHN'S WORT In oil form, St. John's wort is believed to have antibacterial and astringent properties when used topically to treat cuts.

SASSAFRAS The sassafras root is an effective wound treatment. Boil the root in water and bathe your wound in the steam. The volatile oil in sassafras is both a painkiller and an antiseptic.

DANDRUFF

Dandruff is not a disease. It's a normal function of your skin which occurs when your scalp sheds dead cells. White flakes fall as new cells are pushed up from deeper skin layers. This becomes a problem only when the cell replacement cycle isn't working as well as it should, causing excessive flaking.

Unfortunately, medical science hasn't been able to come up with a cause (or a permanent cure) for dandruff, although several theories exist. One points to nervous tension, a theory which is reinforced by the fact that people who are under extreme stress seem to be more susceptible to dandruff. Another suggests that moisture loss kills cells prematurely. This theory also has some merit because dandruff seems to occur more during the drier winter season.

If you suspect that stress may be a contributing factor in your case, take steps to get it under control. Your overall health — not just your dry, flaking head — will improve. (See page 467 for complete information on stress management techniques.) Beyond that, try some of the following widely used natural remedies for dandruff, most of which seem to work by adding moisture to your scalp.

CORN OIL Corn is one of the most abundant food crops in the world. It is not a natural breed of plant, but was cultivated by Native Americans, who crossbred several types of American grasses. Once developed, corn made up 80 percent of the Indian's daily diet.

The Chickasaws, who inhabited various parts of North America, not only ate corn — they used corn oil as a remedy for dandruff. They mashed corn grains and rubbed the resulting oil directly on the affected scalp.

NETTLE In Germany, a hair tonic rub is made from nettle leaves, a few handfuls of nasturtium, and a small handful of boxwood leaves. Nettle rinses (usually brewed like a tea in water) are known to eliminate dandruff and eczema.

TEA TREE OIL Australians believe that tea tree oil has healing and antibacterial properties to treat dandruff. Tea tree oil is a popular ingredient in many commercial shampoos.

VINEGAR Canada is one of the world's top apple-producing countries. And researchers there have discovered that apple cider vinegar is an effective topical remedy for dandruff. Pour the vinegar on your hair, massage it into your scalp, and let it dry for a few minutes. Then wash your hair. Repeat this process daily, and your dandruff should disappear within a few days.

YOGURT An old favorite home remedy for dandruff also adds protein to your scalp. Simply massage plain yogurt into your hair and let it stay on for about 30 minutes. Then rinse and shampoo.

YUCCA A treatment for dandruff once popular among Mexicans has spread to New Mexico and the American Southwest. The yucca plant, also called the desert amole, is used to produce a sudsy shampoo that eliminates dandruff.

Helpful Hints

■ **Choose the right shampoo and hair rinse.** Many commercial shampoos contain detergents which may cause dryness and upset the pH balance of your scalp. Shampoos which have a castile soap or herbal base will be more gentle and may reduce the flaking condition. The list of herbs that help heal and soothe the irritation of dandruff include rosemary, thyme, burdock, comfrey, elderflowers and chamomile.

■ **Use that hair brush.** Many people have found that an easy and pleasant way to condition the scalp is to get into the habit of brushing the hair vigorously each day.

DEPRESSION

Depression has always been recognized as part of the human condition. In fact, as far back as the 3rd century B.C. during the days of Hippocrates, the father of medicine, it was known as melancholia. Though we all have our ups and downs, depression becomes a problem only when it becomes chronic and begins to interfere with the ability to live life to the fullest. Symptoms may include a loss of interest in things which used to have meaning for you, lethargy, sadness, crying jags, self reproach or anything which restricts your happiness and well-being.

When depression becomes severe — when it begins to control your life — you should seek professional help. But, for mild depression — the kind everyone suffers from time to time — there are many safe, natural ways to give yourself a lift.

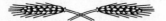

_____ **BORAGE** People in Wales refer to borage as "the herb of gladness." They soak borage in sherry and water, then bring the entire mixture to a boil. They drink it early in the evening or before bedtime.

_____ **DAMIANA** Herbalists recommend damiana to ease depression. Brew a cup of damiana tea by steeping 1 teaspoon of leaves in 1 cup of just-boiled water for 10 minutes. Strain and drink this tea first thing in the morning.

_____ **LAVENDER** Recommended today by aromatherapists to treat mild depression, lavender oil has been popular for centuries. One method of using this therapy is to add 3 drops of essential oil of lavender to a basin of steaming water and then inhale the vapors. You can also add lavender oil to your favorite body lotion.

LEMON BALM The flowers of the lemon balm plant have a pleasant lemony scent. As the great Muslim physician Avicenna said, "It makes the heart merry." Arabs are fond of the scent of the lemon balm and use it to treat depression.

MILKWORT A popular Chinese remedy for depression is a tea of chopped milkwort root mixed with licorice.

PASSIONFLOWER Because chronic sufferers of depression have low levels of serotonin, researchers feel that depression may be relieved by raising the level of that hormone in the blood. One kind of passionflower (*P. quadrangularis*, or giant granadilla) was recently found to contain serotonin. By promoting the transmission of subtle nerve impulses, it aids concentration, alters perception, gently shifts moods and becomes a natural calming agent.

Brew ½ to 1 teaspoon of the dried passionflower leaves and stems into 1 cup of boiling water. You may drink this tea every 3 to 4 hours.

> ## Curiosity Box
>
> *Buddhists believe that depression is caused by the misguided search for constant stimulation. This desire creates an emotional imbalance. Daily meditation — examining the inner self — is thought to be the best way to correct the imbalance and cure the depression. Meditation techniques are discussed more fully on pages 76.*

ROSE GERANIUM BALM Aromatherapists recommend essential oil of rose geranium to soothe anxiety and lift spirits. To make a massage oil, combine 2 drops of rose geranium (or orange oil) in 1 tablespoon of olive oil. You can also use this blend to perfume a warm, relaxing bath.

ST. JOHN'S WORT Originally used to ward off witches and heal deep sword cuts, St. John's wort is now used in Europe as a natural antidepressant. St. John's wort's red color comes from a compound called hypericine, which research has shown to be effective in reducing

---

Helpful Hints

Researchers have found some simple ways that you can help protect yourself from depression.

■ **Eliminate sugars and refined foods from your diet.** Sweeten foods with a limited amount of fructose. And drink fruit juices which have been diluted 50 percent with water.

■ **Avoid alcohol, caffeine, tobacco** and foods which contain chemical additives like colorings, preservatives or artificial flavorings.

■ **Exercise.** Several studies have shown that exercise is an effective method for stimulating the production of powerful mood elevators such as norepinephrine and endorphin. In addition, routine exercises like stretching, swimming and physical games help break the cycle of negative thinking that contributes to depression.

---

depressive symptoms. That's probably the reason this old folk cure helps relieve mild to moderate depression.

Europeans take 1 to 2 drops of the fluid extract mixed with water, 3 times daily on an empty stomach. Alternatively, they brew the herb into a tea.

VERVAIN This herb has been used since medieval times for many purposes, including relief from depression. It also helps stress related problems such as anxiety, lethargy, headaches and migraines. A pleasant way to try this treatment is to brew a cup of vervain tea and either drink it, or use it to scent your bathwater.

VITAMIN B Some researchers theorize that people who are deficient in any one of the B vitamins are at higher risk for depression. The B-vitamin complex includes thiamin, riboflavin, niacin, folate, B6, and B12. Besides supplements, there are many good food sources for B vitamins:

■ Thiamin — sunflower seeds, wheat germ, spinach, pine nuts

- ■ Riboflavin — nonfat yogurt, skim milk, swiss cheese

- ■ Niacin — chicken breast, light tuna in water, swordfish

- ■ Folate — cowpeas, lentils, pinto beans

- ■ B6 — baked potato, banana, chickpeas, prune juice

- ■ B12 — steamed clams, mussels, oysters

DIABETES

The full name for diabetes is diabetes mellitus. Mellitus means "honey-sweet," which is appropriate since diabetes is a condition in which an excess of sugar builds up in the blood and is then spilled into the urine. While all the details are not yet known, it appears that diabetes comes from a combination of hereditary and environmental factors. The contributing environmental factors can include quality of diet, lack of exercise and stress. In addition, some cases may be brought on by infection or made worse by it.

There are two types of diabetes. Type I, or "juvenile onset" diabetes, usually occurs in lean children and adolescents under 25 years of age. With Type I, the pancreas doesn't secrete enough insulin to support the body's needs, and insulin injections are required to control it. Type II, or "maturity onset" diabetes, usually occurs in obese people over 40 years of age. With Type II, the pancreas is capable of making insulin, but the cells are resistant to it. It can usually be controlled by weight loss and proper diet. Type I diabetes is the more serious of the two, but both can lead to hardening of the arteries, nerve damage, kidney damage, loss of vision or even death if left untreated. So it is important for diabetics to follow their doctors' recommendations regarding medication, diet and lifestyle.

The fact that diabetes in the adult may be triggered by external conditions makes onset of the disease somewhat preventable. And because it tends to be hereditary, anything we can do to prevent the onset should be of particular interest to people with family histories of diabetes. Fortunately, diabetes is not the killer it used to be. Because of the discovery of insulin treatment, most diabetics with Type I diabetes can live full, normal lives. Those with Type II can do the same, if they follow the rules.

ALFALFA Arabians use alfalfa to treat diabetes and believe that it can help the body absorb protein, fats and carbohydrates, in addition to purifying the blood. Alfalfa is available in capsule and tea form.

BITTERROOT Native Americans believe Bitterroot clears impurities from the liver and use this herb as a treatment for diabetes. It can be taken as a tincture from the root.

BLUEBERRY A popular European remedy to lower elevated blood sugar is to drink blueberry leaf tea. They drink 1 cup in the morning and 1 cup at night for at least 3 months.

DANDELION American herbologists believe dandelion root tea detoxifies the liver, spleen, blood and pancreas, which may help the body manage

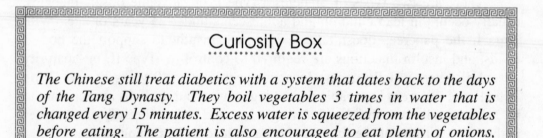

Curiosity Box

The Chinese still treat diabetics with a system that dates back to the days of the Tang Dynasty. They boil vegetables 3 times in water that is changed every 15 minutes. Excess water is squeezed from the vegetables before eating. The patient is also encouraged to eat plenty of onions, bitter melon, tomatoes, pumpkin, white cabbage and celery.

The vegetables are very filling and so suppress the appetite. Because overeating is one of the more common risk factors associated with diabetes, it's easy to see why this ancient treatment is helpful.

In addition, the Chinese recommend these traditional remedies specifically for the relief of diabetic symptoms:

■ *Twice a day, eat a fresh onion soaked in boiling water for 1 minute and seasoned with salt.*

■ *Boil fresh watermelon peel in water and drink 1 glass twice a day.*

■ *Drink fresh guava juice before every meal.*

■ *Boil dried string beans in water and drink as a soup once a day.*

Eat to Manage Diabetes

In both Type I and Type II diabetes, the cells are restricted in their ability to take in sugar. As a result, the sugar is released into the bloodstream, which can cause serious damage. Therefore, the goal of treatment for both juvenile and adult diabetes is to restrict the amount of sugar released into the blood, either by increasing the ability of the pancreas to make insulin, or by reducing the blood sugar level. Attention to diet can be critical in either case.

■ **To help the pancreas produce insulin:** Chromium is a mineral which your pancreas needs to manufacture insulin. In Europe, Asia and the Middle East, raw onions, garlic and common edible mushrooms are favorite natural treatments against diabetes because they contain high amounts of chromium.

■ **To reduce the level of blood sugar:** Modern research has found that by causing slower absorption of sugar into the bloodstream, less of a burden is put on the pancreas to produce extra insulin. Complex carbohydrates, found in many foods, contain natural sugars which are absorbed into the blood at a slower rate. You'll find complex carbohydrates in artichokes, apples, dried beans, peanuts, rice, potatoes, corn, soybeans and other foods.

In Iraq, barley bread is eaten to restrict the absorption of dietary sugar into the blood. And many cultures use cabbage, lettuce, turnips, beans, juniper berries, alfalfa, high fiber wheat grains and coriander seeds to lower blood sugar and/or stimulate the production of insulin.

diabetes. One teaspoon of dried root powder in a pint of boiling water is a traditional remedy.

HONEY One of the most important changes a diabetic must make in his or her diet is to eliminate excess sugar. The Irish, who have a lower incidence of diabetes than we do, have found that an excellent replacement for purified white cane sugar is honey. Though honey is just as high in calories as sugar, it takes the body longer to digest, requiring less insulin all at once. In countries where honey is used more frequently than sugar, the incidence of diabetes tends to be proportionately lower than it is in countries where processed sugar is preferred.

HUCKLEBERRY The Russians drink huckleberry tea as a treatment for diabetes, because they believe it acts as insulin. Use fresh or dried berries and leaves as a tea, decoction or syrup.

MUSTARD Magnesium can help to regulate blood sugar levels, and 1 tablespoon of ground mustard seeds contains 33 milligrams of this mineral. The recommended dietary allowance for magnesium is 350 milligrams for adult men, and 280 for adult women.

SAVORY One of the complications which diabetes sufferers endure is dry mouth. German herbologists believe savory tea prevents this. They recommend 1 cup of savory tea a day.

WATERCRESS Because it is low in carbohydrates and high in iron, this member of the mustard family is believed to be good for diabetics. Watercress contains good sources of vitamins A, B, C and B2, as well as iron, copper, magnesium and calcium. Although slightly bitter, watercress is a tasty addition to salads.

DIAPER RASH

Like all forms of dermatitis, diaper rash is the result of an external irritation to the skin. In this case, a painful rash around the genitals and buttocks is caused by prolonged contact with dirty diapers. Because they have such sensitive skin, just about every baby suffers from diaper rash from time to time. However, you can help prevent it by keeping your baby as clean and dry as possible.

Bathe baby often with warm water, and then make sure every little crease and crevice is completely dry before putting on a fresh diaper. Change baby frequently, using cotton diapers instead of disposables — and because diaper rash can be aggravated by residue from harsh detergents, be sure to use mild soap when you launder those diapers. Avoid plastic pants whenever possible — especially when baby is having a flare-up — and take advantage of the collective wisdom of moms and dads from all over the world to keep baby's bottom soft and smooth.

CALENDULA Calendula is soothing and encourages new tissue formation. A gentle powder can be made by adding crushed calendula to cornstarch.

CORNSTARCH All baby powders help prevent diaper rash by keeping moisture away from baby's skin, but naturalists and pediatricians agree that cornstarch is the safest choice. Unlike other powders, cornstarch is dust free, and that means baby is less likely to inhale particles that can cause lung problems or lead to congestion.

EGG WHITE Some mothers swear by this old home remedy for treating diaper rash. Apply egg whites often to the irritated area to build up a layer of albumin that will protect the skin from moisture while it is healing.

VINEGAR If you use cloth diapers, add ¼ cup of white vinegar to the final rinse water when laundering them. Rinsing diapers in acidic vinegar keeps bacteria in check.

Another home remedy is to use a white vinegar mixture (1 teaspoon of white vinegar per cup of water) in baby's bath — or on a washcloth gently rubbed over baby's bottom between diaper changes. This restores the skin's pH level and reduces itching and inflammation. **CAUTION:** *Don't use vinegar directly on baby if the skin is broken.*

ZINC Thick ointments that protect baby's skin from urine and feces can help clear up and prevent diaper rash. Look for products that contain zinc oxide, which has antiseptic properties.

DIARRHEA

Diarrhea is a symptom, not a disease. It can be caused by many things, including stress, food allergies, overindulgence in rich food, food poisoning, and bacterial or viral infections. Most cases of diarrhea in healthy adults are not serious. However, seek medical attention if the diarrhea lasts longer than 3 or 4 days, or if you are dealing with a patient who is very young, elderly or otherwise chronically ill.

The most serious side effect of diarrhea is dehydration. Losing more liquid than you take in can cause your blood volume to decrease, which will make your blood pressure drop too low — and can affect your heart. So, make sure you drink plenty of clear liquids, such as water, decaffeinated teas, broths and juices. Other than that, the best advice is to simply let your diarrhea run its course — and to try some of the following natural methods to ease the unpleasantness and discomfort.

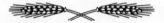

APPLE Early U.S. settlers ate grated raw sweet apples as a remedy for diarrhea. Apples have a high pectin content which is a soluble fiber.

BLACKBERRY Italians drink blackberry juice, wine or brandy to stop diarrhea. This treatment dates back to biblical times. Blackberry leaves contain tannin, an astringent, which stops excess secretion from the intestinal lining. The recommended dose is 6 ounces of juice, or 1 heaping teaspoon of jam, or 2 ounces of wine, or 2 tablespoons of brandy every 4 hours.

You can also make a medicinal tea using dried or fresh blackberry leaves. Steep 1 teaspoon of dried leaves or 3 teaspoons of fresh leaves in 1 cup of boiling water. Sweeten with honey if you like.

BLUEBERRIES Blueberries are used in Sweden to stop diarrhea. Blueberries are rich in anthocyanosides, which kill the bacteria that often cause diarrhea.

CINNAMON The Chinese have a simple cure for diarrhea. They dissolve 4 grams of ground cinnamon in 1 cup of warm water, cover it for 15 minutes and drink it like a tea.

CITRICIDAL Researchers worldwide have tested a substance called citricidal as a remedy for traveler's diarrhea. Citricidal is an extract made from the seeds and pulp of citrus fruits. It is being used effectively in South America, Europe and the Far East.

CLOVES Many travelers carry powdered clove with them to use in case diarrhea strikes. In Uruguay, clove tea and liquor are taken to treat diarrhea. Most South Americans believe that cloves have antibacterial and antiviral properties.

To make clove tea, use 1 teaspoon of powdered clove per cup of boiling water. Steep for 10 to 15 minutes before drinking. You can also help to settle an upset stomach by adding powdered cloves to other herbal teas.

GREEN TEA This brew, popular in China and Japan, contains tannins which are useful to the digestive system when diarrhea strikes.

HONEY South African researchers have found that honey slows the growth of some germs that cause diarrhea, including Salmonella, Shigella and E. coli.

HYSSOP The tannins in hyssop can be helpful in treating diarrhea. Steep 1 teaspoon of ground hyssop in 1 cup of boiling water. Strain and drink.

LEEKS The British prepare a stock from leeks that they use as a remedy for diarrhea. The leek juice contains many minerals, which help to replace those lost in watery stools.

LENTILS The ancient Romans ate lentils to cure diarrhea. Lentils are a good way to replace many of the minerals and nutrients that you lose through frequent bowel movements.

OREGANO This herb is used by the Chinese as a traditional treatment for diarrhea. Oregano contains thymol and cavacol, compounds which are said to help relax the digestive tract.

To brew oregano tea, add 1 teaspoon of the herb to a cup of boiling water, and allow it to steep for 10 minutes. Strain and drink.

SAGE Since ancient times, Greeks have used sage to treat diarrhea, and this herb is still widely used in the Mediterranean and southern Europe. The reason for sage's effectiveness is its antispasmodic properties which can help calm down an upset colon.

To make sage tea, pour ½ cup of boiling water over ½ teaspoon of dried leaves and steep 10 minutes. Strain and drink.
CAUTION: *Sage can be potent, so drink no more than 1 cup a day. And if you're pregnant, stay away from it altogether.*

YOGURT For hundreds of years, Mediterranean people have used yogurt as a remedy for diarrhea, especially for diarrhea caused by bacterial infection. This fermented milk product contains living microbes that hinder growth of the bacteria that cause digestive upsets.

Look for yogurt that contains live lactobacillus acidophilus cultures. These beneficial bacteria re-establish the good bacteria in your intestines that might have been wiped out by the virus or microorganism that caused the diarrhea in the first place. Eat 1 cup of yogurt a day until the diarrhea disappears.

Treating Children's Diarrhea

Broth. Most children willingly sip a cup of clear broth, which makes it an excellent source for replacing lost fluids and nutrients in their systems.

Carrots. In Peru, children with diarrhea are given a mixture of carrots, wheat flour, pea flour and oil. The starch in this mixture helps retain fluids. And researchers at the University of Edinburgh in Scotland have found several additional benefits in the carrots. They not only provide the necessary bulk to get rid of diarrhea, but also replenish the supply of minerals and vitamins lost during an attack. Cooked carrots served as a juice or in soup are an especially effective treatment for infant diarrhea.

Lemon. Add a little fresh lemon juice to baby's water bottle to help calm his or her intestines.

Yogurt. Many parents in Japan, Italy, Russia and the United States include some yogurt in their babies' diets to counteract symptoms of diarrhea. If your baby drinks from a bottle, mix 1 teaspoon of plain, unsweetened yogurt with the formula. And if you breast feed, put some yogurt on your nipple while baby nurses.

DIVERTICULOSIS

Diverticulosis, a disease of the colon which occurs most frequently in people who are over the age of 50, is usually triggered by a lack of dietary fiber or roughage in the diet. The pressure of trying to pass hard, dry stools can cause tiny pouches (or diverticulae) to form. When these pouches trap waste matter, it can cause pain, tenderness and rigidity in the lower abdomen (usually the left side), fever and alternating attacks of constipation and diarrhea.

When the pouches become plugged with debris or inedible foodstuff, bacteria may be formed, causing a disease called diverticulitis. To explain further, diverticulosis is the presence of diverticulae. Diverticulitis is their inflammation. If not treated, diverticulitis can become very serious, sometimes requiring surgery. But diverticulosis can usually be controlled — or prevented — before it reaches this stage simply by making some dietary changes. Here are the best ways we have found to relieve the symptoms of diverticulosis.

- **Avoid seeds.** Nutritionists say that foods which contain nuts, popcorn, poppy, sesame and other seeds should not be included in your diet if you suffer from diverticulosis. These can become caught in the pouches, increasing irritation and pain.

- **Exercise.** Aerobic exercises, such as running, jogging, swimming, walking or bicycling, increase the blood flow through the colon and help overcome bowel irregularity.

- **Increase fiber.** Eat more whole grain breads, cereals, grains, beans, fruits and vegetables. These foods are high in fiber and will help soften your stools.

- **Eat papaya and pineapple.** These fruits are good sources of proteolytic enzymes — which many experts believe can aid digestion and reduce the colon inflammation caused by diverticulosis.

(You can also purchase proteolytic enzymes in capsule form.)

■ **Quit smoking.** Smoking increases the motility, or movement, of the intestines and can aggravate the diverticulosis condition. (One more good reason to quit!)

■ **Drink plenty of water.** Include 6 glasses of water in your diet each day to promote regular bowel movements.

EARACHE

Earaches are caused by an inflammation of either the external or the middle ear, and can be accompanied by overall discomfort, fever and, if left unattended, even a hearing loss. Earaches are fairly common in children because their eustachean tubes (the part of the ear which adjusts pressure and drains fluid from the middle ear) are compressed by reactive lymphatic tissue — the "adenoids," and so have a tendency to get clogged. The result is infection, bacterial or viral, which can quickly spread to the middle ear.

If an earache lasts more than a few days, produces a discharge or is the result of a bacterial infection, you'll need to consult your physician. However, for minor earaches — like those you usually get with a cold — the following remedies have been used for generations.

ALCOHOL Naturalists suggest that you mix equal parts of alcohol and vinegar, and put a few drops in each ear when you come out of the water to prevent "swimmer's ear."

ALMOND OIL A few drops of warm (not hot) almond oil is soothing, although it will not fight an infection.

ECHINACEA Drinking a tea made from echinacea, which is considered to be antimicrobial, is a good remedy to use against infections of the ears, nose and throat.

GARLIC Traditional Chinese medicine recommends the use of garlic for common earaches. Garlic has impressive antibiotic, antifungal and anti-viral properties that effectively treat ear problems. When the ear first begins to hurt, the Chinese place a few drops of garlic oil in the ear canal, followed by a wad of sterile cotton inserted loosely.

Make your own garlic oil by crushing a few cloves of garlic into some olive oil and letting it sit for a few days at room temperature. Strain and refrigerate — but bring back to room temperature before using.
CAUTION: *Do not use this remedy if there is any ear discharge or indication that the eardrum is perforated (difficulty hearing sounds or understanding words).*

Helpful Hints

- **Keep your head elevated** to help the eustachean tubes drain naturally. This is especially important for children, so hold baby's head as upright as possible when bottle or breast feeding. If milk moves into the eustachean tubes — the part of the ear that drains fluid from the ear — it is likely to attract an infection.

- **Drink plenty of fluids.** Swallowing helps open the passageway from the middle ear, and drinking fluids like juices and teas offers a positive way to fight ear infections.

- **Switch to a low-fat diet.** Chronic inner-ear problems may be improved by decreasing the amount of fat and cholesterol in your diet. Some research indicates that ear and hearing problems may be early indications of heart and arterial disease.

- **Keep it warm.** Set your hair dryer at low speed, and hold it a few inches away from your sore ear. Or, do what they did before hair dryers were invented — apply a warm compress.

- **Learn Valsalva's Maneuver.** This is especially helpful to relieve earaches caused by pressure changes (during plane rides, for example). Close your mouth, pinch your nose shut and blow. This will force air out through your middle ear and alleviate the pressure. Scuba divers do this as they descend in the water.
  CAUTION: *If you have circulatory problems, consult your physician before trying Valsalva's Maneuver.*

MUGWORT Don't let mugwort's unattractive name stop you from using this effective pain reliever. Many cultures treat earaches with a poultice made from this flowering plant that's found in the Arctic, North Africa, Siberia, western Asia and the Himalayas.

ONION In several African countries, onions are a popular earache remedy. Because of their natural antibiotic properties, they are effective in fighting infections — like external otitis or "swimmer's ear" — caused by bacteria. To try it, roast an onion thoroughly. After it cools, wrap it in a clean cloth and place it over the ear until the pain stops.

PENNYWORT The juice from the pennywort plant is a common remedy for an earache. Wrap the leaves in a cloth, pound thoroughly and squeeze out the juice. Then place a few drops of juice in the ear canal.

PEPPERMINT The Chinese use fresh peppermint oil to relieve ear pain. Extract and use this natural antibiotic as described above under "pennywort."

ECZEMA

Eczema is an itchy rash that causes the skin to thicken and peel, typically in the creases inside the elbows, behind the knees or under the breasts. It often appears in conjunction with hay fever or an asthma attack. Eczema can also be caused by nutritional deficiencies or by an allergic reaction to detergents, nail polish or other harsh chemicals. Western medicine has always had a hard time treating eczema effectively. Fortunately, there are many natural alternatives.

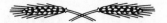

BORAGE Research has shown borage oil to be effective in treating inflammatory skin conditions. Take borage oil capsules, or add cucumber-tasting borage leaves to salad for a healthful change from lettuce.

BURDOCK Burdock root has been used in the treatment of skin diseases over the ages. It is recognized throughout the world as a blood purifier and detoxifier. Generally, burdock is used internally — in powder, tablet or tea form.

CHICKWEED Naturalists agree that chickweed eases irritation and helps wounds heal. The dried herb can be added directly to your bath water, or a chickweed ointment can be applied topically.

COMFREY Treat your eczema with a soothing poultice made by boiling a handful of comfrey (or coltsfoot) root. Let it cool, and then apply the liquid to the affected area with a soft cloth.

EVENING PRIMROSE Proper digestion of fatty acids is needed to maintain healthy skin — and a supplement of evening primrose oil helps your body do just that.

LEMON BALM A compress soaked in warm water and lemon balm oil is soothing for those suffering from eczema.

OATMEAL Oatmeal is an effective skin soother for acne and chicken pox, as well as eczema. (See page 91 and page 447 for recipes for a facial wash and a body wash made from oatmeal.)

TEA TREE OIL A native Australian tree produces tea tree oil, which has been used for hundreds of years to treat skin irritations, including

---

Helpful Hints

■ **When bathing, use warm water** instead of hot water, and add a few drops of soothing lavender or chamomile oil. And after bathing, apply either of these essential oils (mixed with almond or olive oil) directly to the rash.

■ **Wear cotton.** Soft, natural fibers feel good and let your skin breathe.

■ **Exercise.** Getting the blood circulating is beneficial for most skin ailments. Just remember to wash away sweat as soon as possible when you're through.

■ **Eat right.** Help clear your skin by eliminating fried foods and foods with added sugar and artificial color and flavoring from your diet.

■ **Supplement with vitamins and minerals.** If your eczema is caused by a nutritional deficiency, your skin will return to normal once the deficiency has been corrected. Vitamin A and zinc are important for healthy skin, as are vitamins B, C and E. Take supplements, or see page 50 for the best food sources of these nutrients.

eczema. The oil is a powerful natural antibiotic with a strong scent that has recently become very popular in the U.S.

WATERCRESS Next time you buy ingredients for a salad, add watercress to your shopping list. Watercress, a member of the mustard family, is loaded with vitamins A, B and C, and also has a high sulfur content — all of which help eczema.

EYE IRRITATION

Some scientists believe that our eyes need saltwater because we, like most other land animals, emerged from the sea. Whatever the reason, our eyes do need a constant saline bath — which they get every time we blink.

If our eyes don't get enough natural moisture, or if they become dry and irritated as the result of being exposed to high winds or dust, we feel an uncomfortable burning or itching sensation accompanied by redness. Similar symptoms can be caused by allergies and colds — and can almost always be alleviated with some simple home remedies.

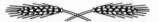

AGRIMONY The leaves of this plant have been used since Saxon times to treat conjunctivitis. To make an eyewash, use 10 grams per 500 ml. of water.

CABBAGE This remedy was very popular with stars of Hollywood's silent screen era. After a long day exposed to bright lights, they applied a poultice of steamed fresh cabbage leaves over closed eyes. To be effective, the cabbage leaves must be boiled until limp, but not thoroughly cooked — and the drained leaves should be comfortably warm to the touch when placed over the eyes.

CALENDULA This herb is known to have antibacterial and wound-healing abilities. For irritated eyes or itching caused by allergies, make a compress by adding calendula to hot water. Allow the water to cool and then dip a cotton cloth in the solution and hold over the irritated eye.

CUCUMBER Ten minutes with a fresh cucumber slice over each eyelid tones the membranes, and cools and soothes tired eyes.

EYEBRIGHT Eyebright, a small plant that grows well in northern Europe and Scotland, gained notoriety back in the 17th century when it was mentioned in John Milton's "Paradise Lost." Since then, it has earned a reputation as a powerful remedy for all sorts of ailments. For eye irritation, eyebright should be used as a compress or eyewash.

Chamomile, calendula and elderflowers are other good choices. See page 82 for instructions on how to make a soothing herbal decoction. **CAUTION:** *When using an eyewash, make sure you wash out your eyecup when you switch from one eye to the other.*

FENNEL Pliny the Elder, an early Greek scientist and physician, observed snakes that had just finished shedding their skins eating the leaves of the fennel plant. He believed that the snakes did this to restore their sight, and assumed that fennel might have some positive effects on humans as well. So, he devised a way to make fennel tea, and his fellow Greeks began drinking it to improve their vision and prevent deteriorating eyesight.

Pliny's observation was a good one. Rutin, a flavonoid found in fennel, strengthens the tiny blood vessels in the retina. And fennel tea makes a soothing eyewash.

GOLDENSEAL Goldenseal has long been used by Native Americans for infections and irritations. To make an eyewash, mix 1 cup of sterile water, ¼ teaspoon of salt, and ½ a teaspoon of goldenseal powder. **CAUTION:** *Discard and replace this solution if it becomes cloudy.*

HONEY An ancient Greek eye remedy — hydromel — is simply a mixture of honey and water. To make it yourself, simmer 1 cup of water and 1 teaspoon of honey for 5 minutes. Dip a clean cloth in the liquid and apply it to your closed eye.

MILK Soothe tired, bloodshot eyes by covering them for 10 minutes with a sterile strip of puffy cotton that has been soaked in cool skim milk.

NETTLE Despite the ominous-sounding name, nettle (also known as stinging nettle) capsules are an effective remedy for itchy eyes.

POTATO An Irish trick to soothe irritated eyes is to apply a poultice made from scraped raw potatoes to closed eyes.

SALINE As anyone who wears contact lenses knows, sterile saline solution soothes dry, irritated eyes.
CAUTION: *Don't try to make it yourself. It must be absolutely sterile.*

SASSAFRAS The Mohawk Indians drew on the antiseptic and pain-relieving properties of an extract of sassafras leaves to make an eyebath. They mixed the extract with water and then dripped it into the eyes. Or they immersed their faces — eyes open — directly into the sassafras water.

TEA The Taiwanese, regular tea drinkers, apply cooled tea bags to itching reddened eyes to get almost instant relief. Scientists attribute this cure to the high level of tannic acid found in tea. Leftover tea bags — especially from herbal blends — make especially good eyebags.

TOMATOES To relieve bloodshot eyes, the Chinese suggest eating 1 or 2 fresh tomatoes first thing in the morning on an empty stomach. Scientists believe that the vitamin C and flavonoids in the tomatoes strengthen blood vessels.

Herbal Relief for Sties

A sty results when one of the oil glands at the base of your eyelashes becomes infected. A combination of heat and herbs is the time-honored remedy for treating them.

A hot tea bag will work, but we prefer a hot compress made from dried calendula flowers to relieve the pain and infection. To make one, pour 2 cups of boiling water over 2 tablespoons of the dried flowers and let the tea steep for 20 minutes Then strain out the flowers and soak a clean washcloth in the calendula tea. Apply the cloth to the eye and keep it there for at least 5 minutes. Repeat this treatment several times a day until the sty is gone.

WITCH HAZEL Herbalists recommend a witch hazel compress to reduce puffiness under the eyes. To make one at home, soak cottonballs in a mixture of witch hazel and distilled water. Place the moist cotton over your eyes, and then lie down for 10 or 15 minutes.

F or information on where to purchase any of the items listed, turn to the glossary beginning on page 523.

FATIGUE

One of the most amazing stimulants in the world is manufactured by your own body. Adrenaline, a hormone produced in the adrenal gland, is the stuff that propels you into action when you are faced with a sudden emotional or physical challenge. It is so powerful that adrenaline-fueled individuals have been known to rip doors off of overturned cars, or force their way through locked doors during fires. Under ordinary conditions, your body produces small quantities of adrenaline every day — the right amount to keep you going. But this natural balance breaks down when you are overloaded with physical or emotional stressors. The result? Fatigue.

There are many natural stimulants that you can use when you need an energy boost. Used correctly, they are not harmful — so long as you don't have heart trouble or high blood pressure, and so long as you're not taking prescription drugs. However, even these safe stimulants are not a substitute for adequate sleep, a healthy diet and regular exercise.

BORAGE Saudis eat raw borage, believing that it strengthens the heart and limbs. And, indeed, research shows that it is a stimulant. Try borage as a substitute for lettuce in salads and on sandwiches.

BORON Grapes and nuts contain boron, a trace mineral that affects electrical activity in the brain. A few grapes and 3 or 4 ounces of peanuts per day will act as a stimulant. Peanuts are also a good source of the B vitamin inositol, which helps the nervous system function smoothly.

CAFFEINE The Chinese emperor Shen Nung wrote in 2727 B.C., "Tea quenches the thirst. It lessens the desire to sleep. It gladdens and cheers the heart." Tea and coffee both contain significant amounts of caffeine,

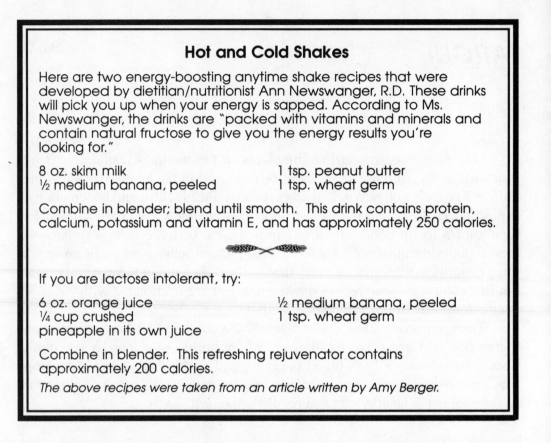

Hot and Cold Shakes

Here are two energy-boosting anytime shake recipes that were developed by dietitian/nutritionist Ann Newswanger, R.D. These drinks will pick you up when your energy is sapped. According to Ms. Newswanger, the drinks are "packed with vitamins and minerals and contain natural fructose to give you the energy results you're looking for."

8 oz. skim milk   1 tsp. peanut butter
½ medium banana, peeled   1 tsp. wheat germ

Combine in blender; blend until smooth. This drink contains protein, calcium, potassium and vitamin E, and has approximately 250 calories.

If you are lactose intolerant, try:

6 oz. orange juice   ½ medium banana, peeled
¼ cup crushed   1 tsp. wheat germ
pineapple in its own juice

Combine in blender. This refreshing rejuvenator contains approximately 200 calories.

The above recipes were taken from an article written by Amy Berger.

but the stimulus provided by tea is much smoother and less aggressive than the caffeine "wake-up" of coffee.

CAUTION: *If you are prone to low blood sugar, it might be a good idea to reduce, or even eliminate caffeine from your diet. You may find you have more energy without it.*

CAYENNE PEPPER Anyone who has enjoyed a bowl of extra spicy gumbo knows that Cajun food can be h-o-t, as well as enlivening. That's because the mandatory ingredient in most Cajun cuisine is cayenne pepper — and all hot peppers contain capsaicin, a powerful stimulant.

DAMIANA In Mexico, damiana leaves are added to liqueurs to enhance the flavor. This known aphrodisiac can also be brewed into a tonic to relieve lethargy.

FIGS Extremely high in natural sugars, figs also rate well for energy-boosting iron, potassium, phosophorus, magnesium and B-complex vitamins. This handy snack is also very low in sodium.

FLORAL WATER A recent study at Duke University found that women between 45 and 60 were refreshed after spraying themselves with a floral fragrance such as lavender or lilac water — something southern women

---

Helpful Hints

■ **Perk up with an energizing massage.** A few drops of essential oil of cinnamon, peppermint, eucalyptus or neroli (made from bitter orange blossoms) can be combined with almond or soybean oil to make an invigorating massage oil. Aromatherapists also recommend dabbing some on your forehead, cheeks and under your nose.

■ **Use a slant board.** The yogis of India use a slant board when they are feeling run down. They lie with their heads at the lower end of the tilted board, allowing blood to rush to the brain and stimulate mental activity and alertness. If you don't have a slant board, lie down and use pillows to keep your feet elevated above your head.

■ **Eat a hearty breakfast.** The Irish, Scots and English all believe in greeting the day with a hearty breakfast. They know, from years of experience, what modern medicine is now supporting with research — breakfast really is the most important meal of the day.

If you think it's okay to start your day with nothing but a cup of coffee, think again. Caffeine causes your pancreas to release insulin, which lowers your blood sugar. Add a sweet roll, and your blood sugar goes up abruptly, calling out even more insulin causing your sugar to drop even more. Instead, make sure your breakfast includes a protein source like an egg, cottage cheese or even meat to help you wake up in a systematic way. Or, follow the lead of our Irish, English and Scotch kinsmen. They eat a breakfast low in sugar and high in carbohydrates. A bowl of thick porridge is a must every morning in most of Great Britain. And porridge is especially good because it is digested slowly, providing a long-term source of energy.

■ **Stock your pantry with energy-boosting foods,** including bananas, cabbage, carrots, dates, figs, oatmeal, onions, peas, prunes, raisins, soybeans, spinach and strawberries.

have been doing for hundreds of years.

GINSENG A Swiss study has shown that ginseng, the best-known ingredient in Chinese medicine, has energy-producing capabilities. In this study, athletes were fed a daily dose of ginseng. Over a period of a few weeks, the efficiency with which their bodies processed oxygen improved dramatically, and the athletes experienced increased energy and stamina.

GOTU KOLA Gotu kola is a long-time energy tonic in traditional Chinese medicine. It is available as a tablet, as a ready-made tonic, or as a powder which can be made into a tea.

EXERCISE

Studies have shown that regular, brisk exercise (fast walking or cycling, for example) boosts energy levels and helps you handle daily stress. Try to exercise at least 30 minutes, 3 times a week.

You'll feel even better if you exercise outdoors. Oxygen stimulates brain activity and enriches the blood by improving the circulation. That's why you feel so good when you walk briskly along a country road or along the beach. Moving water, streams, oceans and rivers generate negative ions, which have a calming effect on the mind. Pollution and air conditioning have the opposite effect, and make you feel irritable and fatigued.

HONEY In ancient Greece, birthplace of the Olympics, athletes believed that eating honey before an event gave them extra energy. Honey is full of vital nutrients and easy-to-burn sugars. Today, some marathon runners use hard candies with liquid honey centers to spur them past "the wall" at the 18-mile marker. Though the honey-induced energy burst is short lived, it's often just enough to make the winning difference.

KELP Mountain guides in Tibet and Nepal must go long distances without rest. To stay alert, they carry pouches of dried kelp. When fatigued, they chew a pinch of it to restore breathing and to invigorate tired muscles. The Japanese, too, use kelp to restore energy. If taken over a long period of time, the iodine in kelp can stimulate the thyroid gland and increase the metabolic rate.

    LITCHI A potent stimulant commonly used in China is derived from the litchi plant. It is considered a source of energy and a mental stimulant. The Chinese prepare litchi by charring or drying it, and then grinding it into a fine powder. It can also be steeped in wine or eaten raw.

    MA HUANG The ephedra plant, known to the Chinese as ma huang, is the source of the powerful drug ephedrine — a potent catalyst that causes the body to release adrenaline. Ma huang is available in cut or powdered form.

CAUTION: *The effects of this plant can be very strong. It should be*

Energy Tonic Soup

Chicken or pork is usually added to this healthful herb soup that is popular in China. It is traditionally served in the fall and winter for extra energy and warmth on chilly days.

8 dried shiitake mushrooms
2 small Chinese or
   American ginseng roots
1 slice dried Chinese licorice root
1 slice fresh ginger
2 cloves garlic, minced
1 onion, chopped
1 carrot, chopped
1 dried hot chili pepper

¾ cup pearled barley
6 cups vegetable stock
1 Tbsp. minced fresh thyme
  (or 1 tsp. dried)
1 tsp. olive oil
2 tsp. red barley miso
minced fresh chives or
   scallions for garnish

Soak the mushrooms in hot water until soft, about 10 minutes. Discard the stems and slice thinly; reserve the liquid. In a large pot, combine first 10 ingredients, plus reserved liquid. If using dried thyme, add it now. Bring the soup to a boil, reduce heat and simmer loosely covered, until the vegetables and barley are tender (about an hour). Remove from heat and add olive oil (and fresh thyme, if using). Scoop the miso into a small strainer and set the strainer into the soup, using a spoon to press the miso through the strainer into the soup. Serve hot, sprinkled with chives or scallions.

Reprinted with permission from The Good Herb *by Judith Benn Hurley, William Morrow & Co., Inc., 1995*

avoided by people suffering from hypertension.

PEPPERMINT Peppermint or peppermint oil is a quick-acting, natural stimulant. The people of Iceland chew a sprig of fresh peppermint to quickly restore alertness. Some cyclists in the Tour de France drink a tea made from peppermint and rosemary before racing. And many truck drivers keep peppermint-flavored candies in their glove compartments to help keep them awake during long hauls.

STAR ANISE The star anise, a small tree that grows in Asia and North America, has been used by Chinese herbalists for centuries. Both the seeds and the oil extract of this tree have powerful stimulant effects. Anise-based teas are beginning to appear on U.S. shelves as remedies for fatigue.

YERBA MATE Yerba mate is a form of holly grown in Paraguay. It is used to brew a tea that is the country's national beverage. Charles Darwin, the famous naturalist, called this beverage "the ideal stimulant" since it contains caffeine, but is less invigorating than either coffee or regular tea. Paraguayan tea is made from finely ground leaves of the yerba mate plant steeped in hot water. Drink 1 cup early in the day, hot or cold, plain or sweetened, with or without lemon or milk.

FEVER

You ache all over. One minute you feel hot and sticky, and the next minute you're icy cold and shivery. Even without taking your temperature, you know you have a fever — a signal that your body has been invaded by a bacterium, a fungus or a virus.

Fever is one of the ways your body fights infection, and is rarely, in itself, harmful. However, if it is accompanied by a stiff neck, or if it lasts more than five days, or goes above 105° — get to a doctor immediately. Be even more cautious if you're dealing with a small child (a fever of 102° can give him or her convulsions) or an elderly person (where a fever can aggravate an underlying medical condition). Fortunately, most fevers in healthy adults last only a few days and do not require medical attention — just a little common sense and "T.L.C." to relieve the discomfort.

APPLE A strong thirst is usually a symptom of a fever. Eating an apple is a pleasant way to ingest vitamins and quench that thirst. Be sure to eat the peel — where the vitamins and minerals are concentrated.

BAYBERRY Bayberry root bark, also known as wax myrtle or candleberry, can be taken as a tea to knock down a fever.

BETEL NUTS Betel nuts contain an aspirin-like substance that is a reliable fever reducer. The nuts grow on palm trees in Malaysia, New Guinea and Normandy Island.

BLACKBERRIES Blackberries are high in vitamin C, which is helpful for the repair process after a fever. A drink of blackberry juice gives you iron and calcium, as well as other essential vitamins and minerals.

BORAGE The French use a hot tea made from the petals and leaves of the borage flower to treat high fevers. Fresh or dried flowers can be used. This remedy works best for fevers brought on by a cold.

CATNIP This feline favorite is effective for humans fighting a fever. A tea made by pouring boiling water over the dried herb promotes perspiration, which, in turn, cools a fever.

CHILI PEPPER The people of Mexico, India, China and Thailand have known for centuries that their spicy cuisines, not only taste good, they make you sweat. So, feed that fever with foods seasoned with hot peppers, cayenne pepper or curry, and help your body sweat out that fever.

DEVIL'S CLAW The tribal people of Africa's Kalahari use the root of the devil's claw plant to fight high fevers. The plant has anti-inflammatory properties similar to cortisone, and may reduce brain tissue swelling that accompanies some bacterial infections. The Africans boil it into a tea or pound it into a powder.

DOGWOOD A rural, down-home South Carolina cure for chills and fever is dogwood bark (which reduces fever) and black cherry bark soaked in whiskey.

EUCALYPTUS The fever tree (also known as the eucalyptus tree and the blue-gum tree) is found in Australia and Malaysia. The oil extracted from its leaves is believed to lower a person's temperature.

FEVERWORT The leaves and flowering tops of the weed-like feverwort (also called boneset) can be steeped into a tea or decoction to promote sweating and, therefore, reduce a fever.

GINGER Both traditional medicine of India (Ayurveda) and modern research in Holland praise the many healing properties of gingerroot — which is eaten to reduce high fevers. It can also be boiled in water and then sponged over the body to induce cooling perspiration.

Helpful Hints

■ **Drink fluids.** Loss of appetite is a common side effect of fever. Solids aren't necessary, but keep those liquids coming in. Drink plenty of water, fruit juices and herbal teas, but stay away from milk (it increases congestion).

■ **Cool, wet compresses** on the lower legs are an effective treatment for fever. Many people prefer this to sponging off the whole body. A cool, moist towel wrapped around the head also brings relief.

■ **Vitamin C.** Soothe a child's fever with rosehip tea sweetened with a little honey. (Don't give honey to children under 1 year old.) This pleasant tasting remedy will help lower his or her temperature, while providing plenty of vitamin C. Another tasty drink that's loaded with vitamin C is red currant juice mixed with water. And, if you have trouble getting your child to drink enough fluids, try freezing fruit juice into ice pops.

LEMON Sipping one or more glasses of hot water with lemon juice before bedtime is a popular European home remedy for fever.

SAGE Sage, which has been taken as a medicinal tea since the Middle Ages, contains antibacterial and antiseptic compounds. It is especially popular among the Chinese and the Dutch, who drink it to reduce body temperature.

SASSAFRAS Many Native American Indian tribes use sassafras tea to reduce fever. Modern research shows that sassafras is an antiseptic.

TEA The Indians and Chinese have used hot tea for hundreds of years to encourage the cooling effect of perspiration.

VITAMIN C The natives of the Middle East, the Orient and Ecuador fight fever by eating fruits high in vitamin C. These include star fruit, pomegranates, acerola cherries, tamarind and citrus (like oranges and grapefruit).

YARROW Used for ages by Native Americans, yarrow is a flowering herb that, once ingested, induces sweating — which reduces fever. To make yarrow tea, steep 1 tablespoon of fresh (or 1 teaspoon dried) leaves and flowers in a cup of boiling water, covered, for 4 minutes. For a fever caused by cold or flu, add 1 tablespoon each of fresh (or 1½ teaspoon dried) elderflower and peppermint before brewing. Drink a cup 3 times a day. (You might enjoy the taste more by adding a bit of honey.)

NATURE'S MEDICINE CABINET

Aspirin is the best-known fever fighter on the market. And though Western medicine recommends this as an effective and safe way to reduce adult fever, natural aspirin — salicin — is an attractive and readily available alternative. Willow trees, birch trees and almonds all yield salicin, and all three of these sources are used by people in parts of Africa to treat fever. **CAUTION:** *Children should take only carefully monitored doses of children's aspirin.*

FLATULENCE

Flatulence, or gas (politely referred to in Europe as "the winds") is usually the result of eating too fast and swallowing too much air. It can also be caused by carbonated beverages, smoking, chewing gum, talking with your mouth full, and by the natural digestive process that breaks down certain foods like beans. Your body forces the excess air in your system out through the nearest opening — and either belching or flatulence is the result.

Gas is characterized by an uncomfortable or painful bloated feeling. The pain can be so severe that it has occasionally been mistaken for symptoms of a heart attack. Though harmless, flatulence is so common, and so unpleasant, that any quick, effective treatment is always greatly appreciated. Here are several for you to try.

ALLSPICE Jamaicans drink hot allspice tea to relieve gas. Also called Jamaica pepper or clove pepper, allspice contains eugenol, which stimulates the digestive enzyme trypsin. To make this tea, add 2 teaspoons of allspice powder to a cup of boiling water, and then steep for 10 to 20 minutes. Drink up to 3 cups per day.

ANISE The Greeks have been chewing these licorice-flavored seeds for centuries to ease digestive problems.

CARAWAY The Pharmaceutical Pocket Book, published by the Council of the Pharmaceutical Society of Great Britain, lists Canamoa tincture as a medicine for upset stomachs. This aromatic oil is extracted from caraway seeds.

CATNIP The Pennsylvania Dutch are well-known for their unique traditions and beliefs. They give catnip tea to children and infants suffering from gas or colic, a remedy that is also popular in many European countries.

CINNAMON The Chinese have a simple cure for flatulence. They dissolve approximately ¼ ounce of ground cinnamon in a cup of warm water, steep for 15 minutes and drink it.

DILL The Chinese have used dill as a digestive aid for centuries, and recent studies show this herb has anti-foaming properties that prevent and break up gas bubbles. To try it, add 2 teaspoons of mashed dill seeds to a cup of boiling water and steep for 10 minutes. Drink 3 times per day.

FENNEL Italians use fennel seeds to prevent gas from forming. The seeds can be sprinkled into soups, stews and other foods. Both the seeds and the roots of the fennel plant are effective in preventing and relieving gas.

GINGER Chinese herbalists use ginger for many remedies, but it's especially good for digestive disturbances. The root can be grated, chopped, shredded or powdered. It is available fresh or dried, and is often added to food and beverages such as ginger ale or ginger beer.

HONEY The writers of the Bible and the Koran both mention honey as a digestive aid. It is widely used in Europe and Asia to prevent gas.

MARJORAM The English often eat fresh marjoram leaves between 2 slices of buttered bread to relieve gas symptoms.

OLIVE OIL Many Italians credit olive oil with preventing gas. They believe it soothes the stomach and aids digestion.

PAPAYA Magellan, Ponce de Leon and Columbus each learned about papayas during their explorations of the New World. This tropical fruit has been used by native islanders for centuries to relieve gastric distress. An effective natural gas reliever, papaya is available fresh, canned and in pill form.

PEPPERMINT The use of mint as a digestive aid dates back to the ancient Egyptians, who cultivated peppermint plants. The Irish put 2 mint leaves in a steaming cup of tea to make a relaxing and effective remedy. Icelanders also favor peppermint tea for stomach relief. And here and abroad, many a desperate parent has soothed a colicky baby with peppermint water.

THYME Wealthy Romans drank thyme tea after overindulging in their favorite heavy meals. One tablespoon of dried thyme added to 1 cup of very hot (but not quite boiling) water makes a good calming drink with a pleasant flavor. Add 1 teaspoon of honey for sweetness.

FLU

It doesn't take long to figure out the difference between a garden variety cold and the flu. If you have a high fever, sore throat, a cough, chills, muscle pain, and you're so weak you can't stand up in the shower — that's influenza. Here are some proven ways to help fight it off and ease your symptoms.

ECHINACEA To prevent colds and flu, some scientists suggest taking echinacea as soon as an outbreak hits your neighborhood. It can also help alleviate your symptoms if the bug has already set in. About 25 to 30 drops of the extract in 1 cup of water or tea, twice a day, is the normal dose for adults. If you don't like the taste, echinacea is also available in capsule form.

Roy Upton, an herbalist, lecturer and executive with the American Herbalist Guild, recommends augmenting the echinacea with hot lemon tea to help sweat out flu symptoms. Simply squeeze the juice of a whole lemon right into a cup. Pour in 1 cup of hot water, add about 25 drops of echinacea tincture, and drink 3 times a day.

GARLIC The ancient Egyptians listed 22 different garlic-based medicines in their pharmacies. A treatment for the flu was one of them. Today, garlic has been shown to stimulate infection-fighting T-cells.

For bacteria and viruses, raw garlic is best. An easy way to take this natural medicine is to chop it into small pieces and chase it down with a glass of water.

NASTURTIUM Nasturtium has been used for centuries by Peruvian Indians as a remedy for coughs, colds and the flu. The traditional cure is a tea made from 2 teaspoons of bruised, fresh leaves steeped in 1 cup of hot water for 10 minutes. Nasturtium leaves, which contain a natural antibiotic, have the peppery-mustard taste of watercress.

PEPPERMINT This menthol-containing plant offers relief for many cold and flu symptoms. To make a cup of plain peppermint tea, steep 1 teaspoon of dried leaves in 1 cup of hot water, covered, for 5 minutes. Aromatherapy advocates also recommend a massage with peppermint oil to help prevent colds and flu.

SHIITAKE MUSHROOMS Japanese researchers claim this fancy Japanese fungus works as well as — maybe even better than — commercially manufactured antiviral drugs. It may be the lentinen in the shiitake that helps it enhance the immune system to fight off colds and flu germs. Try them in the flu-fighting recipe below.

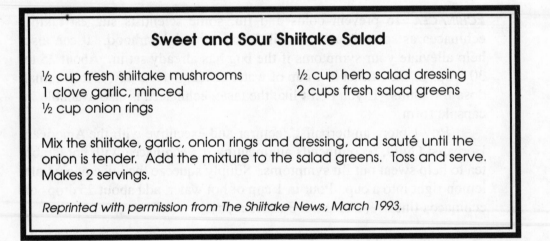

Sweet and Sour Shiitake Salad

½ cup fresh shiitake mushrooms   ½ cup herb salad dressing
1 clove garlic, minced   2 cups fresh salad greens
½ cup onion rings

Mix the shiitake, garlic, onion rings and dressing, and sauté until the onion is tender. Add the mixture to the salad greens. Toss and serve. Makes 2 servings.

Reprinted with permission from The Shiitake News, March 1993.

SORREL Eskimos eat fresh spring sorrel, which they call sour dock, to ease the digestive problems that accompany the flu. Sorrel contains about 38 milligrams of vitamin C per ½ cup of loosely packed raw leaves — about the same amount that's found in ½ an orange. Sorrel adds a lemony flavor to foods and drinks.

Helpful Hints

■ **Buy a new toothbrush.** Exposed to the air and your saliva, a toothbrush can harbor many germs — including flu viruses. To prevent reinfecting yourself, toss your toothbrush 3 days after you feel the first symptoms of flu, and replace it with a new one. (It's a good idea to replace your toothbrush every 2 to 3 months, anyway.)

■ **Drink plenty of fluids.** When congestion forces you to breathe through your mouth, the mucous membranes lining your respiratory tract lose moisture. This creates an ideal environment for a respiratory virus. So drink plenty of hot and cold fluids — at least 6 (even 8) glasses of clear liquids a day. (Avoid milk — it can add to your congestion.)

■ **Drink chicken soup.** Irwin Ziment, M.D., professor of medicine at UCLA, recommends a daily bowl of spicy chicken soup (he adds lots of garlic, onions, pepper and hot spices like curry or hot chilies to his) to prevent or fight flu bugs. Dr. Ziment notes that it's best to sip the chicken soup slowly. The therapeutic effects last about 30 minutes, so the slower the soup is ingested, the longer the results will last. (See page 189 for one chicken soup recipe.)

GALLSTONES

Gallstones are rock-like masses, usually made up of cholesterol crystals. They form in the gall bladder, which is a storage area for liver bile. Bile is used to digest fats. Researchers suspect that the female hormone estrogen is somehow linked to this condition as 75 percent of gallstone sufferers are women.

Symptoms of an afflicted gall bladder include indigestion, nausea and vomiting. In time, when gallstones begin to pass through the bile ducts, inhibiting and sometimes blocking the flow of bile between the liver and small intestine, they can cause severe abdominal pain, jaundice and infection. At this point, surgery is almost always indicated. However, even after gallstones have begun to form, it can take many years before they cause serious problems. And, in the meantime, there are several simple home remedies for relieving the discomfort.

CHAMOMILE Chamomile has a mild sedative power that can relax the stomach, which helps relieve digestive discomfort.

COMFREY The British, French and Greeks use comfrey as an all around digestive aid. They believe that comfrey tea — a good addition to every home herbal pharmacy — is especially effective for treating gallstones.

RADISHES Europeans with gall bladder ailments drink fresh radish juice (a natural antibiotic) — either plain or with a little lemon.

THISTLE Research indicates that milk thistle (also known as holy thistle and St. Mary thistle) may help stimulate regeneration of liver cells. This European remedy is believed to boost the immune system and prevent toxic injury to liver cells. There is also evidence that the milk thistle may gradually dissolve gallstones. The recommended dose of this herb is 2 capsules, 2 or 3 times a day.

GENITAL HERPES

Genital herpes (herpes simplex 2) is characterized by painful, open sores in the genital area. It is highly contagious, passed from person to person through direct intimate contact. An estimated half a million new cases are contracted each year. Condoms offer some preventive protection, however there is no cure.

Once you have been infected, stress is the primary instigator for a flare-up. This makes stress management of major importance in controlling genital herpes. (See page 468 for tips on lowering your stress level.) Acyclovir, which works internally to alleviate the symptoms and dry up the sores, is the medication prescribed most often by doctors. In addition, there are many natural ways to deal with this condition.

ICE An ice cube applied to the infected area is soothing. Wrap the cube in a thin cotton cloth before placing it on the lesions. (And be sure to wash the cloth carefully between uses.)

LYSINE The essential amino acid lysine seems to inhibit herpes outbreaks. Foods high in lysine are seafood, chicken and potatoes. You can also take lysine in capsule form.

TEA The tannic acid found in tea is a natural anesthetic. Soak a tea bag in hot (not boiling) water, wring out the excess water, and place the bag over the irritated area.

VITAMIN E In addition to being good for the immune system when taken internally, vitamin E has healing properties when applied topically.

WHEAT GERM OIL Naturalists recommend dabbing wheat germ oil directly on the affected area. Topical applications of essential oils of lemon balm, geranium or tea tree also speed healing.

WITCH HAZEL To help dry out the sores, apply witch hazel several times a day. Herbalists also recommend salves made with aloe, goldenseal and lavender.

Helpful Hints

■ The amino acid arginine has been reported to aggravate herpes outbreaks. So avoid foods that contain arginine — chocolate, nuts, seeds and coconut.

■ Eat plenty of foods high in zinc and vitamins A, B, C and E to strengthen your immune system. (See page 50 for the best food sources of these nutrients.)

■ Wear cotton underpants and loose-fitting clothing during an outbreak. The cotton will let your skin " breathe," and this will help dry up the lesions.

■ Add echinacea, calendula, goldenseal, nettle or St. John's wort to your bath water to create a soothing environment that promotes healing.

GOUT

Gout is a very painful form of arthritis that usually affects the toe joints. It is caused by an excess of uric acid, a waste product of the kidneys, which lodges as crystals in the joints of susceptible individuals. Gout can also be a secondary disease of people experiencing rapid cell degeneration, such as cancer patients.

Victims of gout are usually overweight, middle-aged men who love meat, eggs and other high uric acid foods. Alcohol consumption also seems to play a role because it interferes with the way the body metabolizes uric acid. And, because gout tends to run in families, it may have a genetic link.

Interestingly, the inhabitants of Scotland who eat meals high in carbohydrates rarely get gout, while Polynesians who eat a diet high in purines (which break down into uric acid) develop it frequently. So it's no surprise that most of the natural remedies for gout focus on nutrition. Treat yourself by eating plenty of green, yellow and red vegetables, by cutting down on fats and animal protein — and by following some of the recommendations we've collected from natural healers around the world. Also, make sure you check out the "arthritis" section on page 111 for even more information on natural anti-inflammatories that help gout as well as arthritis.

ALFALFA The leaves and seeds of this popular plant have been used for hundreds of years to ease gout pain. Drink a cup of alfalfa tea several times a day. Or, try the recipe for alfalfa sprout dressing on page 270.

ASH Throughout Europe, and especially in southern England, a tea of common ash is used to ease gout pain. Infuse 1 ounce of dried leaves in 1 quart of boiling water, dropping in a few mint leaves for extra flavor. For instructions on how to make an infusion, turn to page 82.

CELERY SEED An old German remedy for gout is to chew 1 to 3 teaspoons of celery seed powder mixed with rue, cloves and saxifrage before breakfast. To improve the taste, sprinkle the mixture on bread that has been smeared with quince jelly.

CHERRIES Cherries, which contain magnesium (a natural painkiller) and potassium, have been a Japanese treatment for joint pain for centuries. Fresh, frozen or canned cherries work equally well. They either eat them whole (6 to 8 a day), or boil them down into a delicious syrup.

DANDELION High in vitamins A and C, dandelion leaves are believed to help the body repair tissues damaged by gout. European herbalists have used the following pain-relieving recipes for years:

■ Steam or sauté the leaves, adding a touch of garlic and olive oil.

■ Steep 3 teaspoons of fresh leaves in 1 cup of boiling water to make dandelion tea.

■ Boil 4 ounces of fresh root in 2 pints of water to make a coffee-like beverage. Strain and drink.

Alfalfa Sprout Dressing

Preparation time: 20 minutes   Yields: ¾ - 1 cup

Besides using this on salads, this is great on sandwiches and used as a dip.

1 cup alfalfa sprouts	½ tsp. savory
½ cup mashed avocado	1 tsp. oregano
1 lemon (juice and pulp)	1 tsp. basil
or 3 Tbsp. lemon juice	1 tsp. thyme
¼ tsp. salt	

Blend together. This is thick and may need to be thinned with a bit of oil.

— *from* The Vegetarian Alternative, *edited by Vimala Mc Clure*

FISH Herring, salmon, mackerel, tuna and sardines are good sources of omega-3 fatty acids — substances which are believed to have strong anti-inflammatory and immune system boosting properties. A daily serving of fresh fish will help prevent gout flare-ups. Alternatively, you can supplement with fish oil capsules.

EXERCISE!

One of nature's best all-around remedies, exercise is believed to stimulate the immune system and increase its inflammation-fighting capabilities. Combining a low-fat diet with regular, moderate exercise has helped many a gout sufferers find relief.

GOLDENROD British herbalists recommend tea made from the flowering tops or leaves of European goldenrod as a remedy for joint pain. Because it is believed to stimulate elimination of waste by the kidneys, the theory is that goldenrod helps rid the body of toxins produced by the gouty inflammation.

HAIR CARE

A male lion attracts females with his lush, full mane. Samson found strength in his unshorn locks, and Rapunzel made her golden tresses into a ladder that her prince could climb to rescue her from her tower prison. But Mother Nature had other, more practical, uses in mind. Hair is meant to soften blows to the skull, protect us from the blazing heat in the summer, and trap body heat near the scalp in winter.

The average human head has about 100,000 hairs. Redheads have the fewest hairs, blondes fall somewhere in the middle, and brunettes have the greatest number of hairs. Regardless of hair color, most people lose about 75 hairs a day as part of the natural growth process.

One of the most notable things about hair is that it responds well to outside treatments to keep it clean, soft or colored. Yet it responds even better to inside help from good nutrition. Here, then, are some natural hair care tips to help you keep your hair full and healthy-looking.

■ Use a brush with natural bristles made from keratin. Natural bristles are much softer and rounder than nylon bristles, reducing the possibility that you'll damage your hair while brushing.

■ Give your hair added fullness by bending at the waist and brushing while your hair hangs down.

■ Brush just before shampooing. This helps loosen dirt and dust particles, making your shampoo more effective.

■ Ignore the 100-strokes-a-day myth. More than 20 strokes a day can damage your hair and roots by creating too much friction.

- If you use a blow-dryer, section your hair and dry the lower layers first to add volume. Start at the top of each section.

- During every shampoo, massage your scalp thoroughly with your fingertips.

- Buy only shampoo that is pH-balanced. Avoid any shampoo that contains wax.

- Add kelp to your diet. Popular in Scottish diets, kelp is said to make your hair richer and more full-bodied. The minerals found

Curiosity Box

The Egyptians invented one of the earliest shampoos. They used a mixture of water and citrus juice, and — to get hair truly clean — they added bits of soap and perfume. Although they did not have the technology to study individual strands of hair, the Egyptians stumbled upon two important principles with this combination:

- *Alkaline solutions (most soaps and shampoos) open up the imbrications on hair strands and bind chemically with dirt particles. Soap solutions also bind with water particles and literally pull dirt out of hair during rinsing.*

- *Acidic solutions, (such as lemon juice, vinegar and beer), close imbrications — by sealing in moisture and sealing out dirt. With mild, careful use of acidic solutions, you can increase your hair's fullness and avoid tangles.*

The Egyptian recipe was, indeed, effective, and many of today's commercially prepared shampoos sell the same or similar ingredients — at prices that would have made an Egyptian's hair stand on end.

in kelp, particularly iodine, are also important for hair growth. Members of the kelp family include hijiki, wakame and arame.

Other diet aids to healthy hair include buckwheat and barley, (both high in choline and inositol), brewer's yeast, molasses, rice polishings, liver and yogurt.

■ To add protein to your hair, make a solution of unflavored gelatin and water and massage it into your scalp. Rinse after 5 minutes. Gelatin, which is high in amino acids, strengthens hair and nails.

COLOR

Just about everyone eventually looks in the mirror and sees gray. Friends and relatives comment on how "dignified" you look — and you begin to think about dying your hair.

Or, maybe you want to change your look or just brighten your hair with highlights. Whatever your motive, you should know that there are alternatives to harsh chemicals and lengthy, unpredictable commercial processes.

Dye works best after the hair has been washed, and before it has been rinsed (and sealed) with an acidic conditioner. The most popular natural acidic rinses are beer for brunettes, vinegar for redheads, and lemon juice for blondes. Or, try the following:

■ **For blondes:** Chamomile is recognized by a fragrant aroma that's reminiscent of ripe apples. In fact, the name "chamomile" comes from the Greek word for ground apple. Chamomile is used in perfumes, tobaccos, teas, flavored liqueurs and shampoos. It is particularly effective in shampoos because it has a cleansing and conditioning effect.

Chamomile rinses are easy to find in natural product stores. But if you're interested in making your own, boil a handful of petals in one quart of water. For extra shine, add some marigold petals. Let the solution cool, and then pour it over your hair. This works especially well to renew the brilliant color of blonde hair.

■ **For redheads:** The henna plant, native to northern Africa and southern Asia, is most commonly used today as a hair dye. Commercial products with henna are easily found in drug stores and natural product stores. But to make your own rinse, boil the leaves, fruit and flower petals of the henna plant in water. To bring out red highlights, add red wine to the water. Let the mixture cool and then pour it over your washed, wet hair. Rinse with a mildly acidic solution like vinegar, lemon juice or beer — and then rinse again with clear water.

■ **For brunettes:** Latin Americans have found that strong black coffee is not only good to drink, but also makes an excellent hair dye. To try this beauty secret yourself, shampoo your hair. Then pour cold coffee over your wet hair. Wait 20 minutes, rinse out the coffee with beer, vinegar or lemon juice to seal in the color — then rinse your hair with clear water.

A chamomile rinse, as noted above, is used to bring out natural blonde highlights. But to add beautiful highlights to dark hair, an infusion of chamomile combined with neutral henna works well.

Another way to add shine and color to dark hair is with a rinse of boiled black walnut shells. Make sure you pick up black walnuts — ordinary walnuts are bleached. Boil them for an hour, then cool before using.

CONDITIONERS

Every strand of hair has a cuticle — the same translucent, scaly, outer coating found on fingernails. Oil provided by the scalp, combined with the sealing action of these scales, maintains the moisture level in each strand of hair. (Healthy hair contains about 10 percent water.)

Some people shampoo their hair daily, while others go a week between washings. Neither practice is harmful to your hair, but — whether your hair is oily or dry — you should absolutely condition it if you wash every day. Below are some natural ways to do it.

■ Bananas, strawberries, papaya and avocado all contain

conditioning agents. And they smell good, too! To make your own fruit conditioner, blend one of these fruits with chamomile tea. Apply to wet clean hair, let it sit for 10 minutes, and then rinse thoroughly.

■ To increase your hair's softness, try a rinse made from rosemary. Combine ⅓ cup of fresh rosemary with 2 cups of boiling water. Let steep, covered, until cool, and then strain. Wash your hair with your regular shampoo, rinse it with water, and then rinse again with the rosemary tea.

■ If you have dry, brittle hair, shop for a conditioner that uses one or more of the following herbs: burdock, comfrey, marshmallow, nettle or sage.

■ A remedy for dry, damaged hair that can be done at home once a month calls for either almond, coconut, olive or castor oil. Rub the oil into your scalp and let it soak for at least an hour or two before you wash it out. Another version of this treatment calls for a combination of ½ cup of warm vegetable oil and a teaspoon of cider vinegar. Massage the mixture into your scalp and cover with a plastic shower cap for 1 to 2 hours. If possible, apply heat. (For example, sit under a dryer or wrap your head with a hot towel.) Then wash your hair two or three times.

■ Triggers of oily hair include a high-fat diet, a hormonal imbalance, thyroid problems, stress and fatigue. Herbs that help combat oily hair are lemon balm, yarrow, rosemary or witch hazel. You can purchase shampoos containing these herbs — or make your own infusions. (Turn to page 82 for instructions on how to make an herbal infusion.)

■ You can also add a little sea salt to your shampoo to help cut down on oily hair.

HANGOVER

A hangover is the price too often paid for a night of wanton revelry. Nausea, headache and the infamous "cotton mouth" are the unpleasant hallmarks of a full-blown hangover.

Because alcohol is a diuretic, dehydration — a loss of body water through excessive urination and perspiration — is the main cause of the discomfort. This disturbance in the balance of body fluids also contributes to headaches and nausea, and the excessive urination leads to a loss of many minerals, which further promotes headache. That's why most experts recommend that you drink water — lots of water — before, during and after you imbibe. And if you eat while you drink (especially if you follow the example of the French and Italians and eat starchy foods like breads and pastas), you will slow the absorption of alcohol into your bloodstream. This will allow your body to break down the alcohol at a more reasonable pace.

Of course, the best way to avoid a hangover is to drink in moderation — or not at all. But just in case, keep the following international hangover remedies in mind.

ALFALFA SEEDS Hangover sufferers in Mexico treat their headaches with alfalfa seed tea. They steep a teaspoon of alfalfa seed and a teaspoon of dried orange leaf in a cup of boiling water for 5 minutes — then strain and sip.

BANANA The liquid from a boiled banana peel is a traditional Chinese remedy for a hangover. According to the Chinese, this seems to have a detoxifying effect on the body. And the fruit itself — along with other bland foods like rice, soft-boiled eggs, applesauce and toast — is easy on your system during a hangover and helps replenish lost nutrients.

CAYENNE PEPPER For centuries, herbalists have considered cayenne pepper to be soothing and restorative for the digestive system. Try it yourself by sprinkling a small amount of the pepper into water to make a gargle that will stimulate the production of saliva and other gastric juices to ease hangover-induced stomach troubles.

A Sobering Thought

Though many people think they can offset the immediate effects of too much alcohol with a sobering cup of black coffee and a hot shower, it really doesn't work. At best, this may help "the morning after" by relieving the fatigue and muscle aches that accompany a hangover, but it doesn't decrease the alcohol level in the blood.

KUDZU ROOT A Chinese tea to relieve the symptoms of a hangover is made from equal parts of kudzu root, umeboshi plum and fresh gingerroot. The root of the kudzu vine has been used to treat alcohol abuse for more than 1,300 years. (It reportedly curbs the desire for alcohol.) And all of these ingredients have an antispasmodic effect on the stomach muscles and are helpful in relieving nausea.

ORANGE JUICE Orange juice is an oft-recommended treatment to combat the dizziness and weakness that go along with a hangover. (In China, they prefer fresh tangerine juice.)

4 Good Old-Fashioned Folk Remedies

These 18th and 19th century remedies come from Jon-Erik Svensson's book, Folk Remedies, Recipes, and Advice. Try them all, one right after the other:

■ Suck on a sugar cube drizzled with a few drops of clove oil (which is a painkiller).
■ Chew on a sprig of parsley (to calm your stomach).
■ Drink a cup of lukewarm chamomile tea sweetened with honey (another way to calm your stomach).
■ Take a teaspoon or two of plain honey, and another every half hour for two to three hours.

SPINACH Spinach tea is a popular Oriental remedy for hangovers. To make it, simmer large quantities of spinach, including the roots and the heads, over low heat for 2 to 3 hours. Then drink the liquid. (Spinach contains many of the minerals that are washed out by the alcohol-induced loss of fluids.)

STRAWBERRIES In China, eating fresh strawberries — 8 to 10 throughout the day — is believed to be an effective treatment for hangovers. It probably works because this fruit has such a high mineral content.

HEADACHE

Every year, in the United States, headaches account for:
- 20 million visits to the doctor
- 156 million missed workdays
- Close to $400 million spent on over-the-counter pain-relievers

This common malady can be caused by a wide variety of factors, but is most commonly the result of tension in the head and neck muscles that produces a dull ache. A much more painful and debilitating type of headache, the migraine, is caused by dilation of the blood vessels. (See specific remedies for migraines on pages 367-370.)

Today, over-the-counter painkillers like aspirin, ibuprofen, acetaminophen, and naproxen sodium are the most widely used headache treatments. But, every culture has developed its own ways of dealing with them, and, as a result, there are many natural remedies. Here are some of the best.

ALFALFA SEED In Mexico, headache sufferers ease the pain with alfalfa seed tea.

BIRCH BARK The bark of birch trees is commonly used as a pain-reliever by American Indians. And despite the fact that aspirin is inexpensive and readily available, people in rural parts of Europe and the United States still chew the salicylate-rich bark of the willow and black poplar trees to cure their headaches.

CHINESE ANGELICA A Chinese version of angelica called dong quai is used by herbalists to relieve pounding in the head. Make a medicinal tea by boiling one large slice of dried dong quai root in 2 cups of water, uncovered, for about 10 minutes. Remove the root (save it — you can use it again) and then sip the liquid.

CHRYSANTHEMUM TEA In India and China, tension headaches are soothed by drinking a tea made with dried yellow chrysanthemum. Prepackaged tea bags are available in most health food stores.

COPPER Some researchers believe that a low-copper diet may cause headaches in susceptible people. The theory is that a copper deficiency makes the blood vessel walls constrict — and cause pain. Good food sources of copper include oysters, lobster, liver, nuts, seeds, green olives and wheat bran.

COWSLIP Cowslip, which grows wild in nearly all pastures and meadows, has been praised in the writings of William Shakespeare and Ben Jonson. This gentle pain reliever (a good source of natural aspirin) is common throughout Europe, Siberia, western Asia and North Africa. A tea made of cowslip petals, honey, sugar and lemon juice is a tasty treatment for headaches. Cowslip can be bought in cut or powdered form through most mail-order herb companies and health food stores. The seeds and live plants are also commercially available.

GINGER Ginger tea is used in parts of Africa to treat headaches. You can make it by grating and squeezing gingerroot to extract the juice. Then add about a teaspoon of the juice to a cup of hot water.

Pressure Points

In Asia, healers treat headaches with acupuncture — and self-healers have learned how to treat themselves by applying pressure in very precise ways. For example:

■ In Korea, they tie a kerchief or bandanna tightly around the head, just above the eyebrows. This may work by restricting blood flow and preventing dilation of blood vessels in the scalp that are responsible for some headaches.

■ In China, they massage a spot on the brow bone. Try this yourself by locating the small depression that's just above the pupil of your eye. Then press with your fingertips, rotating clockwise for 30 seconds.

Though we talk about relaxation techniques, in detail, on pages — through — of this book, the following deserve special mention here because they are especially effective for counteracting headache pain.

■ This Lamaze technique that is taught to expectant moms to help them get through the pain of labor and delivery can help you tune out headaches, too: Drop your head so that your chin is on your chest. Slowly turn your head, leading with your chin, to the right and then to the left. Tighten your muscles from the shoulders on up, hold for 15 seconds, then relax.

■ If you tend to get stress-related headaches, try "visualization" to take a short, mental vacation. Whenever you feel the tension start to build, close your eyes and picture a tranquil scene or recall a very pleasant experience. If that image has soothing music associated with it, keep a tape of it handy to trigger an immediate relaxation response.

■ This breathing exercise is not only used to relieve headaches, but is also reported to relieve eyestrain, and neck and shoulder tension — and improve vision: Let your head drop forward and inhale through your nose. Hold that breath as you count to 10. Exhale, open your eyes, and blink quickly 10 times. Move your eyes in a circle — first clockwise, and then counter-clockwise. Then move your eyes diagonally, and up and down, 10 times each. Slowly move your head toward your right shoulder, and then toward your left shoulder. Then rub your hands together quickly, close your eyes, and cover them with your palms. Breathe five very slow breaths, and picture yourself being filled with renewed energy.

■ Since ancient times, the Chinese have used "li shou," or hand swinging, to treat headaches by achieving a relaxing meditative state similar to that brought on in higher forms of yoga. "li shou" supposedly works by reducing the blood pressure and swelling of blood vessels in the head. Here's how they do it: They swing their arms back and forth until blood is shifted from their pounding head to their hands. Once the blood has shifted to the hands, they give off warmth, and are then used to stroke the face gently in a highly stylized pattern of circular massage at points around the eyes.

HONEY Honey, which has natural pain-relieving powers, is a traditional Chinese remedy for headache. Eat the honey straight out of the jar, or mix three large spoonfuls in boiled water and drink. The Chinese also raid the kitchen for fresh radishes, buckthorn berries, licorice, cinnamon, mint leaves, orange peels and gingerroot to ease their throbbing heads.

CAUTION: *Honey is not recommended for people with low or high blood sugar.*

LEMON BALM Europeans use fragrant lemon balm (also known as Mediterranean melissa) to reduce headache tension. One way to do it is to rub a leaf between your fingers and then rub your temples or forehead.

MINT The Chinese and Vietnamese have long used peppermint and spearmint to treat nervousness, which often causes headaches. Since spearmint is an antispasmodic and diuretic, it is also good for headaches related to menstrual problems.

The Chinese make a tea by boiling equal weights of peppermint and crushed scallion heads in water. The Vietnamese opt for straight spearmint tea, or a spearmint soup made by cooking tender, fresh spearmint leaves in water with eggs to make a type of egg-drop soup.

MARJORAM A marjoram massage is recommended by many aromatherapists for headache pain. Add about 10 drops of essential oil of marjoram to a half a cup of skin oil to make your own mix.

ROSEMARY To relieve the dull throb of a stress headache, aromatherapists

Curiosity Box

Stone Age "healers" about 25,000 years ago used flint tools to bore into and remove sections of the skull to alleviate headaches. This earliest form of surgery was called trepanning, and the neurosurgical tools used were called trephines. The practice was continued as recently as 1,000 years ago in the South American Inca civilization.

recommend a massage with the essential oil of rosemary. Herbalists prefer to use the fresh herb as a tea. Rosemary contains soothing rosmaricine, which is non-irritating to the stomach.

VINEGAR The British soak compresses with vinegar, chill them, and apply them to the forehead, temples and neck. You can also ease headache pain by boiling equal parts of vinegar and water and inhaling the rising steam.

VIOLET PETALS The ancient Romans and Greeks used sweet and spicy violet petals to get rid of headaches. They ate the fresh petals, brewed them into a tea, or soaked them in a glass of wine. Violet petal tea is available in health food stores.

YERBA MATE A South American remedy is soothing Paraguayan tea, which is made by steeping the finely ground leaves of the yerba mate plant in hot water. Drink one cup early in the day, hot or cold, plain or sweetened, with or without lemon or milk.

Helpful Hints

Next time you have a headache, try applying a heat pack to the back of your neck — or a cold pack to your forehead. Most people find relief by using one or the other. And many swear by hot, ankle-deep foot baths — for headaches as well as head congestion.

HEAD LICE

Head lice are extremely contagious parasites that spread quickly (most commonly among schoolchildren) and so must be treated immediately. These nasty little creatures attach themselves to strands of hair and get their nourishment by sucking blood. One female louse can attach thousands of eggs, called nits, to hair follicles during its 30-day lifespan. The itching can be extremely irritating, and scratching can lead to infection once the skin is broken.

If your child comes home from school with head lice, try one (or more) of the safe, alternative treatments listed below. At the same time, thoroughly clean all of the clothes, sheets, towels and blankets with which he or she has come into contact. Laundering in hot water or dry cleaning will do the trick. If your child has a favorite stuffed animal, wash that as well. ("Teddy" will keep his nice, fluffy coat if you put him in a pillow case and tie it shut before running through your washer and dryer.)

CINNAMON BARK OIL Cinnamon bark oil is reported to be an effective lice killer.
CAUTION: *Cinnamon bark oil is very strong and should only be used by a competent aromatherapist.*

LAVENDER OIL Herbalists recommend a solution of lavender oil and alcohol for fighting lice. To try it, mix 10 drops of lavender oil in a small tumbler of vodka. Rub this mixture into the scalp at night, and wash it out in the morning. Then comb out the hair with a head lice comb. Repeat as necessary.

OREGANO Spicy oregano oil is a powerful bacteria killer. Europeans use it as a scalp massage to rid hair of lice.

TEA TREE OIL Native Australians have been using tea tree oil for centuries for a host of skin problems. Research has proven it to be effective against lice as well. To try this remedy, massage the scalp with the oil and then shampoo.

THYME A tincture of 4 ounces of thyme, or the essential oil of thyme, can be mixed with a pint of alcohol and applied to the scalp to fight lice. Thyme is considered to be antiseptic and antibacterial.

WARNING: Lindane, a drug in commonly prescribed lice shampoos, has been suspected as being linked to childhood cancer, brain damage and fatal blood diseases, according to the Cancer Prevention Coalition — an excellent reason to first try some of the natural alternatives we offer.

For information on where to purchase any of the items listed, turn to the glossary beginning on page 523.

HEARTBURN

Heartburn has nothing to do with your heart. It gets its name from the location of the burning sensation associated with this ailment — anywhere from the middle of the chest to the back of the throat. You get heartburn when small amounts of stomach acid leak into your esophagus — usually because you ate too much, you ate too fast or the food you ate was too spicy or too greasy.

While usually not serious, heartburn can cause great discomfort. Sometimes the symptoms mimic those of a heart attack. As a result, many a person has left an emergency room embarrassed — but relieved.

Over-the-counter remedies can provide quick relief, but can't be used over an extended period of time because they contribute to chronic discomfort by encouraging an overproduction of stomach acid. Instead, try these natural tips from around the world to help put out the fire.

AGRIMONY In France, agrimony is used as a general tonic for the digestive tract. To make agrimony tea, infuse 5 teaspoons of dried leaves and flowers in a cup of boiling water for 20 minutes. Use a little honey for flavoring.

ANGELICA The European angelica plant yields an oil that is used to treat heartburn. A palatable way of using angelica oil is to boil it in water and drink the resulting syrup.

BLACKBERRY LEAF The high mineral and vitamin C content of the blackberry leaf is probably the reason it is effective when used as a remedy for digestive problems (and as a general tonic) in Great Britain.

CAYENNE PEPPER West Indians prevent stomach trouble with "mandram," a blend of cayenne pepper, thinly sliced cucumbers, shallots, chives or onions, lemon or lime juice, and Madeira wine. Cayenne pepper aids digestion by stimulating the production of saliva and gastric juices.

CHAMOMILE The French prefer chamomile tea as a digestive aid. The herb has antispasmodic properties that make it a soothing treatment.

FIGS Centuries ago, the Romans and Egyptians ate figs to treat a wide range of health problems. And modern research has isolated enzymes (called ficins) in this fruit that have been proven to help digestion.

GINGER Ginger has many uses, but is especially good for digestive disturbances. Chinese herbalists brew a variety of teas with ginger, cloves and ginseng that are believed to have beneficial effects on the digestive system. Here's one traditional recipe: mix 2 grams of cloves, 3 grams of persimmon calyx (available in most Chinese herb shops), 3 grams of ginseng, and 2 grams of dried ginger — then steep in boiling water.

Tea For Stomach Irritation

Heartburn and gastritis (inflammation of the gastric mucosa,) both of which are caused by excess stomach acid, are almost always chronically recurring disorders. Three to five cups of this tea daily will bring gradual but effective relief. It is best to space out the drinking of this tea over the whole day.

8 tsp. angelica root
4 tsp. chamomile flowers
4 tsp. balm leaves
4 tsp. peppermint leaves
2 tsp. caraway seed
2 tsp. fennel seed
1 tsp. wormwood

Reprinted from THE FAMILY HERBAL *by Barbara and Peter Theiss, published by Healing Arts Press, an imprint of Inner Traditions International, Rochester, VT.*

HONEY The Bible and the Koran both mention honey as a digestive aid, and this ancient treatment is still commonly used in both Europe and Asia to prevent heartburn. Honey is especially popular in China, Egypt and India — either added to tea or taken by the spoonful.

LEMON BALM Lemon balm has been used by folk healers for hundreds of years to calm the stomach. The herb contains eugenol which is an antispasmodic, and is most effective for indigestion when taken as a tea.

LICORICE The Greeks have traditionally used licorice and anise seed as effective remedies for many symptoms related to heartburn and indigestion.

Greek wedding guests cap off the festivities by eating anise-flavored cake to counteract the ill effects of overindulging at the reception. And, in fact, it was this Greek practice that established the international tradition of serving wedding cake. Anise is also the flavoring in the popular tummy-soothing Greek apertifs sambuca and ouzo.

KELP In the Orient, people include kelp in their diets to prevent heartburn. Kelp contains alginic acid, which is soothing and aids digestion.

MARJORAM A heartburn remedy popular with the British is to eat a sandwich made by putting a few fresh marjoram leaves between 2 slices of buttered country bread.

MUSTARD The subtle flavor of French mustard enhances a variety of gourmet recipes. However, there is more to this classy condiment than good taste. The French, who often eat very rich foods, rely on mustard to relieve heartburn. And, to avoid heartburn, herbalists recommend cooking gas-forming foods such as broccoli and cabbage with mustard seed.

Mustard and whole mustard seeds sharpen the appetite and stimulate the secretion of digestive juices in the small intestine, speeding up the digestive process. Mustard also stimulates gastric mucous membrane and pancreatic secretions. As a result, the stomach is emptied faster, and the production of excess acid is reduced.

OLIVE OIL A favorite cooking ingredient that Italians credit with preventing heartburn is olive oil, which they say is soothing to the stomach.

PAPAYA Residents of the Caribbean Islands often eat papaya for dessert after heavy meals because papaya prevents indigestion (especially after eating meat or fish).

PEPPERMINT The use of mint as a treatment for indigestion was first discovered by the Egyptians, who cultivated peppermint plants. Peppermint is also used by the people of Iceland. And the Irish put two mint leaves in a steaming cup of tea to make a relaxing and effective remedy.

ROSEMARY Rosemary, another type of mint, was once burned in French hospitals to cover up the stench of disease. However, it was first used as a remedy for digestive disorders by the Hungarians. They distilled medicinal water with rosemary leaves and gave it to their patients. Today, to treat stress-related heartburn and other digestive disorders, aromatherapists recommend a rosemary-oil massage (using about 10 drops of essential oil of rosemary to a half cup of skin oil).

THYME Wealthy Romans drank thyme as an infusion after overindulging in heavy meals. And, indeed, one tablespoon of dried thyme added to a cup of very hot (but not quite boiling) water, makes a good calming drink with a pleasant flavor. Add a teaspoon of honey for flavor.

YOGURT Plain, unprocessed yogurt is a common ingredient in Middle Eastern cuisine that is also used in that area of the world to treat indigestion. Yogurt contains the bacteria acidophilus, which prevents the growth of the harmful bacteria that cause stomach and intestinal illness. Eating yogurt (made with live acidophilus cultures) once or twice a week keeps the flora (the "good" bacteria that help us digest our food) in the intestines healthy.

HEART DISEASE

   Heart disease is the long-reigning killer king in the United States, claiming an estimated 500,000 lives each year. More than 6 million people in this country have some form of heart disease — and an estimated million and a half suffer heart attacks each year. One reason heart disease is blamed for so many deaths is because the term is so broadly applied. Technically, it is only one of many ailments included under the much broader heading of cardiovascular disease ("cardiovascular" referring not only to the heart, but also to the entire circulatory system).

   It's important to understand that heart disease does not develop overnight. It takes decades to get to the point where you're in serious trouble. The problem begins with atherosclerosis, the medical name given to hardening and clogging of the coronary arteries. Substances in the blood (cholesterol and fats) build up on the artery walls. The build-up (called plaque) keeps growing, narrowing the inside of the arteries. This reduces the amount of blood (and, therefore, oxygen) that can get through to your heart. Your heart warns you that it's starving for oxygen if you experience pain when you exert yourself (a condition known as angina pectoris).   And if the coronary artery becomes totally blocked (usually by a blood clot that does not allow blood to make it through the narrowed opening), completely shutting off the blood supply to the heart muscle — that's a heart attack.

   While it's true that you can't do anything to alter a family history of heart disease or change your sex (statistically, men get heart disease at a younger age than women), those are the only things you have no control over when it comes to protecting yourself from this major killer. The fact is, your lifestyle is the most important factor related to your risk of developing heart disease — and lifestyle is something you can control with the diet, exercise and stress-reduction tips we've put together for you.

BARLEY One of the reasons heart disease rates are low in the Middle East could be the high consumption of barley (in cereal and as flour, grits or flakes) in these countries. In Pakistan, barley is even referred to as "medicine for the heart." And it really is. Besides being a soluble fiber, barley also contains a heart-healthy substance called tocotrienol.

BLACKSTRAP MOLASSES The British use blackstrap molasses as a preventive remedy for heart disease and strokes. Since molasses is a good source of iron (which holds the oxygen in red blood cells) — and we know that an iron deficiency can cause heart problems — try adding some blackstrap molasses to your oatmeal or tea.

CALCIUM AND MAGNESIUM The essential minerals calcium and magnesium are found naturally in such foods as beans, tofu, yogurt and leafy green vegetables. It's been reported that a daily supplement of 1,500 to 2,000 mgs of calcium and 750 to 1,000 mgs of magnesium after meals and at bedtime can benefit the heart and blood.

Dietary Fat: What's In a Name?

Are you confused by the different types of dietary fat that you hear and read about? Here's a fat primer that should clear things up for you:

■ **Mono-unsaturated:** This is the healthiest type of fat you can eat. Good food sources of mono-unsaturated fat are olive and canola oils.

■ **Poly-unsaturated:** This type of fat (which is found in safflower, sunflower and corn oils) is worse than mono-unsaturated fat, but not as bad as saturated fat.

■ **Saturated:** This is the worst type of fat — the type of fat that researchers have linked to an increased risk of heart disease. That's because saturated fat (which is found in animal products like butter and lard) is more difficult for the liver to process and keep out of the arteries.

You can judge how saturated a fat is by looking at it. The harder it is at room temperature, the more saturated it is.

COENZYME Q10 The Japanese use the supplement coenzyme Q10 to treat heart disease and high blood pressure. This nutrient is found naturally in mackerel, salmon and sardines.

FISH Studies have shown that people have less heart disease in countries where the normal diet is high in seafood. A recent Dutch study found that eating just one ounce of fish a day, or two to three servings a week, can decrease the risk of heart disease by 50 percent.

The omega-3 fatty acids in fish oil reduce blood vessel constriction, prevent blood clots, and raise good HDL cholesterol. And the best sources of omega-3 fatty acids are mackerel, anchovies, herring, salmon, sardines, lake trout, Atlantic sturgeon and tuna.

FLAXSEED OIL Aside from eating fish, you can get more essential fatty acids in your diet by using flaxseed oil as a substitute for butter. Flax is a phytoestrogen (a plant with estrogen-like qualities) that has been shown to protect against heart disease as well as certain kinds of cancer. Flaxseed oil can be found in the refrigerated section of your health food store.

GARLIC In countries where garlic is part of the daily diet, people have less heart disease. Dr. Arun Bordia, a pioneering garlic researcher in

---

EXERCISE!

Research has shown that regular, moderate exercise really can lower your risk of heart disease. In one study of over 70,000 women, those who were most active had about a 40 percent lower risk of heart attack and stroke than those who were least active. In addition, even modest activity produced significant drops in risk.

In another study, researchers found that physical activity reduces the risk of heart attack in postmenopausal women by as much as 60 percent. And in yet another study, men who reported any leisure-time physical activity at all had a 21 percent lower risk of death from heart disease than did sedentary men.

India, suggests pressing garlic and adding the juice to milk, or eating it boiled (or raw, if you can handle it).

GINGER Some research has shown that ginger, a common ingredient in many Jamaican dishes, may be especially effective in the prevention of strokes and hardening of the arteries.

GINSENG The Chinese use ginseng in hot tea as a heart tonic, and claim it benefits the heart in several significant ways. The most active chemical components in ginseng, the saponins, reduce hardening of the arteries. Ginseng can also protect against injury to the heart due to oxygen deprivation, a condition which can lead to a heart attack.

HAWTHORNE BERRIES The flavonoids in hawthorne berries dilate the coronary arteries, and apparently have a strengthening effect on the heart. Hawthorn berry tea, like most natural remedies, is absolutely safe and

---

The Importance of Diet

There is a great deal of scientific data backing up the idea that paying attention to what you eat is the best thing you can do for your heart. For example, researchers in Italy found that women who eat carrots, fresh fruit, green vegetables and fish have a lower risk of heart attack than women who regularly eat fatty foods. And we know that the Japanese have the lowest rate of heart disease in the world. That is, as long as they eat traditional Japanese food — a diet that typically includes four to five cups of rice, five to eight ounces of fruit, about nine ounces of vegetables, two ounces of beans, two ounces of meat, three to four ounces of fish, a half cup of milk, one egg or less, two teaspoons of sugar, and 1½ teaspoons of soy sauce per day.

One way to prevent the development of hardening of the arteries (arteriosclerosis) is to stop eating meat. By doing so, you eliminate dangerous animal fats from your diet. Then, of course, you'll need to find alternate sources of protein — and many researchers recommend nuts. Nuts are rich in protein and minerals (both good for your heart) as well as fiber and mono-unsaturated fats, and antioxidants that help guard against cholesterol.

can be taken as frequently as desired. Hawthorne berries can be ordered by mail order or the tea can be purchased at health food stores.

L-CARNITINE The amino acid L-Carnitine is reported to lower fat and triglyceride levels. And it's been suggested that its effectiveness can be increased by combining it with vitamins B6 and C. Natural food sources of L-Carnitine are fresh vegetables such as broccoli.

LECITHIN Lecithin is essential to transforming fats in the body — and a lecithin deficiency can lead to high cholesterol, heart disease, kidney and liver disorders. The best food sources of lecithin are brewer's yeast, grains, legumes, fish and wheat germ.

NUTS Dr. Gary Fraser, professor of medicine at Loma Linda University in California advises you to add nuts, especially Brazil nuts, to your daily diet to help protect your heart. Dr. Fraser's research showed that the risk of heart attack decreased by approximately 50 percent in people who ate an ounce or two of these nuts 5 times a week. And related research in the Orient indicates that the fats in walnuts and almonds are healthier than those found in animal products.

OLIVE OIL Olive oil (which is high in mono-unsaturated fat) is a major ingredient in the diets of Italians and Greeks — and these oil lovers have heart disease rates that are among the world's lowest. The best type of olive oil for the heart is extra virgin olive oil, which is extracted by lightly crushing and pressing the olives.

ONION The ancient Egyptians believed that onions purified the blood and were good for the heart. Onions were prescribed by early American doctors for the same reason. Research in England has shown that the common onion has benefits similar to garlic. They help dissolve blood clots, which are a frequent cause of heart attacks and strokes.

RED WINE The French and Italians eat many rich, heavy foods that should indicate a high rate of heart disease. Instead, it is far less than that of Americans. Studies have suggested that the difference might have something to do with their liberal use of red wine, grape juice and olive oil. Researchers found that people who consume all three of these foods had lower rates of heart disease than those who didn't.

_____ **TEA** In a Dutch study, men who drank 2 cups of tea a day had a rate of heart disease a third lower than men who drank less tea.

The Importance of Stress Reduction

Many major studies have examined the negative effects of stress — and the positive effects of various stress reduction techniques — on blood pressure, irregular heartbeat and angina. One study, for example, followed a group of 2,000 people who meditated. They had a heart disease rate of 87 percent less than those who didn't meditate, and saw doctors and needed hospitalization half as often.

In fact, any stress management technique will lower your risk of developing heart disease — whether you choose meditation, yoga, biofeedback, visualization or self-hypnosis. (See pages 73-80 for detailed information on the many benefits of stress reduction.)

HEMORRHOIDS

Hemorrhoids (or "piles") are veins in the anal area which become swollen or varicose — usually as the result of excessive or habitual straining during bowel movements. They can form internally or externally, and are characterized by pain, itching and burning. Though most often caused by chronic constipation, pregnancy sometimes causes temporary problems (especially in the last three months, or for a few days or weeks after delivery).

Hemmorhoids are very common among Americans, but rare in countries like Asia, Africa and parts of Europe where diets include more fiber. Commercial remedies usually contain an anesthetic, which reduces the pain but does not get rid of the condition. However, hemorrhoids (if detected early enough) can be treated effectively without resorting to over-the-counter preparations.

BANANA A Chinese remedy for hemorrhoids is to steam two half-ripe bananas with their peels until very soft, and eat them twice a day — first thing in the morning on an empty stomach, and before bedtime. Bananas are a good source of soluble fiber.

FIGS A traditional Chinese remedy for hemorrhoids is to boil fig leaves in water and either apply or sit in the liquid. (Eating 1 or 2 fresh, unripe figs on an empty stomach first thing in the morning also works.)
CAUTION: *While using this treatment, do not eat pungent or hot foods.*

ONION An Old English remedy is to apply raw, bruised onion to inflamed hemorrhoids.
CAUTION: *If your hemorrhoids have been bleeding, and the tissue is sore, wait until the tissue heals before trying this.*

PILEWORT One of the earliest spring flowers to bloom in Europe, western Asia and North Africa is the pilewort. And for hemorrhoid sufferers, the pileworts don't come a moment too soon. Pilewort tea is a fast-acting remedy for hemorrhoids, but because the tea is unpleasantly acrid, you might prefer to make the pilewort into an ointment and use it externally.

PSYLLIUM This seed is rich in soluble fiber, and taken daily can reduce hemorrhoids by decreasing intro-rectal pressure.

WITCH HAZEL Sitting in warm water can help shrink swollen veins. But before you climb into the tub, soak cotton balls with witch hazel (a natural astringent) and put them in the refrigerator. After your bath, apply the chilled witch hazel to help your blood vessels contract.

HICCUPS

We get hiccups when (for reasons unknown to science — though theories abound) the nerves of the diaphragm and glottis (the slit-like opening between your vocal cords) are abnormally stimulated. Though there are no medical cures for this annoying (but certainly not life-threatening) condition, there are probably as many folk cures as there are families on the planet. Most seem to work because they either increase the level of carbon dioxide in the blood, or because they shut off the nerve impulses. Here are some of our favorites.

GINGER Chinese advice is to slowly chew slices of juicy fresh ginger, swallowing the juice as it accumulates in your mouth. (You might also want to try a mixture of ginger juice and honey.) And a traditional Chinese recipe for hiccup-fighting tea mixes 2 grams of dried ginger with 2 grams of cloves, 3 grams of persimmon calyx (available in most Chinese herb shops), and 3 grams of ginseng. These ingredients — all of which have a soothing effect on the digestive system — are boiled together and sipped.

MUSTARD SEEDS Mustard and whole mustard seeds stimulate the secretion of digestive juices in the small intestine, speeding up the digestive process. As an added, related benefit, mustard seeds are a good remedy for hiccups.

PEANUT BUTTER Put a heaping teaspoon of peanut butter in your mouth. By the time you've managed to swallow the whole thing, your hiccups will be gone.

PEPPERMINT Peppermint tea contains a high proportion of menthol, and is said to be a good hiccup remedy.

RICE WINE VINEGAR The Chinese recommend mixing rice wine vinegar with water as a hiccup remedy. The liquid should be sipped.

SALT Another remedy from China is to lick salt. Let it dissolve in your mouth, and then swallow slowly.

SUGAR British believe in sugar as a remedy for hiccups. They put a half teaspoon of sugar on the tongue and let it dissolve.

Hold Your Breath!

When you get hiccups, probably the first thing you do to try to stop them is take a deep breath and hold it as long as you possibly can. Or maybe you breathe into a paper bag. You know that these methods work (sometimes) — but you may not know that they date back to the earliest days of our country. Both Native Americans and American pioneers treated their hiccups in this way. The scientific explanation seems to be that both methods send a message to your brain that it needs more air. The brain then tells the diaphragm to deepen its contractions, and that (theoretically) breaks the pattern of shallow hiccups.

HIGH BLOOD PRESSURE

Blood pressure is controlled in several different ways in the body — by the brain (which signals blood vessels to constrict or expand), by the kidneys (which regulate salt levels), and by the presence or absence of nutrients like calcium. The main reason for concern about high blood pressure (clinically referred to as hypertension) is because, uncontrolled, it substantially increases the risk of heart attacks, strokes and kidney disease.

High blood pressure is the most common serious ailment in the United States. In light of the standard American junk-food diet, and our work-hard/play-hard attitude, it's no surprise that this disease affects over 40 million Americans each year. However, in addition to pointing the finger at our damaging lifestyles, scientists have established a genetic hypothesis, which indicates that hypertension may sometimes be part of an entire family's health history. Because our chemical makeup is inherited, what really may run in families is the need for higher amounts of certain nutrients. For instance, some families may need more vitamin E in their diets. If they don't get it, heart function decreases, and they have heart attacks at early ages.

If you can't control your blood pressure with diet and lifestyle changes, or if your blood pressure is very high, there are several medications that your doctor may prescribe for you. These drugs work. But they just control the symptoms, they do nothing to eliminate the root cause of the problem. And if you put all your faith in medications, you will probably have to take them — in increasing dosages — for the rest of your life. Obviously, the smart thing to do is reduce your health risk by eating right and exercising regularly — and by heeding the collective wisdom of healers around the world.

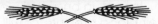

BARLEY Eat more barley muffins and cereal. Barley contains a substance called tocotrienol, which acts much like vitamin E to lower blood pressure.

CELERY You can probably find one ancient Oriental remedy for high blood pressure right in your own refrigerator — celery. Celery contains a pthalide compound that effectively relaxes the smooth muscle lining of blood vessels. This widens the vessels, and so lowers blood pressure.

CAUTION: *The benefit of celery may be partially mitigated by the fact that celery also contains a relatively high amount of sodium, which should ordinarily be avoided by hypertensive patients who are sensitive to salt in their diets. So, eat it only in moderation.*

---

6 Ways to Lower Your Risk of Getting High Blood Pressure

With high blood pressure — as with all serious ailments — "an ounce of prevention is worth a pound of cure." Here, then, are guidelines to help you lower your risk:

- **Aim for a diet that's low in salt and high in potassium** (which decreases salt retention).
- **Increase your calcium intake.** Researchers have linked high blood pressure to calcium deficiencies. They say that supplementing with 1,000 mgs a day can vastly reduce your chances of developing high blood pressure. Good food sources of calcium include canned fish with bones (such as sardines and pink salmon), yogurt, beans, tofu, dairy products, and green, leafy vegetables.
- **Nourish your brain with B vitamins.** The best food sources of B vitamins are fish and legumes.
- **Drink an occasional glass of red wine with dinner.** In England, a highly respected medical journal, *The Lancet*, has indicated that moderate wine consumption is directly associated with lower rates of heart disease.
- **Exercise regularly.**
- **Meditate.** High blood pressure is only one of many conditions that are helped by meditation. In fact, in one study, patients who meditated were able to lower their blood pressure at will. Biofeedback (and other stress-management techniques) have been reported to produce similar results.

DILL A tablespoon of dill seed has 100 mgs of calcium — as much as ¾ cup of cottage cheese.

GARLIC Garlic has been used in China for hundreds of years for many medicinal purposes. It is also used in Germany to decrease high blood pressure. Garlic allows blood vessels to dilate because it has a relaxing effect on the smooth muscles that surround blood vessels. Raw garlic seems to be more potent than cooked garlic.

GINSENG AND GINGER Ginseng and ginger are popular spices in the Orient where their health benefits are well-recognized. And recently, medical research in China and Russia has shown that ginseng and ginger both have the ability to lower blood pressure.

HAWTHORN BERRIES "We nap ish" and "ashnum asho" are Native American names for the hawthorn berry. A report in *British Medical Journal* found that these beneficial berries reduce high blood pressure caused by arteriosclerosis and kidney disease.

LEMON BALM Current research shows that lemon balm tea has properties to slightly dilate blood vessels, helping to lower blood pressure. To make it, put a tablespoon of bruised fresh lemon balm leaves in a cup of warm water. Cover and steep for 20 minutes, then strain and drink (up to 3 times a day).

MACKEREL Because so much of the fat in mackerel is in the form of omega-3 fatty acids, it is considered to be a heart-healthy food. One German study indicated that eating 3 ounces of mackerel a day can lower blood pressure.

MAGNESIUM Swedish researchers think that magnesium works in conjunction with calcium and potassium to help regulate blood pressure levels. (Turn to page 50 for a list of the best food sources of this mineral.)

MULBERRIES The Chinese use mulberries (which they refer to as Hsun or Tian) to make a jam called Sang-hen-kao, which is said to lower blood pressure and prevent heart attacks.

TARRAGON Used in the Middle East for nearly a thousand years, tarragon is high in potassium, which research indicates can help prevent high blood pressure. Try this tasty herb by adding a tablespoon of fresh or a teaspoon of dried tarragon to almost any salad.

YARROW A popular fever buster, yarrow tea also is reported to help lower blood pressure levels by dilating the blood vessels near the surface of the skin. Steep a tablespoon of fresh (or a teaspoon of dried) leaves and flowers in a cup of boiling water, covered, for 4 minutes. If you don't like the taste, try adding honey.
CAUTION: *You can drink a cup of yarrow tea up to 3 times a day, but don't overdo. Too much may keep your body from absorbing iron.*

HIGH CHOLESTEROL

Cholesterol is essential in the body to make cell membranes, sex hormones, vitamin D and bile. It is also used to make protective sheaths for nerve fibers. However, your liver makes all the cholesterol your body needs. You don't need any extra cholesterol. That's why, when you eat too many of the wrong foods, the cholesterol level in your blood can become dangerously high. It builds up on artery walls, clogs your arteries, and restricts blood flow — and this can lead to angina, heart attack or stroke.

The typical American diet is loaded with unhealthy foods, and misleading package labels make it hard to weed them out. For example, some foods currently on the market are labeled "lower in cholesterol." While these foods may have less cholesterol than they used to have, most still have too much. Other foods labeled "low cholesterol" may contain too much for people who have to watch their cholesterol levels. And some that are labeled "no cholesterol" never had any to begin with — like vegetables and grains — but can be bad for your health in other ways. For example, they may contain chemically manufactured hydrogenated or partially hydrogenated fats, which make your liver overproduce cholesterol. And many "no fat" foods make up for the flavor that's lost when the fat is removed by adding a lot more sugar or sodium.

Though changing your diet is clearly the single most important thing you can do to control — and prevent — high cholesterol, it is also helpful to keep your weight down, exercise regularly, take antioxidants — and pay attention to the cholesterol-fighting tips we've gathered for you.

APPLE Studies by Italian, Irish and French researchers all confirm that eating 2 or 3 apples a day lowers blood cholesterol. Apple skin is especially high in pectin, a soluble fiber that binds cholesterol, removing it from the body.

ARTICHOKE According to Japanese, Swiss and American researchers, artichokes have a substance which lowers blood cholesterol.

CARROTS A carrot a day keeps cholesterol at bay. A study conducted at the University of Edinburgh in Scotland found that carrots may help to lower cholesterol levels. Carrots are a good source of soluble fiber, which helps your body get rid of cholesterol.

FISH Like the Japanese, Eskimos and Scandinavians eat a lot of fatty fish. Medical research indicates that the large amount of fish oil in their diets is their secret weapon against high cholesterol and heart disease.

EXERCISE!

To boost your good HDL level, start an aerobic exercise program. It's great for your heart, and it helps cut your cholesterol by reducing body fat.

FRUIT Eat more fruit — a couple of large oranges, one or two grapefruits, or a cup or two of fresh strawberries regularly.

When you peel the oranges and grapefruit, don't throw away the white, fibrous membrane under the rind. This substance contains bioflavonoids, nutrients that help build strong blood vessels. Bioflavonoids — and the vitamins C and E and other antioxidants in the fruit — act as bodyguards for the good HDL cholesterol and help block formation of the bad LDL cholesterol. These nutrients have been shown to slow the development of fatty plaque build-up on artery walls.

GARLIC AND ONION Another natural remedy for high cholesterol comes from France, Italy, Greece and India. All of these cultures are famous for their superb cuisines — loaded with garlic and onion.

A study at Tangore Medical College in Udaipur, India, showed that both garlic and onion help reduce cholesterol levels and make the blood resistant to clotting — thus reducing the risk of heart disease.

GHEE If you can't give up butter, but you still have to watch your

---

The Difference Between "Good" Cholesterol and "Bad" Cholesterol

Your body stores cholesterol in two forms: high density lipoprotein (HDL, the good form) and low density lipoprotein (LDL, the bad form).

High levels of HDL protect your heart — which is why it should measure at least 40 in a man and at least 50 in a woman. To keep your HDL level high, avoid smoking, exercise regularly, keep your body fat down (ideally, no more than 16% for men and 20% for women), and control the effects of stress in your life.

On the other hand, high levels of LDL block your blood vessels, which is why it should be as low as possible — ideally, less than 160. The best way to control LDL is with diet.

---

cholesterol level, maybe you should switch to ghee (clarified butter). Common in Persian and Indian cooking, ghee is made by melting butter, and then straining out the milk solids. Ghee is lower in cholesterol than unclarified butter. It doesn't burn as easily, and it stays fresh longer.

Ghee is used in many dishes — in India's "pilau" and Iran's "polo," for example, two buttery flavored rice dishes that are low in calories and cholesterol. See page 313 for a tasty pilau recipe.

GINSENG For over 5,000 years, millions of Asians have taken 2 to 3 grams of ginseng daily to lower cholesterol.

HAWTHORN BERRIES Hawthorn berry tincture is used in Europe to lower cholesterol levels. The recommended dosage is usually 20 to 40 drops, twice a day. And hawthorn berry tea is widely used to treat all types of cardiovascular problems.

MUSTARD SEEDS The tiny mustard seed contains the mineral magnesium, which is reported to help lower cholesterol. A tablespoon of ground mustard seed contains 33 milligrams of magnesium, about a tenth of the daily recommended dosage.

OAT BRAN Research has shown that 30 grams of soluble fiber a day in your diet can help lower cholesterol. Fiber moves much more quickly through your G.I tract than other foods, and cuts down on the amount of time available for fat to absorb into your system. Just 2 to 3 ounces a day of oat bran or oatmeal can cut your LDL cholesterol levels by 10 to 16 percent.

RED WINE Despite the fact that French food is rich in butter, cream, and red meat, the French have a much lower incidence of heart disease than we do. It may be because the typical Frenchman would not think of having dinner without a glass of wine.

Other Europeans, too, have discovered the secret of wine. In the Mediterranean, doctors prescribe a moderate, daily dose of wine for their patients. The benefits of wine with meals have also been praised by the Italians, Spanish and Greeks, who all indulge. And recent studies show that a moderate intake of red wine (not more than 2 or 3 glasses a day) increases the levels of HDL cholesterol.

5 Ways to Lower Your Cholesterol — Without Medication

Since the best way to control the level of LDL cholesterol in your blood is by modifying your diet, here are some recommendations to help you do it:

- **Cut down on red meats.** Other meats and poultry also contain cholesterol, but not as much.
- **Switch to low- or no-fat dairy products.** You'll still get all the good nutrients associated with dairy products — like calcium and vitamin D — but without the cholesterol.
- **Eat eggs in moderation.** The National Institutes of Health now okays three or four eggs a week. The egg contains a substance called lecithin, which breaks down the cholesterol in the egg and keeps it from sticking to your blood vessel walls. There is enough lecithin in an egg to handle the cholesterol in that egg.
- **Eat mono-saturated fats.** Israeli researchers find that eating avocados, almonds and olive oil — all excellent sources of mono-unsaturated fats — decreases levels of LDL cholesterol. Olive oil also increases the HDL levels. Australian research supports these findings.
- **Take a soluble fiber** such as psyllium in your diet regularly.

SOYBEANS Italian scientists are studying the remarkable effect of the soybean on cholesterol. Soybeans contain the substance lecithin, which breaks down cholesterol. Mixing soybean fiber into an already low-fat, high-carbohydrate diet can really make a difference. Other soy products that you can add to your diet include soy oil, soy flour. soy powder and tofu.

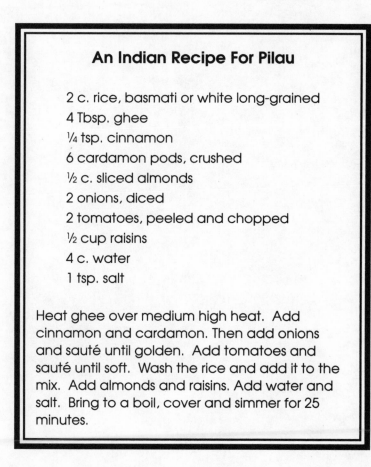

An Indian Recipe For Pilau

2 c. rice, basmati or white long-grained
4 Tbsp. ghee
¼ tsp. cinnamon
6 cardamon pods, crushed
½ c. sliced almonds
2 onions, diced
2 tomatoes, peeled and chopped
½ cup raisins
4 c. water
1 tsp. salt

Heat ghee over medium high heat. Add cinnamon and cardamon. Then add onions and sauté until golden. Add tomatoes and sauté until soft. Wash the rice and add it to the mix. Add almonds and raisins. Add water and salt. Bring to a boil, cover and simmer for 25 minutes.

IMPOTENCE

Nearly all men, at one time or another in their lives, experience impotence (the inability to achieve or maintain an erection, or to ejaculate after erection). Unfortunately, most men equate this loss of potency with a loss of manhood, and the resulting anxiety simply aggravates the problem. Though sexual dysfunction in men can often be linked to stress, research indicates that about half of all impotence problems are physical. A number of underlying medical conditions, such as vascular insufficiency or diabetes, can affect potency. So can drugs like antihistamines and blood pressure medications. And, because men produce a lower level of testosterone as they age, older men often experience a drop in sexual desire. Even so, as long as you are healthy, there's no reason you can't have a healthy, active sex life no matter how old you are. Here are some ways men around the world have learned to rekindle their libidos.

BARRENWORT The Chinese claim that every part of this small plant, except the root, is useful in treating impotence. Barrenwort is most commonly brewed into a tea.

EGGPLANT For generations, Hindus have increased sexual stamina with this tasty recipe: Slice an eggplant. Cover both sides of each slice with butter and minced chives. Brown the slices and serve with a spicy curry sauce.

GINKGO Research indicates that taking 60 mgs a day of ginkgo improves blood flow to the penis. This natural vasodilator is widely available at health food stores.

GINSENG Ginseng was first used by Chinese and Indian healers simply because its root resembles the shape of the human body. It has many medicinal applications, but is most prized for its ability to treat impotence. (Red ginseng is said to be the most effective of all types of ginseng in treating this condition.)

The Atharva Veda, an ancient medical text of India, states, "Ginseng causes an aroused man to exhale fire-like heat." And Korean scientists find that ginseng facilitates mating behavior in rats — interesting, since rats are very prolific even without it.

The medicinal use of ginseng is not limited to the Orient. Early European settlers in America noted that Indians made frequent use of the root, particularly as a powerful sexual tonic.

CAUTION: *Ginseng is a mild irritant and dilates blood vessels, both of which can cause sexual arousal. However, avoid taking it if you have a history of high blood pressure or heart disease.*

MUSSELS The Chinese often cook up a dish of mussels, believing that this shellfish raises body temperature, especially in the genitals.

POLLEN The Burmese share a secret jungle recipe with Cambodians. In both countries, natives restore sexual potency by eating raw pollen and cakes of honeycomb.

Ancient medical texts indicate that pollen was used to treat impotence in China, Babylon, Persia and Egypt. Recent scientific research has demonstrated that pollen contains a form of the male hormone testosterone. And, because it is gathered from many different kinds of medicinal plants, most pollen provides additional natural benefits.

CAUTION: *If you have a history of asthma, stay away from bee pollen.*

PUMPKIN SEEDS Bulgarian mountain dwellers, Hungarian Gypsies, Anatolian Turks, Ukrainians and Transylvanians all eat pumpkin seeds as part of their everyday diets. Originally used to prevent prostate ailments, zinc-rich pumpkin seeds have been found by these people to prevent impotence as well.

VERVAIN Vervain was a prime ingredient in many early medieval love potions. Rubbing the juice of vervain all over the body was thought to be a sure way to increase sexual potency (but maybe that depended on who did the rubbing).

For information on where to purchase any of the items listed, turn to the glossary beginning on page 523.

INCONTINENCE

Incontinence is easily treatable, yet, although it affects 10 to 12 million Americans, few sufferers seek help for this debilitating condition. Problems with bladder control interfere with everything from the ability to take a walk to having sex. And for senior citizens, it's a leading cause of nursing home admissions.

Many foods contribute to incontinence. Watch out for alcoholic beverages, caffeinated carbonated soft drinks, milk and milk products, tea and coffee — even decaf, citrus juices and fruits, tomatoes and tomato-based products, highly spiced foods, sugar, honey, corn syrup, chocolate and artificial sweeteners. Eliminate one item at a time, for several days, to see if that helps. Then, if you still have problems, try some of these other tips.

■ **Drink plenty of liquids**. Six to 8 glasses a day is right for most people. If you don't, you'll produce a smaller amount of urine, but it will be highly concentrated (healthy urine is pale and yellow) and, therefore, irritating to your bladder. That can make you need go to the bathroom more often. It will also make you more likely to develop a urinary tract infection.

The Chinese drink fresh raspberry juice to control frequent urination. And the Greeks like to use a cold infusion of yarrow. They pour 1 pint of boiling water over 1 ounce of dried yarrow leaves and flowers, steep for 5 to 10 minutes, then cool, and drink 1 cup, 3 times a day.

■ **Empty your bladder regularly.** By ignoring nature's call, you can stretch your bladder. This can cause leaking, and possibly infection.

■ **Avoid asparagus.** Not only is asparagus a diuretic, it can cause foul-smelling urine. (Cherry juice and cranberry juice can help control the odor.)

319

■ **Avoid known bladder irritants.** Smoke, caffeine, perfumed soaps and some feminine hygiene products can all irritate the bladder — and cause incontinence.

■ **Try Kegel exercises.** These exercises were developed to help women fight incontinence during and after pregnancy, but they can work for both men and women at any stage of life — and can be done anytime, anywhere, without anyone noticing.

Simply clench your pelvic muscle for a 4 count, and then relax. Repeat for 2 minutes, 3 times a day. To find the right pelvic muscle, practice by trying to stop and restart a flow of urine.

■ **Prevent constipation.** Constipation can affect bladder control because bearing down to pass a hard stool may injure the nerves that help control bladder filling and emptying. Added fiber and exercise will help keep your bowels working well. (See page 195 for a complete discussion of constipation remedies.)

Traditional Chinese Remedies for Bedwetting

As a remedy for bedwetting in children, traditional Chinese medicine suggests mixing ½ teaspoon of ground cinnamon twig with maltose and a little licorice powder as a remedy for bedwetting. Have the child drink this mixture twice a day.

Another Chinese remedy is to have the child eat 2 chicken livers steamed with 3 grams of ground cinnamon and a little water.

INFERTILITY

There's an old story about a Russian peasant who decides to visit an American relative he's only seen in a picture. He hitches a ride from the hinterlands to Moscow, somehow manages to walk onto a plane without a ticket, flies to New York, walks out of the airport and directly onto a bus going to Cleveland, Ohio, gets off the bus, walks into a neighborhood and up to a door. He knocks on the door. A man opens the door and our peasant friend cries, "Uncle Uri!"

If you think that's an incredible series of coincidences, it's nothing compared to conception. Countless factors have to be just right for sperm and egg to meet and hit it off. Smoking, drugs, alcohol, stress and being overweight or underweight can have a big impact on fertility. And, with nature urging us on toward procreation, the inability to conceive can become an incredible source of tension, frustration and resentment for a couple. Still, there are many things both partners can do to increase their chances of conception.

    CALCIUM Most women don't get enough calcium anyway — and you need even more to get pregnant. The recommended daily intake is 1,500 milligrams a day.

    ECHINACEA Herbalists believe that echinacea strengthens the pituitary gland, which controls the female hormones estrogen and progesterone. Echinacea can be ingested in pill or tea form.

    HOT PEPPERS The Japanese believe that hot peppers increase fertility. Since peppers increase circulation of the blood, both male and female reproductive structures could benefit.

MINERALS There's a strong link between trace elements and reproduction. A mineral supplement containing iodine, manganese, copper and zinc may help. In men, the highest body concentration of zinc is found in semen. And because we don't store zinc in our bodies, the more sexually active a man is, the quicker he loses zinc — and needs to replace it.

MUSSELS A classical Chinese dish to promote erections is cooked mussels. Actually, all shellfish improve fertility. Mussels, oysters and other shellfish, such as shrimp, contain high amounts of zinc and iodine. Zinc is reported to have an impact on both number and mobility of sperm.

ONION Indians recommend onion juice and honey to encourage the production of sperm and to raise a man's sperm count. Onions, like garlic, contain the mineral selenium and vitamin E — both of which are needed to develop healthy sperm. To be most effective, this treatment should be taken once every morning.

RASPBERRIES The iron and calcium contained in red raspberry tea has been reported to strengthen the uterus.

VITAMIN A Vitamin A is a must for a healthy uterus. Sterility is one of the symptoms of a vitamin A deficiency.

VITAMIN B You can't do without the B-complex vitamins — riboflavin to enhance sperm count, niacin to keep up your energy, and thiamine for a healthy pregnancy. One of the important functions of B6 is to stabilize female hormone levels needed to conceive. And without B9 (folic acid), there's no cell division. No cell division, no baby.

VITAMIN C Research has indicated that a vitamin C deficiency leads to lower sperm count and abnormally formed, slow-swimming sperm.

Helpful Hints

■ **Wear boxer shorts.** Tight briefs keep the testicles close to the body, where heat can decrease sperm production. Switch to boxer shorts and loose trousers, and stay away from hot baths and electric blankets.

■ **Take a cold bath.** Cold hip baths increase circulation to the reproductive system, and may help increase sperm production.

■ **Use a slant board.** If you want to exercise the uterus, a slant board is considered a good way to eliminate the straining and pulling that gravity exerts on it around the clock.

■ **Watch your diet.** Load up on fruits, vegetables and milk, which are high in alkaline and help give sperm a fighting chance in the cervix. And watch your intake of acidic foods like meat, fish, whole grains, cheese, eggs and seeds — and avoid tea, coffee and alcohol.

■ **Don't smoke.** Research has shown that men who smoke tend to have a vitamin C deficiency, which can lead to fewer, slower-swimming sperm that clump together. (If you can't quit, research shows that daily vitamin C tablets can improve the condition.)

■ **Time it right.** Research has indicated that the egg and uterine lining are at their best in the fall, peaking in November — and a man's sperm count is at its prime between February and May.

　　Increase your chances by abstaining from sex the week before ovulation — and during the week of ovulation, make love only 2 or 3 times to maximize sperm count.

■ **Use the old standby missionary position.** It works best to get the sperm high up into the vagina. Then, the woman should lie still, on her back with her knees raised, for at least half an hour.

■ **Try acupuncture.** In traditional Chinese medicine, using acupuncture on the knees is said to promote kidney energy, which is linked to reproduction. The Chinese also recommend strengthening the knees (and all the joints).

INSECT BITES AND REPELLENTS

Summer rarely passes without at least one attack by a bee, wasp, chigger or mosquito. If you're especially unlucky, you might even suffer a painful spider bite. Some insect bites — like those of the malaria-carrying mosquito of the tropical jungles, the brown recluse spider of the American Southwest, and the black widow spider — can be dangerous or even fatal. Fortunately, most of them are only mildly painful or itchy. But watch for severe swelling, wheezing, difficulty swallowing, nausea and vomiting, and hives — symptoms that can indicate a life-threatening allergic or toxic reaction.

First aid for any insect bite is to wash it with soap and water and apply ice to knock down the swelling and pain. However, since insects live in almost every part of the world, there are many additional home remedies to help you take the sting out.

ALOE Over the centuries, several cultures have discovered the amazing healing properties of the aloe vera plant. On Barbados and other islands of the West Indies, home to what their inhabitants tout as the purest aloe in the world, the juice from this plant is used to treat many things, including insect bites.

To enjoy the benefits of the aloe plant, simply break open a leaf and apply the mucilage to the affected area. This treatment has both an analgesic and a healing effect.

CAUTION: *Some people are allergic to some compounds in the aloe plant. If you are one of them, buy pure aloe liquid or gel instead of using the aloe directly from the plant.*

CORN STARCH Cornstarch has long been used in rural areas of the U.S. as a treatment for insect bites. This remedy probably originated in the kitchens of Europe and was imported to the U.S. by immigrants.

Make a paste of corn starch and water and apply it to the irritated area. A mixture of baking soda and water also works well, and is especially good on bee stings. These preparations are effective because they are alkaline, which neutralizes most venoms, the majority of which are acidic.

ECHINACEA Echinacea, also called purple coneflower and Sampson root, was used by Native Americans to treat everything from snakebites to insect bites. The Indians knew that the plant's roots have wound-healing properties when applied to the skin, and modern science has confirmed these antiseptic properties.

GOLDENROD The crushed leaves of goldenrod were sometimes used by European herbalists for healing insect bites. The plant contains flavonoids that help reduce inflammation.

GRINDELIA Soak the leaves, stems and flowers of the grindelia plant in boiling water and allow to cool. Using a cloth, apply the liquid to a painful bite.

LAVENDER For centuries, lavender compresses have been commonly used in France, Spain and other regions of Europe for soothing insect bites. Lavender oil has antibacterial properties, which can be helpful in preventing infection.

LEEKS The French apply mashed leeks, a natural antiseptic, to insect bites.

MUD Bikers swear by mud for insect bites. So mix some up and slap it on to take the sting out.

ONION Putting a slice of onion on a mosquito bite doesn't sound soothing. However, some English country people still practice this centuries-old remedy. Remedies that add their own "sting" may often work like acupuncture, by masking or interrupting pain signals from the original injury.

PAPAYA Meat tenderizer is commonly used to treat bee stings. Residents of many tropical islands in the Pacific have known about this cure for more than 200 years. They don't use commercially packaged meat tenderizer, however. They go right to the source — the fruit of the papaya. Papaya contains the enzyme papain, which is a primary ingredient in all meat tenderizers. Papain alleviates the sting of bee and wasp venom, as well as the itch produced by many other types of insect bites. The enzyme breaks down the venom proteins, rendering the poison harmless.

PLANTAIN A useful early Native American remedy for bee stings and insect bites was the fleshy leaves of plantain. The leaves contain mucilage, which soothes broken skin. Leaves can be crushed and applied directly to the skin to stop bleeding and pain.

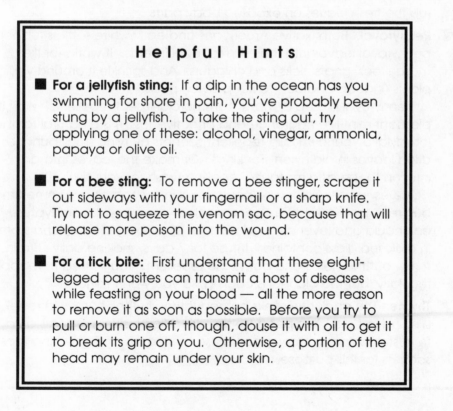

Helpful Hints

■ **For a jellyfish sting:** If a dip in the ocean has you swimming for shore in pain, you've probably been stung by a jellyfish. To take the sting out, try applying one of these: alcohol, vinegar, ammonia, papaya or olive oil.

■ **For a bee sting:** To remove a bee stinger, scrape it out sideways with your fingernail or a sharp knife. Try not to squeeze the venom sac, because that will release more poison into the wound.

■ **For a tick bite:** First understand that these eight-legged parasites can transmit a host of diseases while feasting on your blood — all the more reason to remove it as soon as possible. Before you try to pull or burn one off, though, douse it with oil to get it to break its grip on you. Otherwise, a portion of the head may remain under your skin.

Natural Insect Repellents for General Use:

■ **Essential balm.** Essential balm is a natural repellent made in China. It contains menthol, camphor, and oils of peppermint, eucalyptus, clove and cinnamon. Bugs don't like the odor of these volatile oils. The repellent lasts for about an hour when applied to the hair, forehead, neck, hands or ankles. It also helps prevent itching when bites do occur.

■ **Garlic.** Sardinians rub garlic juice on exposed parts of their bodies to ward off mosquitoes. These insects avoid the garlic, not only because of its strong smell, but also because garlic is fatal to them.

■ **Lavender.** Lavender contains many volatile oils that repel insects, especially mosquitoes and gnats. To use it, dilute oil of lavender with a little ethyl alcohol (1 part alcohol to 2 parts oil).

■ **Parsley, lemon balm and basil leaves.** All keep insects away. Simply rub the fresh leaves on exposed body parts.

■ **Pennyroyal.** Both Native Americans and early white settlers rubbed pennyroyal leaves into their skin to repel insects. It works for flies, mosquitoes, gnats, ticks and chiggers. And sprinkle it around your plants (indoors and out) to keep away pests.

Pennyroyal is used in many commercial insect repellents. With its pleasant mint-like fragrance and effectiveness, it is a natural for the job. Make your own bug-repellent sachets by tying small bunches of dried leaves in old nylon stockings. Or make the leaves into an infusion to use as a mosquito-repelling wash for your skin.

We especially like to use pennyroyal in this soothing, summertime bug repellent: Mix up ¼ ounce each of pennyroyal, eucalyptus, calendula and lavender. Add 2 cups of rubbing alcohol and store in a closed glass container. Infuse for 7 days, shaking daily. Strain, throw out the herbs and bottle the repellent. You'll need to reapply it regularly, but the alcohol is cooling, so you won't mind.

■ **Thyme.** The ancient Greeks burned thyme in their homes to repel stinging insects. And because the dried flowers keep insects away from stored linens, many people use the leaves and flowering tops in sachets for this purpose.

Natural Insect Repellents for the Garden:

■ **Basil.** When planted near tomatoes, basil will repel tomato pests.

■ **Feverfew.** You can protect your herb garden from bugs by planting feverfew, which contains the natural insect repellent pyrethrin.

■ **Window box repellents.** In Europe, window boxes full of easy-to-grow sweet basil, tansy, fennel or bay adorn many homes. Besides being decorative, these plants seem to keep pesky house flies away.

■ **Pest-controlling flowers.** You can control pests and brighten your garden at the same time by planting the right flowers. Angelica, morning glories and yarrow attract ladybugs, which feed on garden pests such as aphids, mealybugs, scales and whiteflies.

TEA Tea leaves are commonly used to soothe itchy bug bites. Few of us realize, however, that the people of Taiwan were the first to discover that the tannin released by wet tea leaves neutralizes the discomfort produced by many types of insect venom.

THYME The Greeks used crushed thyme leaves on bee stings and other insect bites because of the plant's cooling and soothing properties.

WITCH HAZEL Compresses made from witch hazel are a common remedy for insect bites. The herb contains tannic acid, gallic acid and volatile oils, which soothe and help relieve the stinging and itching that come along with a bite.

To Keep Flies Away: Add lavender, mint, bay, mugwort, cloves, wormwood, rue, eucalyptus or elder to potpourri — or hang in bunches.

To Get Rid of Ants: Wipe down surfaces like kitchen counters with a cloth dipped in a solution of vinegar and water, or vinegar, lemon and water. Or put out cucumber peels. Ants are also repelled by the smell of crushed catnip, pennyroyal, rue and tansy.

To Repel Moths: Fill sachets with lavender, rosemary, wormwood, southernwood, woodruff and cloves. Or try cedar wood shavings, ground sassafras root, or a combination of equal parts of dried lavender, tansy and rosemary.

To Repel Roaches: Boric acid is fatal to roaches. Try placing some of the powder in prime locations — in dark corners and under the refrigerator. Roaches are attracted to boric acid, but when they walk through it, they will die.

To Repel Fleas: To keep Rover's bed free from fleas, tuck in a sachet of rue. Fleas also hate the scent of brewer's yeast, which is undetectable to humans. Rub yeast powder directly on the animal once each day or give a tablet by mouth several times a week.

You can also sprinkle regular table salt around your pet's bed and on carpets and other areas where your pet stays. Fleas won't cross a salt path. See page 400 of the Pet Care section for more remedies.

INSOMNIA

For most people, the need for rest is satisfied by following a regular sleep schedule. If that schedule is disrupted, the result may be frazzled nerves, feelings of disorientation or insomnia.

Sleep disorders are probably America's worst and largest invisible medical problem, affecting as many as 100 million people. And tension is often the prime cause. Just as adrenaline is your body's natural stimulant, serotonin — a chemical your brain produces when you are tired — is its natural sedative, slowing or stopping the electrical firings that keep your mind awake. But often, when you're under stress, adrenaline keeps on overpowering the serotonin in your system. And at times like that, the safest way to get some much-needed sleep is with one of the following natural remedies.

ANISE Ground anise seed mixed with honey in warm milk is a generations-old cure for insomnia in Germany and Russia.

CALCIUM Calcium deficiencies have been linked to tension and insomnia. Adult men and women need 800 milligrams daily — and pregnant and nursing women should get 1,200 milligrams.

CATNIP Cats may be onto something when they happily chew on the leaves of the catnip plant. The aromatic oils seem to send them into ecstasy. Catnip can be used by humans as a sleeping aid and effective natural tranquilizer. Make catnip tea by pouring boiling water over dried catnip and letting it steep.

Catnip is available in cut, dried or powdered form through most mail-order herb companies. Live plants can also be purchased.

CHAMOMILE The Germans and the English swear by chamomile tea for its strong relaxing effects to treat insomnia. Drink a cup 1 hour before you go to bed. You can sweeten its taste with a little honey.

Another soothing way to enjoy chamomile's relaxing properties is to add it to your bathwater. Steep the herb in water for 15 minutes, let cool, and then add to your bath.

COWSLIP The cowslip is a flower that grows in the meadows and pastures of England, and in other parts of Europe, Siberia, western Asia and northern Africa. The blossoms of this flower are mixed with sugar, honey, water and lemon juice to make a beverage that acts as a mild sedative that can help you fall asleep.

HONEY A tablespoon of honey just before bedtime may be just the ticket you need to dreamland. It's reported to increase the production of serotonin, our body's own knockout drops.

Or, you might want to try this popular Gypsy remedy for insomnia that is safer and more effective than most tranquilizers. They drink a juice made from honey mixed with hot water, lemons and oranges. It's the carbohydrates in the honey (and the fruit) that make you sleepy.

HOPS Drink a few beers, and you'll find yourself getting kind of mellow and even a little sleepy. Hops, one of the ingredients in beer, is a sedative. In the U.S., hops-filled pillows are an old country remedy for insomnia. And an old English recipe for insomnia is to drink a hops infusion. The hops tea can be flavored with lemon and sweetened with honey. No need for the alcohol.

LETTUCE The English and Irish share a remedy for insomnia. Both make a tea from chopped lettuce leaves that is said to bring on drowsiness. The Irish go a step further and add a sprig of mint leaf, which enhances the taste and encourages digestion. (Indigestion is a frequent cause of insomnia.)

The famous Greek physician, Galen, claimed to cure his insomnia by eating lots of lettuce in the evening. A substance in the lettuce, called lactucarium, is a calming agent.

MILK Drinking milk to encourage sleep is a common practice around the world. Milk works well for several reasons, but primarily because it contains the tranquilizing amino acid tryptophan. Another reason for the calming effect of milk is its high calcium content. Calcium encourages the chemical processes necessary for sleep.

Muslims believe that the brain must be emptied of dreams if you are to be able to enjoy a full night's sleep. Many tranquilizers actually inhibit dreaming. Milk, however, has a reliable sedative effect, yet does not interfere with the dream process.

ONION The Chinese induce sleep by inhaling the vapors of a crushed onion through the nose before going to bed.

THYME Several hundred years ago in Europe, people drank thyme tea to ward off nightmares. An antispasmodic, it can relax muscles to help promote sleep.

TURKEY Did you ever wonder why you get sleepy after Thanksgiving dinner? Well, if you ate a big helping of turkey, you have your answer. Turkey is high in tryptophan, a natural sleeping aid. So chow down, curl up and relax.

Curiosity Box

Some of history's most productive people have seized the day with the help of a short snooze. Some famous nappers include Winston Churchill, John F. Kennedy, Albert Einstein, Wilt Chamberlain and Leonardo da Vinci.

Thomas Edison, who was virtually deaf, developed a novel way to wake himself from a catnap. He would nap sitting in a chair, while holding an iron ball in each hand. Just as he began to fall into a deep sleep, his hands would relax and he would drop the balls. The vibration beneath his feet woke him.

VALERIAN Since colonial times, western countries have used valerian as an insomnia cure. It's still among the most common ingredients in herbal sedatives, usually blended with hops, passionflower and skullcap.

Helpful Hints

■ **Sleeplessness can often be cured simply by altering your sleep habits.** Try this: Don't go to bed unless you are absolutely exhausted. Then, if you don't fall asleep quickly, get out of bed and do something that will help tire you out. In time, your body will associate your bed with immediate sleep — and this may do away with your insomnia.

■ **Limit your intake of caffeine during the day.** Do not have any after noon. To keep caffeine under control, try dumping the first cup of tea brewed with a new tea bag, and drink the second one instead.

■ **Give yourself a foot bath.** Eastern cultures recommend bathing your feet in hot water as a remedy for insomnia. The theory is that the warm water draws blood away from the head, which will help put you to sleep.

■ **Learn and practice the technique of progressive muscle relaxation.** Here's how it works: You isolate each one of your muscle groups, tense it for a 5 count, and then relax for 15 to 20 seconds before moving on. (You feel like Jello by the time you get done.)

■ **Have a snack.** The researchers at MIT tried a variety of munchies out on volunteers, and got the biggest snore for their buck from English muffins and bananas.

■ **Bore yourself.** Recite batting averages, name the states and their capitals or count sheep. Usually insomnia hits when your mind is on overload. So any meaningless, repetitious distraction can help you fall asleep.

■ **Power down.** Give yourself two hours before bedtime to unwind. Read, watch TV or munch a light carbohydrate snack. Carbs increase the production of serotonin, so it might help you nod off.

■ **Plan ahead.** Cut back on liquids after 8 p.m., and you'll lessen your chance of waking up at night with a full bladder.

WHEAT BRAN In China, insomnia is treated by drinking a tea made from wheat bran. Just wrap the wheat bran in a clean cloth and use it like a tea bag.

YERBA MATE Yerba mate grows in Paraguay, where natives use it to treat many ailments, including insomnia. You can make Paraguay tea by steeping finely ground yerba mate leaves in hot water.

ZINC A zinc deficiency may be causing you sleepless nights. The RDA for zinc is 12 milligrams a day, which can be taken as a supplement. You can also find zinc in high protein foods, as well as raisins, dried apricots and figs, and blackstrap molasses.

Diets low in copper or iron may also cause sleeplessness. Turn to page 50 for a complete listing of foods rich in these minerals.

IRRITABLE BOWEL SYNDROME

Considered by some doctors to be as prevalent as the cold, irritable bowel syndrome (IBS) is twice as common among women as men. Also known as a spastic colon or irritable colon syndrome, the condition has a strong link to anxiety and is exacerbated by emotional stress.

Symptoms include intense abdominal pain and bloating, mucus in the feces, excessive gas, chills and sweats, a sense of incomplete evacuation of the bowels, and irregular bowels (constipation and diarrhea, or alternating attacks of both). IBS usually begins in early or mid-adulthood. Symptoms can subside or disappear for periods of time, but usually recur throughout life.

IBS isn't fatal and — unless accompanied by bleeding, fever or weight loss — won't lead to more serious medical complications. If you suspect you are suffering from this condition, see your doctor for an accurate diagnosis. Meanwhile, we offer these tips to help you calm your colon.

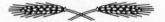

ALFALFA Alfalfa tablets or liquid contain vitamin K, which can re-establish a healthy environment in your intestines by building intestinal flora for proper digestion. Acidophilus cultures also replenish friendly bacteria.

CALCIUM Supplement with calcium — and magnesium. These minerals are said to help "nervous stomach" and the central nervous system.

GARLIC Garlic capsules can aid digestion and help destroy toxins in the colon.

GINGER The Chinese regularly use ginger to treat upset stomachs and regulate bowel movements. Add it to your food whenever possible.

Helpful Hints

■ **Avoid coffee.** The acid and caffeine in coffee can irritate this condition. British researchers reported that 30 percent of IBS sufferers felt better when they gave up their caffeine fix.

■ **Avoid smoking.** Smoking can irritate the linings of the stomach and colon.

■ **Avoid sugar.** Sugars are not digested easily and can cause or worsen diarrhea. Fructose and sorbitol can also aggravate IBS.

■ **Cook your fruits and veggies.** Raw food, especially beans, cabbage, broccoli and cauliflower, are a tough act for your colon to handle. Lightly cooking your fruits and vegetables retains the nutrients and makes them friendlier to your intestines.

■ **Avoid carbonated drinks.** They produce gas that aggravates IBS.

■ **Switch to a high-fiber diet** (35 to 50 grams per day). This will keep your bowels moving regularly, which will reduce constipation and pressure on your intestines.
  CAUTION: *This type of diet can initially worsen symptoms. So gradually introduce more fiber into your diet over a few months.*

■ **Drink plenty of water.** Six to 8 glasses of water a day helps reduce constipation.

■ **Keep a food diary.** This will help you determine which foods trigger an IBS attack. Lactose intolerance, for example, can mimic IBS. And many people are helped by avoiding spicy and fatty foods, like bacon and sausage.
  A British study found that the root cause behind bowel problems was as likely to be food intolerances as IBS. Wheat and corn hit the top of the chart as problem foods, but patients also had trouble with citrus.

■ **Use heat.** Warm baths and a heating pad relieve abdominal pain.

■ **Reduce stress.** Relaxation techniques like meditation, biofeedback, visualization and deep breathing are stress relievers that can ward off an attack of IBS. Exercise is also an excellent way to relieve tension. Turn to page — for more information about stress reduction.

■ **Eat when you're calm.** Because stress and anxiety may cause or worsen this condition, eat slowly in a relaxed environment.

WILD YAM Mexican wild yam is an antispasmodic and anti-inflammatory that helps relieve the symptoms of IBS.

JET LAG

You're standing in front of Buckingham Palace but your body's clock is still on Chicago time. This time warp is caused when you fly across several time zones too quickly. The consequences, known as jet lag, can turn you into a zombie the first few days of your trip. Symptoms are many and varied, affecting both your mind and your body. They can include fatigue, insomnia, fuzzy thinking, headache, irritability, indigestion, loss of appetite, constipation and diarrhea.

Jet lag occurs because your body's biological rhythms are thrown out of synch. These internal pacemakers — which regulate your sleep-wake patterns, and your digestion and hormone levels — have to adapt to your new time zone. It will take about one day for every time zone crossed for your body to fall in step with the new scene if you don't take steps to offset the mental and physical disruption. Fortunately, this is easy to do.

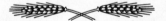

ESSENTIAL OILS Aromatherapists suggest lemongrass, rosemary or peppermint to help you stay sharp. Soak a hankie with a few drops of one of these essential oils and waft it under your nose from time to time during your trip.

FLUIDS Drink plenty of water and fruit juices in flight to keep from becoming dehydrated.

GINSENG The Chinese, Japanese and other Asian people use ginseng to fight off the draining toll exacted by fatigue, stress and disease. They find it has protective and restorative powers which help support all the body's internal systems.

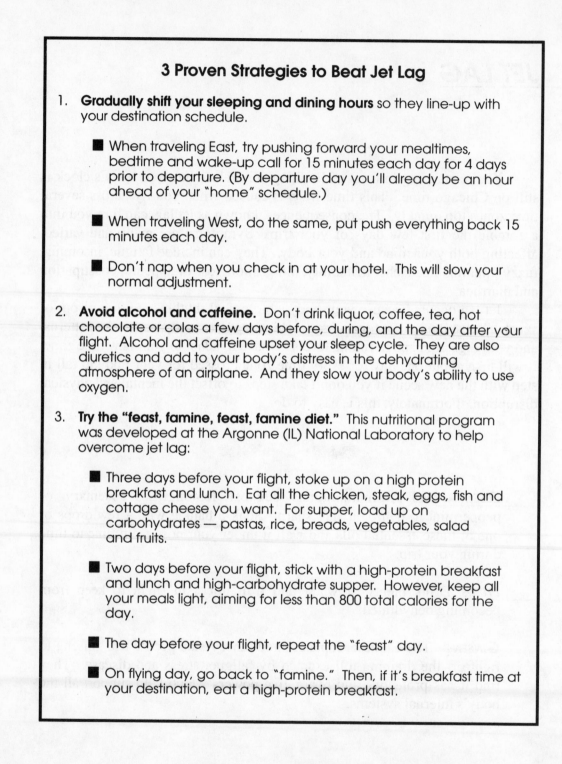

3 Proven Strategies to Beat Jet Lag

1. **Gradually shift your sleeping and dining hours** so they line-up with your destination schedule.

   ■ When traveling East, try pushing forward your mealtimes, bedtime and wake-up call for 15 minutes each day for 4 days prior to departure. (By departure day you'll already be an hour ahead of your "home" schedule.)

   ■ When traveling West, do the same, put push everything back 15 minutes each day.

   ■ Don't nap when you check in at your hotel. This will slow your normal adjustment.

2. **Avoid alcohol and caffeine.** Don't drink liquor, coffee, tea, hot chocolate or colas a few days before, during, and the day after your flight. Alcohol and caffeine upset your sleep cycle. They are also diuretics and add to your body's distress in the dehydrating atmosphere of an airplane. And they slow your body's ability to use oxygen.

3. **Try the "feast, famine, feast, famine diet."** This nutritional program was developed at the Argonne (IL) National Laboratory to help overcome jet lag:

   ■ Three days before your flight, stoke up on a high protein breakfast and lunch. Eat all the chicken, steak, eggs, fish and cottage cheese you want. For supper, load up on carbohydrates — pastas, rice, breads, vegetables, salad and fruits.

   ■ Two days before your flight, stick with a high-protein breakfast and lunch and high-carbohydrate supper. However, keep all your meals light, aiming for less than 800 total calories for the day.

   ■ The day before your flight, repeat the "feast" day.

   ■ On flying day, go back to "famine." Then, if it's breakfast time at your destination, eat a high-protein breakfast.

342

SUNLIGHT If you've flown eastward, take a walk in the late afternoon sun. If you've flown westward, take a walk in the morning sun. This will help your body accept your new schedule. Sunlight helps synchronize life's rhythms. So proper exposure to Old Sol's rays will help reset your body's internal clock.

EXERCISE!

On a long plane ride, periodically do simple seat-bound calisthenics. Flex your feet, rotate your ankles, shift your legs, shrug your shoulders and stretch your arms. Walk around. Exercising stimulates circulation and digestion while it eases muscle spasms and swollen joints. As a result, you'll be less lethargic upon arrival.

For information on where to purchase any of the items listed, turn to the glossary beginning on page 523.

KIDNEY STONES

About 3 percent of all Americans will undergo the excrutiatingly painful passage of at least one kidney stone. What's more, half of these victims will endure recurring bouts, some suffering through 10 or more stones a year.

There are several types of kidney stones. The most common are caused by a build-up of calcium salts and can grow to be as big as golf balls. Whatever the size, the stone's journey out of the wide open spaces of the kidney and down the narrow ureter is sorely felt, triggering stabbing spasms in the lower abdomen and back. Attacks can last minutes, or continue for days — as long as it takes for the stone to reach the bladder.

While doctors are unclear exactly why stones form, they have identified some factors that increase a person's chances of becoming stone prone. For example, kidney stones are apt to run in families. And 4 out of every 5 patients are men between 30 and 50 years old. If you are in this at-risk group, here are some dietary choices you can make to help reduce your chances of developing kidney stones.

APPLE JUICE The acidity in apple juice helps change your blood's pH balance, reducing the chances of stone formation.

BARLEY WATER Herbalists believe that barley water helps flush out stones. Make your own by simmering 2 ounces of barley in 1 quart of water. Strain, cool and drink.

CARBOHYDRATES Whole grains, rice, pasta, and most vegetables and fruits are high in fiber — which keeps stone development from gaining momentum. People who follow an Oriental, Mediterranean or vegetarian diet, all of which rely heavily on carbohydrates, are much less stone prone.

CITRUS FRUIT Researchers found that drinking citrus juice or eating oranges, tangerines or grapefruit causes the citrate level in urine to rise. This inhibits stone formation.   On the other hand, when citrus consumption and citrate levels drop, salt levels soar. And a high salt level boosts urinary calcium and promotes the build-up of stones.

CRANBERRY JUICE Juice from cranberries neutralizes Escherichia coli (the bacteria responsible for most bladder, kidney and urinary tract infections), thus creating an inhospitable environment for stone growth.

NETTLE TEA In Germany, people drink nettle tea to ward off stones. To make it, put 1 teaspoon of dried nettle in a teapot and add 1 cup of boiling water. Steep for 5 minutes, strain and drink.

PARSLEY AND CLOVER TEA Mennonites in Pennsylvania Dutch Country favor a special herbal mix of parsley and clover as a preventive against kidney stones. Brew your own by steeping ½ teaspoon each of dried parsley and red clover in a cup of boiling water. Strain and drink.

WALNUTS The Chinese pan-fry unsalted walnuts in vegetable oil until crunchy, and then blend with water and sugar. They take this syrupy potion until the pain and stones have passed.

WATER The many benefits of drinking at least 8 glasses of water a day are well-documented. Among other things, this helps flush out tiny stones and dilute concentrated minerals (preventing them from crystallizing).

I t's not just what you eat, but what you don't eat that affects the formation of kidney stones. Here are some preventive steps you can take to protect yourself.

Reduce calcium. Dairy products (including milk, cheese and ice cream), mackerel, salmon, collards, sardines, dried figs, turnips, okra, chickpeas, dried figs, tofu and many antacids are loaded with calcium, which increases your risk of forming kidney stones.

Reduce oxalate. Spinach, rhubarb, peanuts, chocolate and tea are rich in a substance called oxalate, a dietary factor which contributes to stone formation.

Reduce protein. Studies have shown that kidney stones plague people who eat a lot of high-protein foods. Men should keep their consumption of meat, chicken and fish to under 7 ounces a day. And women should cut back even more.

Reduce salt. Salt fuels the chemicals which cause stones. So go easy on sodium-laden cold cuts, salamis, smoked meats and fish, hot dogs, bacon, olives, pickles, canned soups, sauerkraut and frozen and canned foods.

LARYNGITIS

When you find that you are literally at a loss for words, your silence could be the result of laryngitis — inflammation of the larynx or "voice box." It can be caused by bad weather, dry air, a cold, an allergy, chemical fumes, pollen, tobacco smoke — or by too much partying, hooting and hollering. It is characterized by a hoarseness which often progresses to a sore throat, pain when swallowing and a dry cough. When it is a symptom of a viral infection, you may also run a fever and feel sick and achy.

Laryngitis can last a few days, or persist and become chronic. Though not serious, it is uncomfortable — but easily treated. Here are some soothing international remedies we've uncovered.

CABBAGE The English make a "cabbage syrup" to fight hoarseness and coughs. If you'd like to try it, liquefy red cabbage in a blender. Then strain and weigh the juice, and add honey until the total weight increases by 50 percent. In other words, if you have 8 fluid ounces of cabbage juice, add enough honey to bring the total weight to 12 fluid ounces. Simmer this mixture until it reaches a syrupy consistency. Take 2 teaspoons several times a day. (Cabbage is rich in vitamin C and honey is a soothing lubricant.)

CHERRIES The Chinese find that cherries help relieve the discomfort and lessen the symptoms of laryngitis. When they suffer from a sore throat, they treat it by slowly chewing about 10 cherries twice a day. (Cherries contain magnesium which is a natural painkiller.)

GINGER The Western world has been using fresh ginger as a source of "good medicine" for over 2,000 years. The Chinese have used it for medicinal purposes even longer. To make a tea that is soothing and healing for laryngitis, simmer fresh gingerroot in boiling water for approximately 10 minutes. (Honey and lemon add a nice flavor.)

OAK BARK Highly tannic and famed for its astringent, anti-inflammatory and antiseptic properties, oak bark effectively clears up larynx-irritating phlegm.

PINEAPPLE JUICE Hawaiians make a soothing drink to treat laryngitis. They add fresh grated ginger and spearmint to fresh pineapple juice.

SAGE While ancient Chinese herbalists believed that sage gave spiritual clarity, modern herbalists believe that the antiseptic properties of this herb soothe laryngitis. To try it, steep sage leaves in boiling water. Cool, strain out the leaves and then gargle with the water.

THYME Herbalists have known for many years that thyme is antiseptic and antibacterial. That's because it contains "thymol," a substance that is now a popular ingredient in commerical cough syrups and mouthwashes. To sooth your strained vocal cords, try adding thyme leaves to boiling water and inhaling the steam.

WATER Drink 8 to 10 glasses of water every day. This will keep your mucus thin and fluid — the right consistency to properly lubricate your vocal cords.

Helpful Hint

Keep the humidity in your house at 40 to 50 percent. Use a humidifier or steam treatment to give your vocal cords some TLC.

Soothe your sore larynx — and keep chronic laryngitis from recurring — by steering clear of known irritants.

- **Avoid alcohol.** Liquor is corrosive, harsh, hypertonic and burning. It strips vocal cords of lubrication, drying and further inflaming them.

- **Avoid caffeine.** Coffee, tea, colas and chocolate dehydrate and strain vocal cords.

- **Avoid dairy products.** Milk, cheese, ice cream and yogurt thicken mucus and muffle the voice.

- **Avoid smoke.** Don't stand downwind of tobacco smoke, eat in a smoke-filled restaurant or hover over a barbeque grill. Smoke irritates and dehydrates vocal cords.

- **Don't clear your throat.** This stresses your larynx. Instead, gently cough or swallow hard a few times.

- **Don't eat in bed.** Eating while lying down, even if it is just a bedtime snack, is apt to cause reflux burping and flood your larynx with corrosive gastric juices.

- **Don't talk.** Give your sore throat and inflamed vocal cords a rest to lessen stress and speed recovery.

MEMORY LOSS

For most adults, an occasional episode of forgetfulness is merely annoying, but for the elderly, it is an unwelcome sign of aging. In the extreme, memory loss can be very serious — bordering on amnesia. While this type of debility can often be attributed to stress, fatigue or poor nutrition, it can also be a symptom of Alzheimer's disease or a potentially fatal brain tumor, and should always be checked out by your doctor. However, if you just want to give your brain a quick boost, there are several simple steps you can take on your own.

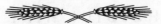

GINKGO Many people believe that ginkgo, a popular herbal remedy in Europe and in the U.S., has the ability to improve memory. Research conducted in France and all over Europe indicates that the herb acts by increasing blood flow to the brain and improving the oxygen supply to the heart and other organs. This boosts mental alertness.

LEMON Japanese scientists dispersed lemon oil around a room and found that it helped people concentrate. Typing mistakes, for example, were reduced by 54 percent. The scent apparently works by activating the hippocampus, an area in your brain that regulates smell, emotion and behavior.

Easily used with an aroma lamp, lemon oil also lessens psychological or emotional stress, which can interfere with memory.

ROSEMARY In ancient Greece, students often wore rosemary garlands to improve their memories. And rosemary tea improves blood circulation, which helps the brain function.

___ZINC___ Researchers theorize that a lack of zinc in your body may impair your memory. Studies conducted by Dr. Harold Sandstead of the University of Texas Medical Branch in Galveston show that adequate dietary zinc levels may improve the ability to recall words and visual designs. Food sources high in zinc include oysters, legumes, cereals, whole grains and dark-meat turkey.

Helpful Hint

If you want to remember something, write it down on a piece of yellow paper. According to Dr. Alexander Schauss, director of the American Institute for Biosocial Research in Tacoma, WA, his research into color therapy shows that yellow is the memory color.

MENOPAUSE

Menopause generally occurs between the ages of 45 and 55. During pre-menopause — the period before a woman's menses cease completely — the menstrual flow can be very irregular, ranging from excessively heavy to barely noticable, and PMS can become markedly pronounced. Symptoms include hot flashes, cramping, mood swings, depression, fatigue, night sweats and vaginal dryness. Less common symptoms include loss of muscle tone, puffy eyes, swollen ankles, loss of sex drive, and soreness in the back, hips, legs or feet.

The complaint most commonly associated with menopause is hot flashes — warm tingling sensations spreading upward through the body into the face, often accompanied by redness or sweating. Another common problem is vaginal dryness, which is caused by hormonal imbalances. Because the body produces less estrogen during menopause, the vagina produces fewer secretions. This starves the good bacteria in the genital area and allows an overgrowth of drying yeast to take over.

Although some women get through "the change" without any problems, most women do experience at least some discomfort. Only one thing is for sure when it comes to menopause — no two women are exactly the same. But, no matter how serious or how mild your symptoms are, you'll find relief by taking advantage of the international secrets we've gathered together in this section.

ALOE The juice of the aloe plant is readily available in bottled form at most health food stores. Try drinking some twice a day (some women add it to their favorite fruit juice) to help relieve the overall symptoms of menopause.

CHOLINE If mental sluggishness and forgetfulness plague you during menopause, supplementing with this mineral may solve the problem.

DONG QUAI The root of the plant known as dong quai (or tang kwei) is used by Chinese women to ease the general symptoms of menopause. Because it tastes good — sort of like celery — it is often included in Chinese recipes. Dong quai is also available in capsule form. Take 1 capsule, 3 times a day — or open the capsule and sprinkle the powder on your salad or soup.
CAUTION: *The Chinese say dong quai should never be taken with fruit or fruit juices. Also, be aware that stomach acidity affects this herb and can make it more potent.*

FENUGREEK Fenugreek is very safe — and it appears to have properties similar to estrogen. Fenugreek tea is a popular American folk remedy that can help alleviate menopausal symptoms. Just add 2 teaspoons of mashed seeds to 1 cup of boiling water and simmer for 10 minutes. Since fenugreek is an acquired taste, chances are you will want to add honey, lemon or mint.

NUTMEG A Jamaican recipe for easing excessive bleeding during menopause is to grate 1 ounce of nutmeg in 1 pint of white rum. Take 1 teaspoon 3 times a day as long as necessary.

FOR MOOD SWINGS, TRY:

CALCIUM This mineral is a calmative — and it helps prevent osteoporosis, a major concern for postmenopausal women.

CATNIP The natural sedative properties of catnip are as beneficial during menopause as they are during menses. Try combining equal parts of catnip and passionflower in a cup of boiling water for several minutes to make a relaxing, de-stressing herbal tea.

CHASTE BERRY Some menopausal women have found that a tea made of chaste berries helps fight off their fatigue. It also seems to have a balancing effect on the hormones that affect PMS symptoms.

CAUTION: *If you're going to try chaste berry tea, you need to drink it consistently once menopausal symptoms appear — and continue for the duration.*

GINSENG A general remedy for menopausal women, Siberian ginseng helps with symptoms as diverse as abdominal cramps and emotional imbalances.

LEMON BALM Add this soothing herb to a cup of St. John's wort tea. Just mix the two in equal parts in boiling water.

PASSIONFLOWER Combine this herb with chaste berries in a cup of tea to alleviate both fatigue and emotional imbalances during menopause.

ST. JOHN'S WORT St. John's wort tea has been used to treat menopausal mood swings for generations. The herb contains hypericin which is effective in treating depression.

SESAME OIL Don't eat it, rub it in. Sesame oil massaged into the pelvic region is reported to lessen the mental and emotional angst of menopausal PMS.

WILD YAM Indigenous to Mexico, the wild yam is used to balance raging hormones during menopause. For fastest absorption into the system, use creams or oils made with this plant.

FOR HOT FLASHES, TRY:

GINSENG Many women report that ginseng tea helps control hot flashes.

MOTHERWORT The minty taste of motherwort tea strengthens the uterus and nervous system. The herb helps lower blood pressure, lessen heart palpitations and reduce hot flashes.

PEPPERMINT Because of its ability to stimulate those nerve endings that sense cold, peppermint tea is a useful herb for balancing out the

Eat to Beat Menopause

■ **Clean up your diet.** Cut down on red meat, dairy products and carbonated beverages. Same goes for spicy foods, alcohol, very hot drinks and fatty foods, all of which increase your body's temperature.

■ **Avoid refined sugar.** The nervousness and anxiety associated with menopause is aggravated by sugar. Use fructose if you must use a sweetener — but it's really best to stick to fresh fruit to satisfy your sweet tooth.

■ **Avoid caffeine — especially chocolate.** Between the sugar and the caffeine content, chocolate is one of the worse things you can put in your body when you're going through menopause. Remember, you want to do everything you can to keep yourself "unwired."

■ **Eat yogurt.** During any hormonal change, yeast can overgrow in your system and cause painful cramping, severe PMS, gastrointestinal discomfort and many other problems. The acidophilus in yogurt (made with live cultures) helps the body keep yeast colonies under control. If you prefer, take acidophilus in tablet or powdered form.

■ **Take advantage of ancient Chinese wisdom.** Because the kidneys are responsible for detoxifying the body, Chinese healers have traditionally instructed menopausal women to eat black beans, chicken liver, oysters, clams and mussels, because they aid kidney function.

temperature of the body during hot flashes.

SAGE The earthy taste of sage tea will please your taste buds, while its medicinal properties take the fire out of your hot flashes.
CAUTION: *Too much sage tea can make you anemic, unless you supplement with iron.*

VITAMIN C Because it helps prevent flushing, vitamin C is recommended to stave off hot flashes. Eat plenty of fresh citrus fruit — and take a supplement. Since vitamin C is water-soluble and is eliminated from the body if not used immediately, it is best to take small quantities several times a day. Stick with the buffered tablets — vitamin C in the form of ascorbic acid can be irritating to the stomach when taken in these large quantities.

VITAMIN E Take an extra supplement of vitamin E if you're going through menopause, even if you're already taking a multivitamin. Vitamin E is said to help regulate body temperature, so it could minimize your episodes of hot flashes.

CAUTION: *Do not take vitamin E without your doctor's approval if you have any type of heart disease, high blood pressure or diabetes.*

WATER Water keeps your body cool, so have a big, icy glass of bottled or distilled H_2O beside you at all times.

FOR VAGINAL DRYNESS, TRY:

CALENDULA Creams containing calendula can help heal the irritated or cracked walls of the vagina if it becomes excessively dry.

COMFREY A poultice made of comfrey ("the healing herb") can soothe vaginal dryness when applied directly on the sore area.

VITAMIN E Vitamin E oil can be applied right from a capsule into the vagina to help soothe dryness and irritation.

WHEAT GERM OIL A natural lubricant, wheat germ oil can be inserted into the vagina to help heal soreness.

WARNING! Stay away from goldenseal if you suffer from vaginal dryness. This herb dries mucous membranes and will make the problem even worse.

Helpful Hints

■ **Exercise.** Even a brief walk every day will help get your blood circulating and kick up some endorphins to make you feel better. A regular aerobics class would be a better choice, especially if you combine it with some light weight-training.

■ **Stop smoking.** This unhealthy habit can upset your hormonal balance even further. (See page 451 for tips to help you quit.)

■ **Enjoy sex.** It keeps the vagina elastic and encourages blood flow to the area.

■ **Maintain a regular routine.** Go to bed at the same time every night, wake up at the same time every morning, and go for an after-dinner walk every evening.

■ **Keep yourself busy.** Take a class in something fun, start a hobby, do some volunteer work, or find something else to keep your days busy and your mind occupied.

■ **Relax.** Don't overdo, keep stress to a minimum — and be good to yourself.

■ **Meditate.** Try Transcendental Meditation (TM), T'ai chi, meditation tapes (either audio or video) — or even something as simple as watching the sun rise or set every day.

■ **Try yoga.** Yoga stimulates the entire body, from the mind to the muscles to the internal organs. By improving your circulation and breathing, yoga washes away the fatigue and depression that often accompany menopause. We recommend the Tree Pose, the Sun Salutation and the Bridge to energize, revitalize and balance your system.

For more information on yoga and step-by-step instructions for doing the Sun Salutation, turn to page 6.

MENSTRUAL PROBLEMS

Studies suggest that more than half of all women suffer from some sort of menstrual discomfort, making it the most common chronic female health problem. Symptoms include depression, irritability, abdominal cramps, headaches, nausea and diarrhea.

Cramping, the most common symptom, can range from mild uterine contractions to full-blown spasms of the pelvis that can be so severe they require bedrest. One recent theory is that an overgrowth of yeast (a fungus known as candida) in the body may cause or aggravate this situation. So, if you have lengthy, severe cramping episodes during your period, you may want to check out whether a yeast infection might be causing some of your discomfort. And always keep in mind that debilitating or unbearable pain should never be endured. If you're losing sleep or work every month, see a doctor immediately to rule out any serious complications.

Some researchers believe there is a link between menstrual problems and an overproduction of prostaglandins in the body that regulate (among other things) muscle contractions, digestive processes and the release of sex hormones. Western medicine offers many manufactured drugs that slow or stop the body's production of prostaglandins — ibuprofen and naproxen sodium, for example. But there are many other, more natural ways to deal with the painful symptoms of menstruation.

ALLSPICE This tasty spice from Jamaica provides relief from cramps when taken as a hot tea. Just add 2 teaspoons of allspice powder to a cup of boiling water. Steep at least 10 minutes and enjoy the aromatic smell of cloves, cinnamon, pepper and juniper while you wait for this tonic to take effect.

ALOE The soothing juice of the aloe vera plant helps relieve cramping for some women. Add the juice to your favorite fruit juice or mix it in water.

AMARANTH Amaranth, a 3-foot-high plant with bright red and purple flowers, is a natural astringent (which inhibits bleeding). In France, the highly nutritious leaves are cooked and eaten like spinach to prevent cramps and heavy bleeding during menstruation.

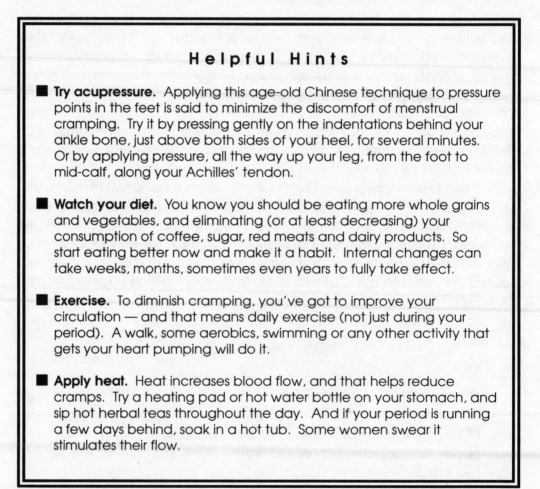

Helpful Hints

■ **Try acupressure.** Applying this age-old Chinese technique to pressure points in the feet is said to minimize the discomfort of menstrual cramping. Try it by pressing gently on the indentations behind your ankle bone, just above both sides of your heel, for several minutes. Or by applying pressure, all the way up your leg, from the foot to mid-calf, along your Achilles' tendon.

■ **Watch your diet.** You know you should be eating more whole grains and vegetables, and eliminating (or at least decreasing) your consumption of coffee, sugar, red meats and dairy products. So start eating better now and make it a habit. Internal changes can take weeks, months, sometimes even years to fully take effect.

■ **Exercise.** To diminish cramping, you've got to improve your circulation — and that means daily exercise (not just during your period). A walk, some aerobics, swimming or any other activity that gets your heart pumping will do it.

■ **Apply heat.** Heat increases blood flow, and that helps reduce cramps. Try a heating pad or hot water bottle on your stomach, and sip hot herbal teas throughout the day. And if your period is running a few days behind, soak in a hot tub. Some women swear it stimulates their flow.

BLACKBERRY The juice of this berry is reputed to slow down a heavy blood flow during menstruation.

BLACK COHOSH Black cohosh is a cramp-relieving herb that dates back to colonial days. Native Americans brewed the herb into a tea.

BROMELAIN Found naturally in pineapple plants, this enzyme works as an anti-inflammatory against menstrual cramping. Women who take bromelain in capsule form prior to the start of their periods report a reduction in swelling and pain.

CALCIUM In addition to its highly touted use for preventing osteoporosis in aging bones, calcium is beneficial to the muscles. Because it is a natural relaxant, it eases cramping.

CARAWAY Greek women drink caraway tea to relieve menstrual cramps. To brew the tea, grind or crush 1 teaspoon of seeds and steep in 1 cup of boiling water.

CATNIP Relaxing catnip tea is a good tonic for cramp relief. Boil a cup of water, add 1 teaspoon of catnip and steep for 5 minutes.

CHAMOMILE French women swear by chamomile tea to relieve their menstrual symptoms. They claim it not only works on cramps, it also lessens the emotional stress. The Greeks and the Romans, too, believed in the ability of chamomile to soothe the cramps of painful periods. And, indeed, chamomile does have antispasmodic action.

CHASTE BERRIES This herb (which has been around since the time of the ancient Romans) is known for helping a variety of menstrual problems — from irregular cycles to irregular blood flow. It is available as a tea or tincture, and in capsule form.

CHINESE ANGELICA A 2,000-year-old Chinese medical book, *Shen-nung Pen Ts'ao Chingar*, describes a time-tested remedy for menstrual difficulties using Chinese angelica or "women's ginseng" — and the plant is still used today to relieve a host of gynecological problems. It has antispasmodic action that eases painful cramping. It is most effective, though, in the treatment of menstrual irregularity.

CRAMP BARK Cramp bark is a muscle and nerve relaxant that prevents (you guessed it!) menstrual cramps. Native Americans called it squaw bush and used it for that very purpose. To try it, drink 2 cups of cramp bark tea daily, starting a week before your period is expected to begin. Prepare the tea by steeping a teaspoon of the herb in a cup of boiled water for about 7 minutes. Strain and drink.
CAUTION: *The berries of the cramp bark tree are poisonous.*

DONG QUAI This herb (which is also called Chinese celery) is used by Chinese women to regulate their periods and relieve menstrual cramps.
CAUTION: *Don't use dong quai when you're eating fruit or drinking fruit juices. And be forewarned that changes in stomach acidity can change the properties of this herb — and make it more potent.*

FEVERFEW In Ancient Greek times, feverfew was used to ease childbirth. More recently, people learned that this medicinal herb can also alleviate menstrual cramps when taken regularly.

GINGER The Chinese treat menstrual pain with a tea made from dried gingerroot boiled in water, along with equal amounts of brown sugar and seeded red dates. Ginger increases blood circulation — and that can relieve spasms in the uterus.

LEMON BALM Lemon balm tea helps menstrual cramping. It relaxes the body and has a sedative effect on the nervous system. Simply add 2 teaspoons of chopped lemon balm to 1 cup of boiling water. Drink as needed.

RASPBERRY The Chinese were the first to discover that the leaves of the raspberry bush have medicinal value. Centuries later, the English found that these leaves can be brewed into a tea that relieves menstrual cramps.
An added benefit: Raspberry leaves are an excellent source of

calcium, iron, phosphorous and vitamins A, B, C and E. A woman's body is often depleted of these important nutrients during menstruation, and drinking raspberry-leaf tea is an excellent way to restore them.

SAGE Sage tea was believed by the Ancient Greeks to slow heavy bleeding during menstruation.

VALERIAN Valerian is a medicinal herb that is usually prescribed for muscle relaxation, stress or insomnia. The fragile pink and white flower of the plant contains a natural antispasmodic that also helps reduce cramping. Valerian was used for thousands of years by people in ancient Greece and China. It was then introduced in Europe, Canada, Australia, New Zealand and (most recently) the U.S.

VITAMIN A An antioxidant, vitamin A not only speeds healing, it also regulates and controls heavy bleeding.

VITAMIN C Vitamin C, which is essential for a healthy body, is said to help regulate menstrual cycles and lessen heavy blood flows. This could be because menstrual irregularities sometimes result from poor nutrition.

VITAMIN E In addition to its many other healing benefits, vitamin E helps minimize cramping. Not only does it help circulation, it also inhibits the development of prostaglandins.

WILD YAM Do as they did in Colonial times and make yourself some wild yam tea to relieve menstrual cramping. Simply steep 1 teaspoon of wild yam root in a cup of water for 30 minutes.

MIGRAINE HEADACHES

Migraines are excrutiatingly painful headaches that can last for a few moments or a few days. They tend to surface between the ages of 10 and 30 — twice as often in women as in men — and then mysteriously stop around age 50. During an episode, the eyes are very sensitive to light, and hearing seems heightened. Migraines can also be accompanied by nausea and vomiting, diarrhea, or a tingling sensation in the arms and legs. Many migraine sufferers say they can "feel one coming on" because they see flashes of light or get blind spots. Others say they slip into a negative frame of mind that can range from sadness to anger to just plain lethargy.

Roughly one-third of all migraines are thought to be caused primarily by food allergies. Other factors include low blood sugar (hypoglycemia), stress, genetics, strong odors or smoke, and pollutants and chemical irritants. Identifying — and then avoiding — the "trigger" that causes your migraine is the best thing you can do for this condition, because once the headache is in full force, little can be done. Still, we have some suggestions that can help prevent, or at least lessen the intensity of, a flare-up.

AGRIMONY This liver-detoxifying herb may help prevent migraines.

ALMONDS Indigenous to North Africa and western Asia, almonds are readily available in American markets. These tasty nuts have a pain-relieving ingredient in them — similar to aspirin — that can be used to ease migraines.

BEE PROPOLIS This brown resin is loaded with vitamins, minerals, amino acids and enzymes — a whole lot of nutrition in one package that can help prevent some migraines.

Helpful Hints

■ **Eat balanced meals at regular intervals** — or suffer the agony of a migraine brought on by nutritional deprivation. Your system is very delicate, and you simply can't skip meals or eat poorly.

■ **Exercise.** Everyone benefits from aerobic exercise. And if you are subject to migraines, it must be incorporated into your daily routine to strengthen your cardiovascular system.

■ **Keep a journal.** Keep track of your day-to-day habits, and you may find that you can prevent your headaches simply by making a few simple lifestyle changes. Write down what you did, what you ate, when you ate it, what kind of mood you were in, etc. — and, chances are, you'll notice a pattern that will identify your migraine trigger. For most people, that trigger is food — at least one of the following:
• Monosodium glutimate or MSG — a flavor enhancer widely used in Chinese restaurants and in many commercially packaged foods
• Yeast
• Aspartame ("Nutrasweet"), or cane sugar
• Sodium nitrate (used in most aged, cured or deli meats, such as hot dogs, cold cuts, bacon, etc.)
• Alcohol (especially wine, beer, Scotch and cognac)

CALCIUM Calcium is an important supplement even for people who don't get migraines. It is best taken at night, because calcium has a calming effect on the body and helps promote sleep. That same calming effect helps migraine sufferers by relaxing muscles in the head and easing tightening in the temples.

CHROMIUM If you suffer from low blood sugar or hypoglycemia, you are a likely candidate for a migraine — and a chromium supplement can help you.

EVENING PRIMROSE Herbalists say that the oil of the evening primrose, when taken in capsule form twice a day, can help loosen the tight muscles that accompany a migraine.

- Caffeine (in coffee, tea, caffeinated sodas and chocolate)
- Tyramine (in over-ripe bananas, avocados, chicken livers and fava beans)
- Plums, pineapples, apples, grapes, oranges or tomatoes
- Potatoes, eggplant, cabbage, corn or onions
- Dairy products
- Nuts
- Soy products, including tofu and miso
- Eggs, fish, beef or pork
- Some grains (like wheat, oats and rye)

■ **Try a little color therapy.** Blue and green lights seem to be the most soothing colors for migraine sufferers.

■ **Use heat.** Some migraine patients claim that immersing their hands in extremely hot water seems to minimize the pain.

■ **Try an acupressure massage.** This ancient Chinese remedy for treating migraines has proven effective for countless people. It relieves tension while it loosens tight muscles and encourages the release of endorphins (natural de-stressers) in your system.

FEVERFEW This member of the daisy family has been used extensively in Europe to treat migraines — and studies in both Europe and the U.S. have shown that this herb unquestionably relieves the pain. Feverfew has an anti-inflammatory agent that helps dilate the tight, constricted blood vessels that are characteristic of migraines. It also contains a compound that stops blood vessel spasms from occurring.

Feverfew is most effective if taken in capsule form every day as a preventive. However, it is still helpful during a flare-up — and its healing properties are multiplied if it is combined with the tincture of a natural sedative like valerian or Jamaican dogwood.

CAUTION: *Although you can chew 1 small feverfew leaf every day to prevent migraines, some people develop sores in their mouths from this practice. You may want to try the capsule form, instead. Also, stay away* *from feverfew if you're on the medication Warfarin.*

___**FISH OIL** Omega-3 fish oils have natural anti-inflammatory properties that ease the pain of a migraine headache without the need for aspirin (which can actually aggravate the condition).

___**GINGER** Ginger has an agent that relaxes muscle spasms and lessens the tightness that is brought on by a migraine attack.

___**LAVENDER** Not only does this flower have a delightful scent, it is a natural sedative, analgesic and antispasmodic. So make yourself a soothing rub of 1 part lavender oil mixed with 2 parts of virgin olive oil, and massage it on your throbbing temples.
CAUTION: *Lavender is also effective when taken as a tea — but don't drink too much of it if you're pregnant.*

___**MAGNESIUM** Many migraine sufferers may be victims of a magnesium deficiency. So try supplementing with this essential mineral if you're prone to this condition.

MOTION SICKNESS

Motion sickness is caused when the body's equilibrium becomes unbalanced while riding in some sort of a vehicle — a car, a boat, an airplane, etc. This is usually due to an ear infection, or to a reaction to conflicting sensory information — confusion between the brain and body as to the source of the motion. The resulting discomfort can be as mild as lightheadedness, dizziness or a queasy stomach, or as severe as nausea, vomiting or cold sweats.

There are many over-the-counter remedies for motion sickness. However, they do not offer relief without the risk of side effects. Dramamine, for example, can make you groggy. That's why it's much better to counteract motion sickness with the following safe, natural alternatives that we've rounded up for you.

CRACKERS If you're nauseated (a common symptom of motion sickness), the bicarbonate in soda crackers will absorb the stomach acid that's upsetting your stomach.

GINGER In one recent study, ginger effectively eliminated or reduced motion sickness in approximately 75 percent of the cases. So try one of the following methods to take advantage of the ability of this amazing root to help you avoid — or eliminate — the symptoms of motion sickness.

■ The Chinese prescribe ginger powder mixed with water to keep sea-sickness at bay during long voyages.

■ In Hong Kong, sailors munch on dried gingerroot when on board.

■ If you're prone to motion sickness, plan ahead. Suck on a few pieces of crystallized ginger about 2 hours before you're scheduled to travel by boat, plane or car — and pop another piece into your mouth, as needed, throughout your journey.

■ If you don't like the taste of ginger, take it in the form of gelatin capsules (which are available at most health food stores). Take one 2500 mg. capsule just before you embark on your trip.

Helpful Hints

■ **Avoid alcohol.** In fact, if you tend to feel queasy when riding in a vehicle, avoid all liquids except for ginger ale or raspberry juice.

■ **Eat small meals while traveling.** Big meals and heavy foods can aggravate motion sickness.

■ **If you're riding in a car, sit in the front seat** or in the middle of the back seat — and focus on the horizon instead of looking off to the side.

■ **If you're riding on a boat, the middle of the deck** has the least motion. If you start feeling nauseous, don't go below deck. Stay up top in the fresh air and focus on the horizon.

■ **If you're riding on an airplane, sit near the front** so you won't feel as much motion during take-off and landing. Some people who suffer from motion sickness find that they are most comfortable if they sit between the wings, in the middle aisle.

■ **Try acupressure.** At the first sign of nausea, acupressure can help squelch the feeling. Press the area on your hand between the thumb and the forefinger for several minutes and then switch hands. Also try massaging the tendons between the second and third toes on the top of each foot.
  Modern Chinese doctors prescribe a type of acupressure wristband that uses no medication. Here's how it works: When motion sickness starts to set in, you press a button on the band that applies pressure to a point on your wrist, giving you immediate relief.

■ Make ginger tea by mixing ½ teaspoon of dried ginger in a cup of hot water. Or, use 1 teaspoon of fresh ginger juice (made by grating fresh gingerroot and squeezing out the liquid).

■ Drink ginger ale. This therapeutic beverage soothes every kind of stomach distress.

OLIVES

An early sign of motion sickness is excessive salivation, which in turn upsets the stomach. Early Americans found that eating olives dries the mouth and effectively wards off nausea.

RASPBERRIES

Drink the juice of freshly squeezed raspberries just before — and while — traveling. This should help prevent dizziness and curb the frequent urination that often accompanies motion sickness.

MUSCLE ACHES

Though achy, tender muscles can be the result of a nutritional imbalance or pure physical exhaustion, they are more often caused by simple overexertion. (Lactic acid can build up in your muscles and cause soreness when you exercise.) Your best bet is to use common sense while exercising, by getting enough rest and by eating properly. Even so, you're bound to overdo it from time to time — and when you do, you'll find that pain relief is easy using our natural approach to healing.

_____ **ARNICA** Used externally, arnica can soothe sore muscles when rubbed directly on the area in pain. Either purchase tincture of arnica or make your own by soaking whole decimated plants in alcohol.

_____ **BUTTERMILK** In Bulgaria, the treatment for sore muscles is hot compresses soaked in buttermilk. If buttermilk is not available, Bulgarians use sour milk, which they claim is almost as effective. Both are non-acidic and soothing to the skin.

_____ **CAMPHOR** Italians combine equal parts of olive oil and camphor and rub it in. This simple home remedy is the basis for many over-the-counter preparations available in the U.S. Camphor works by increasing blood circulation to the skin.

_____ **CHAMOMILE** Used medicinally since the 16th century, chamomile is one of the top 5 best-selling herbs in the U.S. It is an antispasmodic when taken internally and makes a wonderfully soothing bath — and, when prepared as an oil-based rub, is excellent for muscle aches.
  Here's the way they do it in many Mediterranean countries: Fill a

glass jar with chamomile flowers and add enough olive oil to fill the jar. Screw down the cap tightly and leave in the sun for 3 weeks, adding more olive oil and flowers as the mixture settles. Strain off the oil, pressing the flowers to extract the last drop.

CHINESE TIGER BALM In China, muscle aches are relieved with a preparation called Chinese Tiger Balm. This healing ointment contains oils of camphor, menthol, peppermint, clove and cajeput.

GINGER In Japan, they use ginger to heal aching muscles and relieve tightness by making ginger oil and applying it directly to the sore area. Just grate some fresh gingerroot and squeeze the juice into a bowl. Mix with an equal amount of olive oil and massage into the skin.

Many Asians also use ginger in the bath. To try it, grate about 1 teaspoon of fresh ginger and squeeze the juice directly into your bathwater. Soak until the water cools. The aromatic scent will delight your senses, while the healing liquid soothes your pain.

LAVENDER OIL A massage with lavender oil will relax muscles and ease soreness.

Hot baths help soothe muscle aches. Add dried rosemary, peppermint or chamomile to the bathwater for an even more relaxing experiense. (Use a tea ball to avoid clogging the drain.)

_____ **ONION** Russians recommend a mixture of chopped onions and honey to soothe muscle aches. (No, you don't have to eat it — just smear it on.)

_____ **POTASSIUM** This important mineral is readily found in many common fruits and vegetables. So when you're achy or sore, up your consumption of bananas, which have one of the highest potassium levels of all foods. Other good food sources of potassium include cantaloupes, oranges, avocados, raw spinach, raw cabbage and raw celery.

_____ **TEA TREE OIL** Australian tea tree oil is often used as a rub for sore muscles. Massaging the oil into the sore area increases blood flow to the underlying muscle.

_____ **VINEGAR** The British consider vinegar compresses to be the best way to relieve muscle aches.

MUSCLE CRAMPS

Though physical exhaustion, improper nutrition and poor general health can cause muscle tightness and cramping, it usually occurs as the result of overexertion. Other contributing factors include smoking, drinking alcohol, or working out when the weather is too hot or humid.

The most common reason for cramping is muscle fatigue combined with an imbalance of salt and water in the body. This is why athletes drink plenty of water and drinks like Gatorade, which help restore proper levels of salt (and other minerals) to the body.

So always take a water bottle with you when you're going to be working under high-heat conditions or exercising vigorously. And take advantage of the rest of the cramp-busting secrets we've gathered below to protect yourself from these painful spasms.

CALCIUM Calcium, an essential nutrient for your muscles, helps prevent cramping.

CHAMOMILE When prepared as an oil-based rub, chamomile helps alleviate muscle cramps. Try the same recipe we gave you on page 375 of Muscle Aches.

CHINESE TIGER BALM In China, muscle cramps are relieved with the herbal ointment known as Chinese Tiger Balm.

CRAMP BARK Also used for alleviating menstrual cramps, this herb is a good muscle relaxant. Apply straight tincture of cramp bark directly to the cramped area. Or, if you prefer, mix it with some skin cream first.

_____ **GINGER** Not only does ginger help soothe muscle aches, it can also relieve cramping.

_____ **HONEY** In Scotland, people with cramps in their legs and feet eat honey to curb the pain. Honey contains magnesium, a natural painkiller.

_____ **NIACIN** A member of the B-family, niacin helps promote blood flow and can minimize muscle cramping. Start with small quantities — less than 250 mgs per day — and be sure to take with food to avoid possible side effects like flushing and itchy skin.

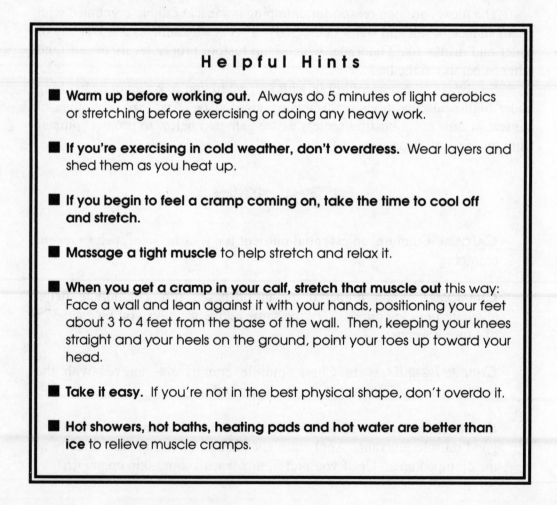

Helpful Hints

■ **Warm up before working out.** Always do 5 minutes of light aerobics or stretching before exercising or doing any heavy work.

■ **If you're exercising in cold weather, don't overdress.** Wear layers and shed them as you heat up.

■ **If you begin to feel a cramp coming on, take the time to cool off and stretch.**

■ **Massage a tight muscle** to help stretch and relax it.

■ **When you get a cramp in your calf, stretch that muscle out** this way: Face a wall and lean against it with your hands, positioning your feet about 3 to 4 feet from the base of the wall. Then, keeping your knees straight and your heels on the ground, point your toes up toward your head.

■ **Take it easy.** If you're not in the best physical shape, don't overdo it.

■ **Hot showers, hot baths, heating pads and hot water are better than ice** to relieve muscle cramps.

ONION Try an onion poultice applied directly to the cramp. Simply mix some chopped onion with some salt, wrap the mixture in a piece of thin, soft cloth, and apply it to the sore area.

WITCH HAZEL A remedy used by American Indians for muscle cramps is extract of witch hazel bark. They mix this natural astringent with sunflower oil and rub it on their muscles until the pain goes away. This stimulates blood circulation without causing irritation to the skin. Witch hazel extract is available at health food stores.

NAIL CARE

In every culture around the world and throughout history, society has dictated the way nails should look. For example, in both ancient Egypt and China, different nail colors were used to signify social status. No ancient Egyptian dared to wear the colors reserved for the king and the queen. And Egyptian military leaders prepared for battle by having their hair curled and lacquered, and their nails painted to match their lips.

Fashion sometimes calls for us to wear our nails long, pointed, and/or brightly colored. Other times, it has us trim them short and square and coat them with clear or natural polish. But, whether they are long, short, plain or fancy, nails must first and foremost be strong and shiny. And the only way to achieve this is with a healthy diet.

BARLEY The Chinese eat fried, ground barley seeds to keep their nails strong. Barley seeds contain vitamins and minerals that are important building blocks for healthy nails.

BLACK CURRANT A Scottish study showed that black currant oil is very effective for healthy nail growth. Weak and brittle nails can be strengthened by the gamma linoleic acid found in the oil. A supplement of 500 milligrams twice a day is recommended. You should see results within 2 months.

HONEY According to Dr. Alfred Vogel in his book, The Nature Doctor, you can treat inflammation around the fingernails and toenails with honey (which has antibacterial properties) mixed with a dash of horseradish. This natural remedy is also good for nail molds and other conditions of the skin that usually take a long time to heal.

KELP Nails are almost 97 percent protein. When healthy, they are highly resistant to tearing or breaking. However, dietary deficiencies can make nails brittle. The Chinese, Japanese and Scottish all avoid brittle nails by eating lots of mineral-rich kelp, which provides nutrients vital for strong nails.

MILK Milk is loaded with vitamin D, B12 and protein — all necessary for healthy nails.

SWEET POTATO Because sweet potatoes are loaded with B-vitamins and beta-carotene, eat them to help restore damaged nails.

TEA TREE OIL Australian tea tree oil is often used as a rub for sore muscles, but it is even better as a natural treatment for fungal infections of the skin, toenails or fingernails. The clear liquid is very aromatic with a smell similar to that of eucalyptus, another medicinal Australian plant. And, unlike conventional drugs that are used to treat nail fungus, tea tree oil is not toxic and has no unpleasant side effects.

Just paint a light coating of the oil on the affected area 3 or 4 times a day. Even if the fungus seems to have disappeared, continue treatment for 2 weeks. It may take a while for a healthy nail to start growing in. (Take zinc with this treatment to make it even more effective.)
CAUTION: *When you purchase tea tree oil (available in most health food and herb stores), make sure the label says that it is pure.*

VITAMIN A Vitamin A supplements or eating foods rich in beta-carotene have helped some people improve dry, damaged nails. Carrots and dark-green, leafy vegetables are good sources of this nutrient.

VITAMIN B A study conducted recently in Switzerland found that nails become stronger with the help of the B vitamin biotin.

VITAMIN D Ten minutes of sunlight a day is an easy, inexpensive way to get all the vitamin D you'll ever need. If you live in a cold, rainy climate, get your vitamin D from dairy products, canned salmon or fortified whole-grain cereals.

Home Care for Ingrown Toenails

Most people suffer from an occasional ingrown toenail, a condition that is far from serious, even though it feels like it ought to be. Though any toe can be affected, the problem usually strikes the big toe. The tenderness, swelling, pain, redness and infection can be caused by many factors — shoes that are too tight, an impact or injury to the nail, cutting into the skin when trimming toenails, or a misshapen nail.

Most ingrown toenails can be easily treated at home, although they often take several days to heal. Only rarely is surgery required to remove either part or all of the afflicted nail — and this should be considered only if the condition is chronic and is caused by a permanently deformed nail.

To avoid ingrown toenails:

■ Wear loose-fitting shoes, preferably open-toed, as often as possible. And if you're prone to ingrown toenails, avoid high heels, especially those with pointy toes. Wearing socks helps too.

■ Keep your toenails clean and dry.

■ Keep your toenails trimmed, but don't cut them down too short or your skin may grow over the top of the nail. Never round your toenails. Cut them straight across with a nail clipper.

If you do get an ingrown toenail:

■ Stay off your feet as much as possible.

■ Dry, brittle nails are more painful, so soak your feet several times a day in warm water to keep them soft and supple.

■ Watch for symptoms of serious infection. Excessive pus or excruciating pain are signs that you need to see a doctor immediately for treatment. This is especially important if you are elderly, if you have circulatory problems, or if you're diabetic.

VITAMIN E Vitamin E helps skin and nails retain moisture, so it's effective in keeping nails from becoming brittle.

WHEAT GERM Nutritionalists often advise people to put some wheat germ into just about anything they eat or drink. The B vitamins and vitamin E in wheat germ will help strengthen your nails.

Helpful Hint

■ To keep your nails in good condition, treat your fingertips like skin — from the tip of your nail to the cuticle base — by gently washing and moisturizing regularly.

■ Remember that dry nails (and cuticles) break, crack, tear and split more easily than wet ones, so, before doing any grooming or cutting, be sure to soak them in warm water.

■ To help heal damaged or brittle nails, soak them nightly for about 15 minutes while relaxing or watching TV. Then, apply your favorite moisturizer.

   Here's a good moisturizing lotion for nails that you can make at home: Warm ½ cup of olive oil over low or medium heat and then add 2 tablespoons of dillseed and 1 teaspoon of wheat germ. Pour into a bottle and keep the bottle in a cool, dark place for a week or so, and then strain.

■ When you work on your cuticles, don't use metal tools. Instead, push them back with your fingers (making sure that you have first softened them thoroughly by soaking in warm water).

NAUSEA

Nausea can be caused by a number of things — a virus, overindulgence in food or alcohol, or even stress. When you're nauseated, there is little else you can think about. Your stomach feels queasy, your breath feels hot, and you can't even stand the thought of food, let alone the sight of it. Fortunately, this unpleasant condition is almost always short-lived and usually goes away without requiring any medical treatment.

Because nausea and vomiting (which can cause serious dehydration) are early warning signs of many serious diseases, see a doctor if your nausea lasts an especially long time, or is accompanied by faintness, fever or severe pain. However, most cases of nausea do not require professional attention and can be relieved without using expensive, foul-tasting, store-bought remedies. Ease your discomfort with the simple home remedies listed below. And, for additional ways to deal with nausea, see Vomiting on page 503, Motion Sickness on page 371, and Morning Sickness on page 413.

ARROWROOT There probably aren't many poisoned arrows zinging around the jungles of Central and South America these days. Which means that there's no longer much of a need for an antidote for arrow poison. Yet arrowroot, which once served this purpose for the Mayans, is still used by the residents of these regions in baking.

Arrowroot provides a rich source of natural calcium and carbohydrates, and is also excellent for soothing the stomach. Sometimes the powder is dissolved in a beverage to treat nausea, vomiting or bowel troubles.

BAKING SODA Women who live in the South and Southwest drink water mixed with baking soda to relieve nausea. This reportedly works by neutralizing stomach acids.

CINNAMON A recipe still used today to treat nausea in the Near East harks back to the time of King Solomon. The king's herbalist ground 3 small cinnamon sticks or one 6-inch stick of cinnamon bark with 1 tablespoon (about 8 seeds) of cardamom seed. He probably used a mortar and pestle, but you can use a nut grinder, coffee grinder or blender. Place the mixture in a labeled jar, and use 1 teaspoon in a cup of hot tea for relief.

GINGER Chinese cooks chew gingerroot to reduce the feeling of nausea caused by being exposed to cooking fumes all day. You can make ginger tea by mixing ½ teaspoon of dried ginger in 1 cup of tea. Or, you can take ginger in the form of gelatin capsules, available at most health food stores.

GINGER ALE Americans invented ginger ale to treat nausea — probably inspired by Chinese immigrants who brought ginger with them by boat to the western coast of the early U.S., and used ginger tea to soothe upset stomachs.

GRAPEFRUIT A Chinese remedy for nausea is to drink tea made from fresh grapefruit peel. Tangy or bitter tasting foods or liquids often relieve nausea.

MUSTARD SEEDS The French eat whole mustard seeds to treat nausea.

OLIVE Early Americans consumed olives at the first hint of nausea — which is usually excessive salivation. Tannin, the primary component in olives, helps to dry the mouth and minimize this excess liquid that adds to stomach queasiness.

PEACH The Chinese drink peach tea to relieve nausea. They have revered the peach tree for its medicinal value since the fifth century, when Confucius mentioned it in his writings. In fact, the Chinese character that represents the peach tree is one of the oldest in the Chinese alphabet — and is often seen on ancient Chinese sculptures.

PEPPERMINT Peppermint, which is useful for treating indigestion, provides a volatile oil that the British use as both a flavoring agent and a medicine for nausea.

RASPBERRIES To curb morning sickness and nausea, the British and Chinese both recommend a daily dose of raspberry leaf tea. One Chinese tea recipe calls for 1 pint of boiled water poured over 2 rounded teaspoons of dried raspberry leaves. Steep, strain and drink throughout the day.

SODA CRACKERS Soda crackers are a saving grace for those experiencing nausea. Made with bicarbonate of soda and cream of tartar, which neutralize and absorb stomach acid, soda crackers also help minimize dry heaves. For the best, fastest relief possible, don't drink anything with them — not even water.

VINEGAR An old New England nausea remedy is to drink a glass of water with a teaspoonful of slightly acidic apple cider vinegar mixed in.

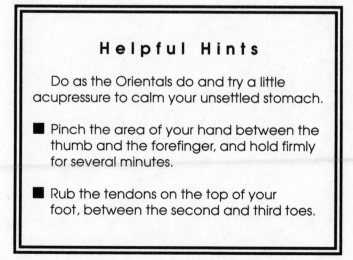

Helpful Hints

Do as the Orientals do and try a little acupressure to calm your unsettled stomach.

■ Pinch the area of your hand between the thumb and the forefinger, and hold firmly for several minutes.

■ Rub the tendons on the top of your foot, between the second and third toes.

NOSEBLEEDS

A nosebleed is generally caused by the rupture of a blood vessel or capillary inside the nose. It can be the result of an infection or a blow to the nose — or even the result of a strong sneeze.

If your nosebleed is profuse or does not stop after about 30 minutes, call your doctor. You should also consult your doctor to rule out a serious underlying medical problem if you have recurring nosebleeds. And if headache, dizziness, fever, unconsciousness or the possibility of a fracture accompanies the bleeding, go to the emergency room immediately. However, in most cases a nosebleed can be easily and simply treated with the following natural remedies.

BANANA A Chinese antidote for nosebleeds is to boil 40 grams of banana peel and corn silks in water, and then drink the potion when it cools slightly.

CALENDULA Dab a bit of calendula oil onto a cottonball and gently sniff while you're experiencing a nosebleed.

CHIVES Squeeze the liquid out of fresh chives and drink a small cup twice a day if you have a tendency to get nosebleeds.

ONION Chinese doctors report that inserting a cottonball soaked in onion juice helps stop nosebleeds. Just take an onion leaf and cut it open. Then, rub a cottonball onto the leaf until it becomes moistened with the juice. Squeeze the liquid out of the cottonball and into the nose for instant results.

St. John's wort This multi-purpose root is an effective astringent that will halt nosebleeds when sniffed from a cottonball.

Vinegar To stop a nosebleed, drinking a bit of vinegar water is reputed to help.

Helpful Hints

■ **Lean forward.** In order to keep blood flow from draining back into your throat, bend forward.

■ **Apply cold compresses.** While bending forward, apply an ice pack or some other cold compress to the back and sides of your neck.
Since cold helps to constrict blood vessels, an ice pack or cloth filled with ice cubes placed directly on the nose can also help.

■ **Don't blow.** The worst thing you can do during a nosebleed is blow your nose. This could dislodge any clotting that has occurred as part of the natural healing process. The same goes for inhaling — so sniff anti-nosebleed remedies very gently.

■ **Don't pick.** Nose picking is one of the foremost causes of nosebleeds — especially in children. So teach yours to gently blow their noses to keep them clean.

■ **Hold your nose.** Sometimes just pinching the sides of your nostrils for several minutes will stop the bleeding. Hold your nose firmly just beneath the boney part for at least 5 minutes — maybe as long as 15 or 20 minutes — to encourage clotting.

■ **Humidify.** Dry air can cause nosebleeds. So use a humidifier to put moisture back in the air when conditions are dry — especially during winter months when your heater is running full blast.

■ **Sit up.** During a heavy nosebleed, it's easier to control the blood flow and keep it from getting into your throat (and possibly choking you) if you sit up straight.

_____**VITAMIN C** If you have recurring nosebleeds, increase your intake of vitamin C.

_____**WITCH HAZEL** Saturate a cottonball with this natural astringent and sniff it to stop a nosebleed.

_____**YARROW** Soak a cottonball in yarrow and then take as many whiffs as necessary to stop the bleeding.

OSTEOPOROSIS

Osteoporosis (porous bones) is a debilitating condition that we generally associate with elderly women. However, though it strikes many more women than men, it has become fairly commonplace in both genders. Osteoporosis is usually the result of years of poor nutrition and lack of exercise.

Though it is not the only culprit, lack of calcium is cited as the main cause of osteoporosis. According to Dr. Robert Willix, a recent study by the National Institutes of Health found that half of all Americans are literally starving their bones of calcium — they're not even getting half the amount their bodies require. As a result, there are 25 million cases of brittle bones seen every year in this country that cause 1.5 million fractures and lead to annual health-care costs of $10 billion.

Protecting your bones is not simply a matter of popping a calcium supplement every day. To minimize bone loss as you age, you need to follow a complete program that includes a healthy diet along with regular exercise. Remember, the best remedy for osteoporosis is prevention — and there are many sensible, natural ways to achieve this goal.

- **Eat dairy.** Eat plenty of calcium-rich foods, especially milk products (unless you have an allergy or candida problem).

- **Eat your greens.** Load up on lots of green, leafy vegetables. They're not as excellent a source of calcium as dairy products, but they're still pretty good. To give you an idea of how they measure up, 2 ½ cups of broccoli is roughly equivalent to a glass of milk.

- **Avoid sugar.** A lack of phosphorous inhibits calcium absorption — and an excessive amount of refined sugar in your system will wreak havoc with your phosophorous level.

- **Avoid alcohol.** When consumed in excess, alcohol affects the

EXERCISE!

It's never too late to start exercising. One of the best ways to build new bone is to get moving. Walking, running, jogging, cycling, climbing stairs, dancing, playing tennis, jumping rope and playing racquetball are all bone-building and strengthening aerobic exercises. The recommended workout is 3 times a week, for 30 minutes each time.

■ Supplement your aerobic workouts with 2 days of light-weight training — a great way to increase your bone mass. Start light, and build up to comfortable weights for all parts of your body. The stronger the muscles around the bones, the stronger the bones will be to support the muscles.

Studies have shown that women who did weight-bearing exercises 3 times a week increased their bone mass significantly. As reported by Dr. Robert Willix, one study found that one exercising woman boosted her bones mass by 5.2 percent, while her sedentary sisters lost 1.2 percent of their bone mass during the same period.

■ If you have arthritis, choose an exercise that's gentler on your joints. Though not as effective as a combination of aerobics and weight-training, exercycling or using a NordicTrack machine can provide fairly good bone-building activity. You can also do pool exercises. You weigh only about 15 percent of your land weight when you're in the water, so you can do a whole workout regimen in a pool without damaging your joints — but greatly improving your bones.

gastrointestinal tract and limits its ability to absorb nutrients such as calcium. Alcohol also impairs liver function, limiting the production of vitamin D, which is essential for healthy bone mass.

■ **Supplement with boron.** This trace mineral appears to play an important role in the body's assimilation process of not only calcium, but also magnesium, phosphorus and vitamin D. Boron can be purchased in tablet form at health food stores.

■ **Limit animal protein.** Most Americans eat twice as much animal protein as they should. Because this kind of diet makes your body release an increased amount of calcium into your urine, switch to tofu or beans as your main protein source.

When you do eat animal protein, make sure you get every bit of benefit from the calcium in that food. The best way to do this is to make soups or stews, adding bones to the stock along with the meat. Then, add a small amount of vinegar to help pull all the calcium out of the bones.

■ **Avoid salt.** Like protein, salt causes your body to lose some of its calcium supply each time you urinate.

■ **Limit caffeine.** You urinate more often because of caffeine's diuretic properties. Even a cup of coffee or tea a day can interfere with calcium absorption.

■ **Eat berries.** Add some purplish-colored berries to your daily fare. Cherries, raspberries and blueberries contain phytochemicals that have special healing properties and may help to stabilize collagen structure, which is calcium's foundation for building strong bones and teeth.

■ **Try Oriental healing herbs.** In the East, herbs such as dong quai, licorice, black cohosh and fennel have been used for centuries to help prevent osteoporosis.

■ **Eat wild yam.** Bone loss is accelerated in women after menopause, when estrogen levels drop. And because the herb wild yam has natural hormonal properties, it is considered by many to be useful in preventing and mending osteoporosis.

■ **Season your food with Asian fish sauce.** This concoction that is made of ground-up fish (including the bones) is loaded to the proverbial gills with calcium. In fact, about 4 tablespoons equals the RDA for calcium, so add this mineral-rich remedy to your soups, sauces, stews or stir-fry.
CAUTION: *Asian fish sauce has a high sodium content, so don't use it if you have high blood pressure.*

■ **Don't be too weight conscious.** Being too thin is just as damaging as being too fat, so eat up. Proper hormone levels, which are necessary to maintain adequate calcium deposits, are created to some degree by fatty tissue. Some studies have indicated that the lack of proper nutrients in excessively thin women is responsible for their marked susceptibility to osteoporosis.

PET CARE

It is estimated that pets are part of the family in more than 50 percent of American homes. Though dogs were long the favored household companions, according to some surveys, cats are now number one. They are joined by a growing number of birds, fish, rodents and reptiles.

Whether we're "dog people" or "cat people," we all want the best for our furry friends. And for those of us who believe in taking the natural approach when we deal with our own health, that means choosing from the following safe, alternative ways to prevent and treat disease in our pets.

CONSTIPATION

Because dogs have very short intestines, they need to be able to go outside at least twice a day to move their bowels. If made to wait too long, constipation can result. In addition, all pets need lots of bulk in their diets — and exercise — to maintain regularity. When your pet needs a little help to get things moving, here are a few natural remedies you can use.

__MILK__ Milk is a natural laxative — for dogs and cats.

__MINERAL OIL__ Some vets suggest adding a teaspoon to your pet's food to help alleviate constipation.
CAUTION: *Don't use this treatment for more than a few days.*

__RAW MEAT__ Raw meat is a natural laxative — and a natural food for dogs and cats.

CUTS

Frisky pets are bound to get cut now and then. It's usually enough to simply clean the wound thoroughly. However, if your pet has a cut that's serious enough to require a bandage, do it this way: Make a solution of 2 drops of calendula tincture to 1 ounce of water. Moisten some gauze with this solution and wrap it around the wound. Also, see page 84 for instructions on how to make a tincture.

DIARRHEA

If your pet's diarrhea is accompanied by vomiting or blood in the stool, or if it lasts longer than 48 hours, call your vet immediately. However, most cases of diarrhea are not serious — just the result of a little too much "people food" — and should respond to the following remedies.

CAROB POWDER Feed your pet a mixture of carob powder, water and honey.

GARLIC Try adding a little garlic juice to your pet's food to help heal the digestive tract.

RICE Feed steamed rice alone, or mixed into your pet's regular food.

YOGURT A little plain yogurt or acidophillus milk will help replenish the natural digestive bacteria in your cat's or dog's intestinal tract.

FLEAS AND TICKS

Fleas and ticks can make a meal out of most living things, though they prefer dogs, cats and people. It is impossible to eradicate these pests entirely, but there are a number of natural ways to control the infestation.

BORAX Sprinkle borax on your carpet and leave it there. The main chemical component in this powder dries out flea larvae, preventing them from hatching.

BREWER'S YEAST Fleas hate the scent of brewer's yeast (which is undetectable to humans). Rub yeast powder directly on your dog or cat once a day. Brewer's yeast is also effective when given orally — sprinkled on food or in tablet form.

GARLIC Feed your pet deodorized garlic tablets or mix fresh or powdered garlic in the animal's food. Garlic is believed to be a natural flea killer.

HERBAL REPELLENTS To keep fleas away, herbalists recommend adding a few drops of pennyroyal or eucalyptus oil to your dog's bathwater. Or, use natural flea powders made from aromatic herbs like rosemary, rue, pennyroyal, eucalyptus, citronella and wormwood to discourage fleas.

Rosemary, rue, pennyroyal and wormwood are also recommended for repelling ticks.

MANGE

Mange, an infection caused by mites, makes the skin irritated and sore. Your pet's fur falls out in clumps, making your pet look and feel miserable. The following remedies offer relief.

ECHINACEA This herb is soothing to the skin. Mix a few drops of echinacea tincture into a cup of warm water and sponge it on the affected area.

LEMON JUICE Rub the juice from a freshly cut lemon on sore spots — or use the lemon tonic recipe in the box on page 402.

ZINC Zinc can help restore a "mange-y" coat. Either give a supplement, or grind a teaspoon of pumpkin seeds directly into your pet's food.

WORMS

Dogs and cats can get worms from insects, from wild animals and from eating infested feces. Good nutrition, adequate exercise and the following treatments will help kill the worms and prevent them from returning.

_____ **BRAN** Add ½ to 2 teaspoons of bran to your pet's food. The roughage

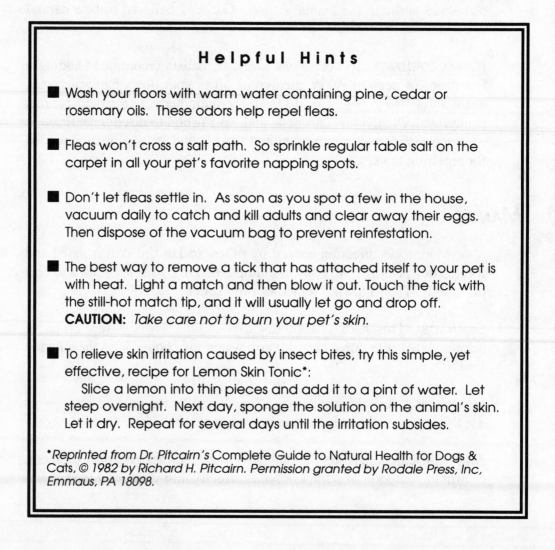

Helpful Hints

■ Wash your floors with warm water containing pine, cedar or rosemary oils. These odors help repel fleas.

■ Fleas won't cross a salt path. So sprinkle regular table salt on the carpet in all your pet's favorite napping spots.

■ Don't let fleas settle in. As soon as you spot a few in the house, vacuum daily to catch and kill adults and clear away their eggs. Then dispose of the vacuum bag to prevent reinfestation.

■ The best way to remove a tick that has attached itself to your pet is with heat. Light a match and then blow it out. Touch the tick with the still-hot match tip, and it will usually let go and drop off. **CAUTION:** _Take care not to burn your pet's skin._

■ To relieve skin irritation caused by insect bites, try this simple, yet effective, recipe for Lemon Skin Tonic*:
   Slice a lemon into thin pieces and add it to a pint of water. Let steep overnight. Next day, sponge the solution on the animal's skin. Let it dry. Repeat for several days until the irritation subsides.

*Reprinted from Dr. Pitcairn's Complete Guide to Natural Health for Dogs & Cats, © 1982 by Richard H. Pitcairn. Permission granted by Rodale Press, Inc, Emmaus, PA 18098.

will help carry the worms out of the intestinal tract.

_____ **GARLIC** Mix ½ to 2 cloves of garlic in the animal's food every day as a preventive.

_____ **VEGETABLES** Feeding your pet carrots, beets or turnips will increase intestinal action — and help eliminate worms.

NUTRITION TIPS

Many of the food preservatives and additives that are harmful to humans have the same effect on our pets. That's why it's best to feed your animals — and yourself — foods that are free from artificial dyes, preservatives and added hormones. Your veterinarian can recommend a good commercially prepared pet food — or you can make your own.

The recipes printed on pages 404-405 have been reprinted from Dr. Pitcairn's *Complete Guide to Natural Health for Dogs & Cats*, © 1982 by Richard H. Pitcairn. (Permission granted by Rodale Press, Inc, Emmaus, PA 18098.)

GROOMING TIPS

Cats take care of most of their own grooming. In fact, the first rule of cat etiquette seems to be, "When in doubt, groom!" However, if you have a dog, you'll need to bathe it regularly. And whether you have a dog or a cat, it's a good idea to pay extra attention to the eyes, ears, nose and anal area.

■ If your pet's nose is swollen, blocked, gritty or infected, keep it clean with a cloth dipped in warm water. Hold the cloth on dried matter until it softens and comes off easily. Then, once the nose is clean and dry, apply a balm made from petroleum jelly mixed with a few drops of almond or calendula oil.

■ Clean crust and dried secretions from eyes with a mixture of

Lean Meat Menu for Cats

⅓ cup cooked oatmeal
½ cup (¼ lb.) chopped organ
   or lean meat

1 Tbsp. grated or chopped vegetables
2 tsp. butter
¼ cup whole milk

Warm the oatmeal in a 1-quart pan, and add the meat and vegetables. Mix in the butter and supplements, heat and serve. Place a little milk on the side. This recipe is appropriate for a cat weighing 9 to 10 lbs. For smaller or larger cats, adjust the recipe as indicated below.

Cat feeding guide:

If Your Cat Weighs	Multiply Recipe by
5 to 6 lbs.	⅔
7 to 8 lbs.	¾
11 to 12 lbs.	1⅓
15 lbs.	1½

Daily supplements:

   1 tsp. cat powder mix
   1 tsp. cat oil mix
   30 to 50 I.U.s vitamin E (or 20- to 40-minim capsule or capsules of wheat germ oil)

Cat powder mix:

   ½ cup nutritional yeast   ¼ cup kelp powder
   ¼ cup bone meal

Mix ingredients together well and store in a sealed jar on a dark shelf.

Cat oil mix:

   ¾ cup vegetable oil   ¼ cup cod-liver oil
   20 to 40 I.U.s of vitamin E (to prevent spoilage)

Shake the ingredients together well in a sealed brown bottle and store in the refrigerator. Olive oil is the preferred vegetable oil.

Dog Meat and Grain Menu

2 cups cooked brown rice	½ cup lean meat 2 tsp. oil	¼ cup grated or chopped vegetables

Mix all the ingredients together and serve. Some dogs like their food warm, so try heating it slightly before serving. This recipe is appropriate for a dog weighing 25 lbs. Adjust the recipe to meet your dog's weight as follows:

Dog feeding guide:

If Your Dog Weighs	Multiply Recipe by
5 lbs.	¼
10 lbs.	½
40 lbs.	1½
60 lbs.	2
85 lbs.	2½
105 lbs.	3

Daily supplements:

Dog powder mix	Dog oil mix	Vitamin E supplement

Note: Since dogs vary greatly in size, there is no single required amount of supplementation, as there is for cats. Instead, the recommended amount increases with the size of the dog.

Dog powder mix:

2 cups nutritional yeast	½ cup kelp powder
1½ cups bone meal	

Mix the ingredients together well and store in a sealed jar on a dark shelf.

Dog oil mix:

1¾ cups vegetable oil	¼ cup cod-liver oil
50 to 100 I.U.s of vitamin E (to prevent spoilage)	

Shake the ingredients together well in a sealed brown bottle and store in the refrigerator. The best vegetable oil for dogs is probably safflower, but soy, corn and sunflower oils are good, too.

WARNING! Do not give dogs chocolate or onions. Both can be very toxic. And do not feed them cat food — it contains too much protein.

warm salt water. Add a rounded ½ teaspoon of sea salt to a pint of warm distilled water. Mix well and apply to the area with a clean cloth. A few drops of this solution will soothe irritated eyes, too.

■ If your pet's ears are secreting a waxy substance, treat the problem with warm (not hot) olive oil. Use an eye dropper to drip the oil into the ear opening. Let the oil sit in the ear for a few minutes, then hold the ear flap down over the ear opening and massage the area directly behind and under the ear to soften and lift the wax out of the ear canal. Use a tissue to remove the excess oil and wax that has worked its way to the surface.

> ## A home remedy for ear mites
> Mix ½ ounce of olive oil and the contents of one 400 I.U. capsule of vitamin E, and draw into an eye dropper. Immerse the dropper in warm water, being careful not to squeeze out any of the mixture. When warm, remove the dropper from the water and slowly squeeze a few drops into the ear canal.
> Use once a day for 3 days, refrigerating the unused contents.

CAUTION: *Never insert a cotton swab into your pet's — or your — ear canal.*

■ Diarrhea is the main cause for irritation around the anus. So if your dog is ill, be sure to wipe (do not rub) this area with a cloth dampened with warm water after each "outing." When dry, apply a few drops of calendula ointment to help the skin heal faster and reduce the irritation. Use this treatment 2 or 3 times a day until the diarrhea has passed.

DENTAL CARE

Pets get cavities, too — and a diet of table scraps and foods that are too soft can lead to gum disease. Treat minor dental problems with these natural remedies.

■ A fresh bone or a hard vegetable (like a carrot) acts like a natural toothbrush. So make sure your dog gets one at least once a week.
CAUTION: *Any bone you give your dog has to be big enough and sturdy enough so the dog won't choke. Poultry bones are too small and too soft.*

■ For infected teeth or gums, make this brew for your pet: Boil 1 teaspoon of echinacea in 1 cup of water for 10 minutes. Cover and let steep for at least one hour. Strain and swab on the animal's gums. Your pet may drool, but don't worry — drooling is a natural reaction to this potion.

■ Because it is antiseptic and believed to promote tissue growth, goldenseal makes a good mouthwash. Add 1 teaspoon of the herb to a pot of boiling water. Let sit until cool, and apply to your pet's teeth and gums with a cotton swab.

PHLEBITIS

Phlebitis, or more precisely thrombophlebitis, occurs when a blood clot lodges in a vein, usually a leg vein. It can be caused by an injury, birth control pills — or it can have a genetic link. If the clot is in a vein close to the surface of the skin, the condition is called superficial phlebitis. Though painful, this condition is not serious. If, however, the clot is in one of the larger, deeper veins, it can be life-threatening. If the clot begins to travel (becomes an embolism), it can block the flow of blood to the heart or lungs.

Whether the clot is superficial or deep, all cases of phlebitis require medical attention. Here are some natural remedies to help the treatment.

- **Exercise.** Sitting is bad for phlebitis, so get up and take a walk several times a day. Walking keeps the blood flowing through the veins at a good pace, lessening the likelihood that blood cells will stick to a vein wall. It also relieves the pressure and ache.

- **Put your feet up.** Elevating your feet above your heart for an hour or so several times a day helps relieve the pressure in the vein.

- **Wear support hose.** This provides almost instant, as well as long-term, relief for phlebitis sufferers. Available anywhere pantyhose are sold, support hose relieve internal vein pressure and may prevent additional clots from forming.

- **Try moist heat.** This remedy is comforting and soothing. Wet a cloth towel with water and heat it in the microwave for a minute to a minute and a half. The towel should be very warm, but not burning. Wrap the cloth snugly around the phlebitis leg and leave it there until cool. Repeat 3 or 4 times a day.

■ **Take vitamin E.** Evidence suggests that vitamin E may relieve the ache of this condition. The recommended starting dose is usually 1,000 I.U.s per day for 3 days, then 400 I.U.s for another 3 or 4 days until the leg stops hurting.

■ **Use zinc.** If your leg itches as well as aches, a little zinc oxide ointment may help. Apply a light coat of the white ointment as needed.

POISON IVY

Poison ivy — and poison oak and poison sumac — are not really "poisonous." However, the sap of these plants contains a resin (called urishiol) to which most people are highly allergic.

Your first contact with urishiol won't be serious. However, each time you are exposed to it, your allergic reaction will become more immediate and more intense. You will develop a streaky red, itchy, blistering rash which can last for weeks. Though the rash will eventually disappear on its own, there's no reason to suffer through the discomfort when there are so many effective remedies to help you.

ALOE Aloe's antibacterial properties make it an excellent natural remedy for poison ivy. In addition to being very soothing, it helps repair skin tissues.

BURDOCK This herbal staple has been used since the days of King Henry III for skin irritations, including poison ivy. Fresh, crumpled leaves can be applied directly to the inflammation.

CLAY The healing properties of clay and mud have been known for centuries. This simple recipe works for any type of itchy rash — and for insect bites, too. Mix together:
>   2 tsp. salt
>   5 drops peppermint oil
>   5 Tbsp. water (more if necessary)
>   ½ cup red or green volcanic clay (available at most health food stores or by mail order)

The clay should have the same consistency as paste. Spread it on the rash and leave it there until it dries completely.

GRINDELIA For more than 100 years, folk healers have used a poultice of grindelia to ease the itch of poison ivy. Steep the plant (leaves, stem and flowers) in boiling water. When cool, soak a clean cloth in the mixture and apply it to the afflicted area.

PLANTAIN Popular among early American settlers, this weed is still used to treat bee stings and poison ivy. And recent research indicates that when applied directly to the skin, the crushed leaves of the plantain really do help relieve the itching.

SASSAFRAS The antiseptic properties of this plant help make it an effective remedy for poison ivy. To try it, boil the leaves and apply the cooled water directly to the sores.

SWEET FERN Gay Head Indians used sweet fern to cure poison ivy. They made a poultice by boiling the leaves and applying them to the rash.

Helpful Hints

■ The best way to deal with poison ivy, poison oak and poison sumac is to learn to recognize these plants — and then avoid them. If there's any doubt in your mind, test a suspicious plant for urishiol by crushing a leaf on a piece of white paper. If it contains urishiol, it will turn black within 5 minutes.

■ If you think you've come in contact with one of these plants, wash your skin, clothing, camping gear — everything — thoroughly with soap and water.

■ Once the rash breaks out, stick with cold showers and baths. Hot water will make the itching worse.

PREGNANCY

Though pregnancy is a perfectly normal, healthy process, it carries with it a host of problems — especially for a first-time mother. Fortunately, there are plenty of support groups, classes and other resources that you can tap into for help. The library offers dozens of books on every aspect of pregnancy and parenting. Even more valuable are secrets born of personal experience that have been passed down from generation to generation throughout the world — secrets that we've gathered together to share with you here.

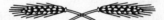

MORNING SICKNESS

Though we don't know exactly what causes morning sickness, some researchers believe it has something to do with a Vitamin B6 (pyridoxine) or zinc deficiency. There is also evidence that low blood sugar and the increased protein requirements of the developing fetus contributes to the problem. Whatever the cause, you'll find many simple, effective ways to ease that awful feeling in this section. (See also the Nausea section on page 387.)

**BAKING SODA** To treat morning sickness, women who live in the South and Southwest drink a glass of water mixed with a teaspoon of this natural antacid.

**BANANA** Bananas are an excellent source of Vitamin B6 and potassium. Eat one daily to help lessen your nausea.

**CARBOHYDRATES** Research shows that foods high in complex carbohydrates (pasta, potatoes, rice and whole grains) minimize and, in some cases, prevent morning sickness.

_____ **GINGER** Laboratory studies reveal that this digestive aid is also an excellent anti-nausea agent. Brew a cup of ginger tea by adding ½ teaspoon of powdered ginger and 1 teaspoon of honey to 1 cup of boiling water. Or, if fresh ginger is available, squeeze the juice from about 1 tablespoon of the root and add to 1 cup of hot water.

_____ **GRAPEFRUIT** A Chinese remedy for morning sickness is to drink tea made from fresh grapefruit peel. Tangy or bitter tasting foods or liquids often relieve nausea.

_____ **PEACH** The Chinese, and many Europeans, believe in the soothing effect of peach tea to calm morning sickness.

_____ **RASPBERRY** A great tasting, nutritious drink, raspberry tea relieves many of the discomforts of pregnancy, including morning sickness. Make the tea by steeping 2 teaspoons of raspberry leaves in 1 cup of boiling water. Strain and drink immediately or freeze to make raspberry tea ice cubes.

_____ **VINEGAR** In New England, 1 cup of water with 1 teaspoon of apple cider vinegar is said to help relieve morning sickness.

BREAST-FEEDING

Nature designed it. It's delicious, it's nutritious and it's baby's best defense against infection. It's mother's milk. But, as wonderful and beneficial as breast-feeding is, it does have its drawbacks. Because lactation is affected by stress as well as diet, mothers often fear they aren't producing enough — and sometimes they aren't. In spite of this, women around the world have successfully nursed their babies for centuries — depending on the following natural remedies to help with the process.

_____ **ANISE** More than 2,000 years ago, anise tea was used to help new mothers maintain the flow of breast milk. To try it, crush 1 teaspoon of anise seed and mix with 1 cup of boiling water. Steep for 10 to 20 minutes, strain and drink.

BORAGE Eating borage leaves is a favorite way for Saudi Arabian women to stimulate milk production. Borage leaves, which have a taste similar to cucumber, can be added to salads or used in place of lettuce on sandwiches.

CHASTE BERRIES In the 1950s, German researchers verified the milk-producing and energy-building properties of chaste berries.

FENNEL Popular in India and other parts of the world, a brew of 1 teaspoon of fennel seeds boiled in barley water is thought to increase milk production.

FENUGREEK In Greece many women rely on the milk-producing properties of fenugreek seeds. Eaten boiled with honey, they are full of vitamins A, B, C, calcium and other vital nutrients.
CAUTION: *Fenugreek may stimulate uterine contractions and should not be used in the early stages of pregnancy.*

GREENS European folklore suggests that greens like watercress, chicory, dandelion, alfalfa and spring onions can enhance the breast's ability to produce milk.

NUTS AND SEEDS In folk medicine, walnuts and almonds are believed to stimulate milk production — along with sunflower, sesame, celery and pumpkin seeds.

RASPBERRY To increase the flow of milk, new mothers in China drink 1 cup of raspberry tea made by pouring a pint of boiling water over 2 rounded teaspoons of dried raspberry leaves. Brew for a half hour; then strain and sip throughout the day.

SAW PALMETTO American Indian women know that saw palmetto berries promote milk production and keep the breast functioning normally. They eat a few each day during the last month of pregnancy and while nursing.

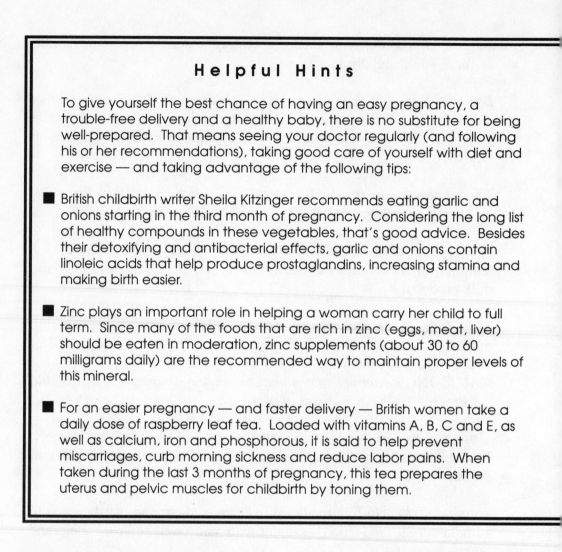

Helpful Hints

To give yourself the best chance of having an easy pregnancy, a trouble-free delivery and a healthy baby, there is no substitute for being well-prepared. That means seeing your doctor regularly (and following his or her recommendations), taking good care of yourself with diet and exercise — and taking advantage of the following tips:

■ British childbirth writer Sheila Kitzinger recommends eating garlic and onions starting in the third month of pregnancy. Considering the long list of healthy compounds in these vegetables, that's good advice. Besides their detoxifying and antibacterial effects, garlic and onions contain linoleic acids that help produce prostaglandins, increasing stamina and making birth easier.

■ Zinc plays an important role in helping a woman carry her child to full term. Since many of the foods that are rich in zinc (eggs, meat, liver) should be eaten in moderation, zinc supplements (about 30 to 60 milligrams daily) are the recommended way to maintain proper levels of this mineral.

■ For an easier pregnancy — and faster delivery — British women take a daily dose of raspberry leaf tea. Loaded with vitamins A, B, C and E, as well as calcium, iron and phosphorous, it is said to help prevent miscarriages, curb morning sickness and reduce labor pains. When taken during the last 3 months of pregnancy, this tea prepares the uterus and pelvic muscles for childbirth by toning them.

CHAPPED, SORE NIPPLES

Nursing can make your nipples sore and tender. They can crack and bleed — and even become infected. But not if you use these natural soothing balms.

ALOE The women of Barbados apply the sap from the stalks of the aloe plant to relieve sore nipples.
CAUTION: *Since aloe is very bitter tasting and a known laxative, do*

■ As the birth approaches, your baby's weight will press down on your genitals. Massaging the vagina, vulva and peritoneum with wheat germ, coconut, almond, olive or vitamin E oil will increase elasticity, improve circulation and help prevent tearing during delivery.

■ Many flower oils have the power to relax, refresh and energize you after delivery. So treat yourself to a warm bath with your choice of rose, frankincense, neroli, geranium or fennel oil added to the water. In addition to being soothing, these oils are antiseptic.

■ Wine has long been credited with restorative powers. Italian women add equal amounts of clove, ginger and cinnamon to sweet wine and sip it to increase energy and stamina after delivery.

■ After childbirth, many women suffer from fatigue that can last up to 2 years. They may also have trouble losing the extra weight they put on while pregnant. Both of these problems can be blamed on an exhausted thyroid gland (which regulates body metabolism). Eating seaweed (kelp or dulse) once or twice a day can provide the iodine and other minerals needed for normal thyroid function. According to Oriental tradition, kelp will also help get the uterus back into shape.

■ Aromatherapists tell new mothers to put a few drops of lavender on their wrists and temples for an invigorating lift.

not feed baby from the treated breast.

GOLDENSEAL European mothers use a compress made from goldenseal, comfrey and curly cabbage to relieve soreness.

MOLASSES An early American folk remedy calls for molasses to be applied to the sore nipple after baby is done feeding. To remove the molasses, bathe the nipple with a solution of brandy and water, and then rinse with clear water.

PAPAYA Tahitian women like to put fresh papaya juice on tender nipples. It speeds healing and is safe to use prior to nursing.

STRETCH MARKS

During pregnancy, every woman winds up with stretch marks as her body swells to accommodate the growing fetus. At first, these stretch marks look like purple or red streaks on the skin. Then, over time, they fade to a silvery white. Though there is no way to avoid stretch marks completely, there are things you can do to increase and maintain your skin's elasticity to minimize their effect.

CALENDULA Soak a handful of calendula flowers in wheat germ oil for 2 to 3 weeks. Massage this mixture into your skin wherever signs of stretch marks appear.

WARNING! There are some otherwise valuable herbal remedies that are best avoided or used only with professional supervision during pregnancy:
- Angelica, dong quai and yarrow are used to bring on menstruation.
- Black cohosh, blue cohosh and pennyroyal may increase the strength of contractions.
- Comfrey and tansy may have a harmful effect on an unborn baby's liver.
- Since ephedra is an antihistamine and uterine stimulant, it may interfere with the normal growth and development of the fetus.
- Feverfew is sometimes used to bring on menstruation.
- Ginseng may increase the general discomfort associated with pregnancy.
- Because goldenseal is believed to cause uterine contractions, it should be avoided in the early stages of pregnancy.
- Because licorice affects the hormonal system, it should not be used at all during pregnancy. It also causes salt retention.

LAVENDER This fragrant oil mixed with neroli is particularly helpful to maintain normal skin function and elasticity. Make a lotion of 20 drops of lavender oil and 5 drops of neroli in 2 ounces of almond oil. Massage your breasts, abdomen and thighs daily.

VITAMIN E Stretch marks may be minimized by rubbing with vitamin E oil during pregnancy. Not only does the oil help prevent stretch marks, the massage itself is a soothing way to ease tension.

You can also massage with wheat germ, coconut, almond or olive oil.

PREMENSTRUAL SYNDROME (PMS)

The symptoms of PMS are as individual as the women it affects. However, 2 days to 2 weeks before the onset of menstruation, most women experience some degree of bloating, headaches, cramping, irritability, muscle soreness, back pain, insomnia and/or an overall feeling of uneasiness. And it is estimated that about half of all women between the ages of 15 and 50 are plagued with severe PMS at some point during their lives. The culprit? Low hormone levels — especially estrogen and progesterone — which normally drop after ovulation.

Though symptoms associated with premenstrual distress usually subside once the flow begins, relief from PMS has been sought for centuries. As a result, many natural remedies have been discovered.

***

CALCIUM It's a known fact that calcium levels drop just about the time PMS begins — and this could have a tendency to increase cramping. Eat broccoli or kale to add this important mineral to your system.

CHASTE BERRY Ancient Romans believed this herb (also called vitex or monk's pepper) lowered a woman's libido — hence the name. Modern research shows that chaste berry works on the pituitary gland to stimulate the production of progesterone and moderate the symptoms of PMS.

CRAMP BARK Europeans take 1 dropperful of cramp bark tincture in a little bit of warm water for relief from PMS symptoms. This is safe to take as often as needed.

DANDELION Dandelion tea is a natural diuretic that prevents your body from storing excess water. To make dandelion tea, add 2 teaspoons of

dandelion root to 1 cup of boiling water. Steep for 15 minutes, covered.
Drink 2 or 3 cups every day to relieve PMS symptoms.

LEMON BALM Lemon balm tea is used in the Middle East to relieve

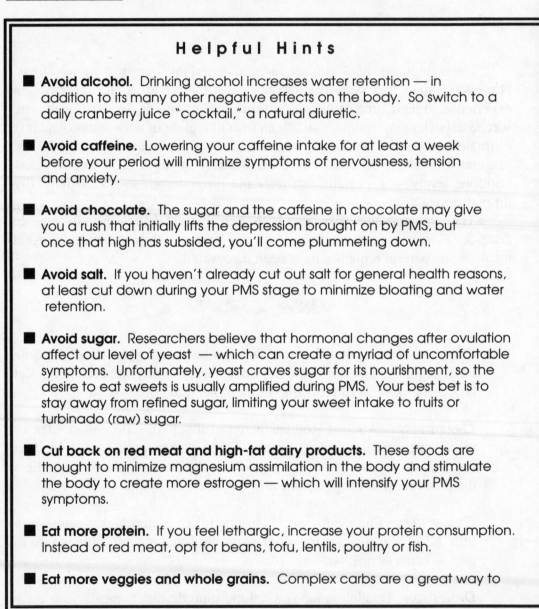

Helpful Hints

■ **Avoid alcohol.** Drinking alcohol increases water retention — in addition to its many other negative effects on the body. So switch to a daily cranberry juice "cocktail," a natural diuretic.

■ **Avoid caffeine.** Lowering your caffeine intake for at least a week before your period will minimize symptoms of nervousness, tension and anxiety.

■ **Avoid chocolate.** The sugar and the caffeine in chocolate may give you a rush that initially lifts the depression brought on by PMS, but once that high has subsided, you'll come plummeting down.

■ **Avoid salt.** If you haven't already cut out salt for general health reasons, at least cut down during your PMS stage to minimize bloating and water retention.

■ **Avoid sugar.** Researchers believe that hormonal changes after ovulation affect our level of yeast — which can create a myriad of uncomfortable symptoms. Unfortunately, yeast craves sugar for its nourishment, so the desire to eat sweets is usually amplified during PMS. Your best bet is to stay away from refined sugar, limiting your sweet intake to fruits or turbinado (raw) sugar.

■ **Cut back on red meat and high-fat dairy products.** These foods are thought to minimize magnesium assimilation in the body and stimulate the body to create more estrogen — which will intensify your PMS symptoms.

■ **Eat more protein.** If you feel lethargic, increase your protein consumption. Instead of red meat, opt for beans, tofu, lentils, poultry or fish.

■ **Eat more veggies and whole grains.** Complex carbs are a great way to

cramps and headaches. To make it, add 2 teaspoons of the herb to boiling water. Steep for 5 minutes and drink several times a day.

MAGNESIUM Some herbalists believe the chocolate craving many

---

keep your energy level constant, so load up on brown rice, potatoes, whole grain breads, pastas and veggies. Eggplant and asparagus are especially good because they are natural diuretics

■ **Eat less — more often.** A good rule of thumb — even when you're not PMS-ing — is to eat smaller meals throughout the day. The constant influx of food every few hours keeps your blood sugar level consistent, which prevents fatigue from setting in.

■ **Try aromatherapy.** Aromatherapists treat the symptoms of PMS with a combination of the essential oils of chamomile, lavender, sage, neroli and geranium. Add equal quantities of these oils to boiling water. Then, as the water continues to boil, inhale the scent.

■ **Take a daily multivitamin.** And make sure your multivitamin includes minerals like zinc, iron, manganese, copper and aluminum. These natural mood-modifiers help prevent the emotional imbalances often experienced during PMS.

■ **Exercise.** Everyone should exercise a minimum of 3 times a week for 20 minutes. And if you want to exercise even more during "that time of the month," go for it. Exercise not only alleviates stress, it helps create endorphins in the brain — which gives you a mental lift that can counteract the depression some women suffer during PMS.

■ **Have sex.** This is a natural, pleasurable way to exercise and release mood-lifting endorphins.

■ **Practice some form of stress management.** Stress exacerbates PMS symptoms. So meditate or do yoga regularly — especially before your period. (See page 467-476 for complete information on stress management.)

women experience during PMS is related to a magnesium deficiency. Make a sandwich on crusty whole grain bread, add a little mustard — and your magnesium level will be back where it belongs.

NETTLE Nettle tea helps alleviate water retention. To make it, add 2 teaspoons of nettle to boiling water and steep for 10 to 15 minutes. Drink 2 to 3 cups daily.

PARSLEY To relieve bloating, steep 1 teaspoon of dried parsley in 1 cup of boiling water for 4 minutes. Add lemon or honey to improve the taste and drink as needed.

PRIMROSE OIL Rub a little evening primrose oil on your breasts or abdomen to help improve blood flow and relieve premenstrual tenderness.

SESAME OIL Practitioners of Ayurvedic medicine recommend rubbing sesame oil on the abdomen and back to ease cramping and abdominal pain.

VALERIAN A recognized sleep aid since Shakespearean times, valerian helps relieve a number of PMS symptom. One teaspoon of valerian tincture or a cup of valerian tea taken once a day is the recommended treatment for insomnia, back and breast pain, cramps, irritability and bloating.

VITAMIN A Vitamin A capsules are recommended for women who are affected by PMS-related skin problems or excessively oily skin. It also helps to eat plenty of orange veggies like carrots and squash, which are loaded with beta-carotene (which turns into vitamin A in the body).

VITAMIN B All the B vitamins are important, especially B6, which has a calming effect that soothes the irritability that often accompanies PMS.

VITAMIN E Vitamin E supplements have been found to decrease many symptoms of PMS, according to researchers at Johns Hopkins University. It eases physiological symptoms like bloating and swelling, as well as emotional symptoms like anxiety, depression and irritability.

YAMS Many doctors across the country agree that the natural progesterone found in yams (and soybeans) helps rebalance the body's hormone levels after ovulation — a direct link to all menstrual problems.

For information on where to purchase any of the items listed, turn to the glossary beginning on page 523.

PROSTATE DISEASE

Enlargement of the prostate gland — a condition known as benign prostate hypertrophy (BPH) — is normal as a man ages. No one knows exactly why this happens, but it certainly has something to do with hormonal changes. As long as the growth is outward, away from the urethra, there are few, if any, symptoms. But when the growth spreads inward, it begins to interfere with urination. And when the growth gets to the point where it severely restricts the urinary flow — a condition known as obstructive BPH — it becomes painful and serious.

In a worst-case scenario, this condition can lead to incontinence, impotence and infertility. On the other hand, in many cases, symptoms come and go — often improving spontaneously. Though surgery is sometimes necessary, it should be used only as a last resort. Most cases of BPH can be successfully managed with close medical supervision — and with the help of the following natural remedies.

BEE POLLEN In Cambodia, natives believe that eating raw bee pollen and honeycomb keeps the prostate gland healthy, and scientific studies back them up. It is an excellent source of the vitamins and minerals needed to sustain glandular function.
CAUTION: *If you are asthmatic, stay away from bee pollen.*

CORN SILK American Indians believe in the healing power of corn silk — eaten fresh or brewed into a tea. To soothe the inflammation of an enlarged prostate, they combine it with couch grass, yarrow root or saw palmetto. Brew your own tea using 3 ounces of fresh (or dried) green silk per cup of boiling water. (Don't use corn silk that has oxidized and turned dark red.)

COUCH GRASS Since colonial times, couch grass has been prescribed to treat infected or enlarged prostates. A diuretic with antimicrobial action, it cleans the prostate from the inside, carrying infection out with the urine flow. The recommended dose is 1 cup of couch grass tea, 3 times a day.

GINSENG This staple of Chinese medicine is believed, to have a positive effect on the male reproductive system. Herbalists recommend that you either chew on a pea-sized piece of ginseng, or drink ginseng tea made by brewing ¼ teaspoon of powdered ginseng in 1 cup of boiling water for 10 minutes. **CAUTION:** *If you have high blood pressure, don't use ginseng.*

NATURE'S MEDICINE CABINET

On the southeastern coast of the U.S., saw palmetto bushes produce dark purple berries the size of olives. Centuries ago, natives of the region ate these berries to normalize prostate function.

These natives were familiar with the symptoms of an ailing prostate — and they knew that the saw palmetto berries helped them when those symptoms flared up. But they didn't know that the berries contain saponins, hormone-like compounds found in many medicinal plants that reduce inflammation.

PARSLEY The men of Holland prevent prostate troubles by drinking parsley tea. This treatment is said to be effective for almost any ailment that affects the urinary tract. Parsley is a good source of vitamin A and is also a diuretic, which promotes urine flow.

PUMPKIN SEEDS Studies performed at Vienna University have revealed that swelling of the prostate is almost nonexistent among the men of Transylvania. And research done by the Szekler group in the Transylvanian Alps has hinted that this phenomenon may be attributed to the Transylvanian passion for pumpkin seeds. Pumpkin seeds contain large amounts of magnesium, which French physicians have proven to be effective in the treatment of prostate ailments. The seeds are also an excellent source of zinc (which has also been linked to prostate health).

PSORIASIS

Psoriasis is a skin condition that has plagued mankind since before biblical times. It is characterized by a well-defined, thick, patchy area of skin, usually covered with white scales that are probably caused by an overproduction of skin cells. Though psoriasis appears to be hereditary, a flare-up can be brought on by severe sunburn, stress and several types of prescription medications.

Though there is no cure for psoriasis, there are plenty of readily available ways to ease the symptoms.

CAPSAICIN Capsaisin is a natural chemical found in hot peppers. Research at eight medical centers in the U.S. found that when this chemical is applied to the scaly patches of psoriasis, patients noticed improvement in 4 to 6 weeks.

COD LIVER OIL A few drops of cod liver oil or linseed oil taken every day is a popular folk remedy for psoriasis. Because they are so high in fatty acids, these oils may work to decrease the swelling and itching.

LECITHIN Psoriatic skin shows high levels of cholesterol, and lecithin can clean the cholesterol out of the skin to help restore normal skin function. Lecithin is found in soya and sunflower oils, and is also available as a supplement.

TEA TREE OIL The oil from the Melaleuco alternifolia tree is used by Australians to treat psoriasis and other skin conditions. A few drops of the oil applied topically several times a day relieves the itch and softens the scales.

Lubricating your skin with lavender, chamomile, almond or olive oil is also effective.

RHEUMATISM

Unlike arthritis, which seems to be an inevitable result of the natural aging process, rheumatism is most often diagnosed in women between the ages of 20 and 35 (though it can affect people of all ages and both sexes). This inflammation of the lining of the joints is considered an auto-immune disease because it is caused by a malfunction of the body's own immune system. Symptoms include fatigue, body aches, joint tenderness and lack of flexibility.

Modern medicine offers powerful drugs — and surgical joint replacement — to relieve the pain of rheumatism. For a better, safer alternative, first try the following natural remedies, some of which are as old as civilization. (And check out the "Arthritis" section beginning on page 111 for even more recommendations.)

ALFALFA For generations, folks living in the Blue Ridge Mountains have picked fresh alfalfa to brew a homemade pain reliever. It seems to work especially well on the hands and fingers, and so is recommended for people who spend a lot of time at a typewriter or computer keyboard. If you don't have access to fresh alfalfa, you can buy prepackaged alfalfa tea bags at your local health food store.

BLACK CURRANT A rheumatism remedy that is very popular in Europe — especially among the mountain people of eastern Europe — is black currant tea. They brew a tea from the leaves of the black currant bush.

CELERY The Germans and Japanese both believe in the pain relieving effects of celery. They recommend eating cooked or raw celery daily for 1 to 2 months. Alternatively, you could substitute a daily glass of celery juice. Celery is a diuretic, and the loss of excess fluid can reduce the inflammation associated with rheumatism.

CHINESE TIGER BALM In China, the pain of rheumatism is treated with Chinese Tiger Balm. This healing ointment contains aromatic oils of camphor, menthol, peppermint, clove and cajeput. When massaged into a painful area, it increases blood flow.

COMMON ASH People in Europe and southern England prepare a tea of common ash to ease rheumatism. They drink it 3 times a day before meals. To make it, infuse 1 ounce of dried leaves in 1 pint of boiling water. Add a few mint leaves for flavor.

DEVIL'S CLAW Desert African tribes have known of the healing power of devil's claw for hundreds of years. And recent studies conducted in France and Germany show that the plant contains cortisone-like properties which relieve inflammation and swelling.

EUCALYPTUS In tropical climates, many people swear by the healing properties of eucalyptus. Eucalyptus ointment along with

Curiosity Box

A therapy that may sound more like a punishment was discovered 2,000 years ago by Hippocrates. For centuries, Europeans used live bee stings as the leading cure for rheumatism, arthritis and gout. More recently, scientists in Switzerland, France, Germany and Great Britain took this traditional cure one step further and devised a treatment that employed a series of injections of the venom — using either a hypodermic needle or a live bee!

Bee venom, like many toxic substances, stimulates the immune system to release anti-inflammatories into the bloodstream. (This is one example of the way counter-irritation theory works.)

For additional information about bee therapy, write to the American Apitherapy Society, Inc., 252 B Road, Red Bank, NJ 07701, or call (908) 842-5700.

a warm compress is used to relieve the stiffness that accompanies rheumatism. You can easily duplicate this treatment at home because many commercial ointments contain eucalyptus.

GINGER Recent medical research in Holland has indicated that eating ginger can help alleviate rheumatism. Ginger increases blood circulation which carries inflammatory substances away from the sore joints and warms the area.

ICE An ice pack placed above and below rheumatic knees relieves the pain and eases the stiffness. Apply 2 or 3 times a day for 20 minutes. **CAUTION:** *Ice should never be applied directly to the skin.*

PRIMROSE OIL A teaspoon a day of primrose oil is believed to help regulate the immune system, the underlying cause of both rheumatism and arthritis.

QUINCE St. Hildegard, a German mystic, believed that raw or cooked quince helped alleviate the soreness and inflammation of rheumatism. The versatile fruit can be stewed in water or wine, baked in pastry or made into jelly and candy.

ROSEMARY In Europe, it's popular to sprinkle a few leaves of crushed rosemary into the bath. This treatment eases the pain of rheumatism — and is also very relaxing.

SPIKENARD The Cherokee Indians make powdered spikenard into a tea to treat rheumatism. The root also can be applied directly to the painful area in a poultice.

STRAWBERRIES A Swiss botanist made a case for strawberries as a remedy for rheumatism after a steady diet of strawberries helped relieve his own joint pain — probably because strawberries help eliminate uric acid from the system.

TOMATOES The English believe that a glass of tomato juice daily will do much to relieve rheumatism. They like carrot juice for the same reason.

YUCCA Native Americans in the southwest use yucca to relieve rheumatism. Like devil's claw, yucca contains cortisone-like properties that help alleviate pain and swelling. Yucca can be boiled or baked — just like a potato.

For information on where to purchase any of the items listed, turn to the glossary beginning on page 523.

SHINGLES

Shingles is a painful, itchy, blistery outbreak of the herpes zoster virus. It attacks the nerves just beneath the skin surface, usually on the chest, legs and thighs. Although no age group can be entirely excluded from contracting this often serious malady, it most frequently afflicts the elderly. Shingles are in the same family as chicken pox, and it is thought that the virus may lie dormant in people who contracted chicken pox as children, only to attack again once their immune systems have weakened with age.

Though the best remedy for shingles is prevention — through proper diet and nutrition, adequate rest, moderate exercise and minimal stress — there are many home remedies that can help bring relief. The most important thing to remember is that the sooner you take steps to lessen an oncoming attack, the less pain you'll feel and the quicker you'll heal.

BASIL In England, the fragrant oil of sweet basil has been found to provide helpful treatment in a number of skin conditions — including shingles.

CAYENNE PEPPER Capsaicin, the active ingredient in cayenne pepper, relieves the pain of shingles and other external ailments when applied directly to the skin. This natural chemical affects the sensory nerves (which are directly affected in a shingles attack), while it stimulates blood flow to the area (which reduces inflammation). Capsaicin is available in a cream or ointment.

ELECAMPANE Although it is primarily ingested in tea form as a treatment for several respiratory ailments, elecampane oil may also be applied externally to skin lesions such as those present with shingles.

GOLDENSEAL Herbalists recommend applying goldenseal tea directly on shingles blisters, either with a wet tea bag or with a tea-saturated cloth.

HONEY Honey mixed with vinegar is said to be helpful in eliminating shingles. You can drink it, but most people prefer to apply the mixture directly on their sores.

LEMON BALM German researchers have studied this common plant and found that it has a calming effect on some of the symptoms of a shingles outbreak. The combination of lemon balm and rose oil seems to benefit most herpes conditions when it is applied directly to the blisters.

LYSINE Don't wait until you have a full-blown case of shingles to take lysine tablets. An ounce of prevention is worth a pound of cure, and lysine has been known to keep most strains of the herpes virus at bay.

ST. JOHN'S WORT St. John's wort offers relief from shingles — whether taken internally or applied externally. When ingested, the herb acts as an antidepressant, a stress-reducer and a calmative for frayed nerves — all of which may help speed recovery from herpes zoster. Furthermore, thanks to its antimicrobial properties, the oil of St. John's wort is soothing when applied to the inflammation and blistering.

Eat to Beat Shingles

There is evidence to suggest that arginine is the chemical agent responsible for triggering herpes outbreaks in those who carry the virus. So, if you're prone to shingles, stay away from arginine-rich foods completely — chocolate, nuts and gelatin — or at least stay away from them when you sense a flare-up coming on. You may be able to lessen the severity of the eruption.

VITAMIN E To promote healing and lessen the pain of a shingles outbreak, apply the oil from vitamin E capsules directly to the sores.

SHIN SPLINTS

    An irritation of the connective sheave that binds together lower leg muscles and bones is called a shin splint. It is caused when there is a strength discrepancy between the muscles that allow you to flex your foot up (dorsiflexors) and the muscles that allow you to flex your foot down (plantarflexors). Sharp pains in the lower leg are the result, stopping many amateur runners in their tracks.

    This is another affliction where an ounce of prevention is worth a pound of cure. Below, we offer both.

■ **Wear the right shoes** — walking shoes for walking, running shoes for running, tennis shoes for tennis, etc. And never exercise in worn-down or overly stiff shoes.

■ **Stick with familiar territory.** A great deal of lower leg pain is caused by walking or running on new terrain or on unfamiliar tracks — especially where there are quick changes in the running surface. It's also best to avoid uphill running, overstriding on a downhill run and running on sand.

■ **Always warm up.** Do 10 minutes of stretching exercises before you walk or run.

■ **Don't overtrain.** Work gradually toward your exercise goal.

■ **Build up the muscles** surrounding the shin by biking with toe clips, climbing hills or doing the following exercises:
1. Standing upright, near a wall or table for balance, pull your

toes upward while balancing on your heels. Repeat this for 3 sets of 10.

2. Sitting with your legs straight out in front of you, pull your toes back toward you and hold for a count of 8, then extend your toes so they are pointed and hold for a count of 8. Do this 10 times.

■ **When you feel pain — stop.** Immediately! Then apply ice first for 20 minutes and then heat. Ice will reduce pain and inflammation. Heat is soothing and will decrease muscle spasms.

SKIN CARE

Although we're not accustomed to thinking of skin as an organ, it is. In fact, the epidermis is the largest organ in the human body. One third of the blood pumped by the heart courses through the skin. Every day, thousands of dead skin cells are shed, and thousands more take their places. Skin is the first line of defense against infection and also keeps us from dehydrating. Skin is not simply a pliable shell holding the body together. It is a complex, self-replenishing, breathing, life-preserving membrane.

Healthy skin is smooth and clear, and retains a glowing vitality even as we age. Yet our obsession with skin care has more to do with vanity than good health. Though we know that "beauty is only skin deep," and we understand that good character endures far longer than good looks, every culture in history has prized perfect skin as a symbol of youth. Because of this, the skin care secrets that have been handed down throughout the ages have been among the most guarded in the world.

The best thing you can do for your skin is keep it clean. Wash your face (at least) twice a day with plain water and a mild soap — and remember to apply all skin care products gently, especially around the delicate eye area. Most skin care experts recommend that you use a toner and moisturizer after washing, a deep-cleansing mask once a week, and a face scrub or exfoliant about once a month. And we recommend that you choose from the many natural preparations we've gathered together in this section instead of spending hundreds of dollars on commercially manufactured alternatives.

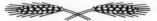

NATURAL CLEANSERS

ALMONDS Finely grated almonds make a gentle natural cleanser for oily complexions. Try adding buttermilk, rosewater or cucumber juice for a soothing wash.

Good Skin Begins With Good Nutrition

The Chinese know that putting things on the skin is not the only way — or even the best way — to preserve beauty. So they feed their skin by eating plenty of fried, ground barley seeds, which are loaded with minerals and B vitamins, and lots of yams, which are an excellent source of beta-carotene. Take a tip from the Chinese and nourish your skin from the inside with the following skin-healthy foods and supplements:

Beta-carotene. Beta-carotene (which your body converts to vitamin A) is especially important for your skin. It — along with vitamins C, E, riboflavin and selenium — is a powerful antioxidant, a nutrient that can protect your cells from damage caused by natural oxidation in your system. A chart listing the best food sources of beta-carotene can be found on page 50.

Carrot juice. You don't have to buy an expensive skin cream that contains retinal to get the benefit of vitamin A. You can drink a glass of fresh carrot juice. For added flavor, mix in apple or beetroot juice — also good for the skin. If you don't have your own juicer, seek out a nearby fruit and vegetable juice "bar" where you can buy these healthy mixtures.

Kelp. Seaweed — rich in iodine — is common in the Scottish diet. While kelp is the most common, there are more than 400 varieties in the world, most of which work just as well to maintain skin tone. The iodine in kelp nourishes the thyroid gland and ensures normal body metabolism and good blood circulation.

ALMOND OIL Never scrub make-up off with just soap and water, especially around the extremely delicate eye area. Use sweet almond oil to gently dissolve it. Wipe off the excess oil with a cool infusion of elderflowers or chamomile.

APRICOT OIL Another good cleansing oil is apricot oil, which can remove particles of dirt and leftover makeup while leaving the skin soft and moist. Mix with warm water, apply and rinse.

CUCUMBER To help keep oily skin under control, make a cleanser by grating a cucumber into a pint of milk and boiling for 3 minutes. Allow the liquid to cool, strain it through a piece of muslin and refrigerate. After a week — or if the milk has soured — discard any remaining

Lemon. There is evidence that lemon may actually preserve the youthful look of your skin. (CBS anchorman Mike Wallace drinks 3 glasses of hot water with lemon each morning — and no one would guess his skin is 76 years young.)

Selenium. Supplements of chelated selenium, or at least a good multi-vitamin including this mineral, are essential for the the health of your entire body — including your skin. You can also get selenium by eating onions, tomatoes, cabbage, broccoli, tuna and bran.

Vitamin C. To maintain healthy, wrinkle-free skin, you need to supplement with plenty of vitamin C. (Natural vitamin C is preferred to ascorbic acid, which can be hard on the stomach.) The best food sources of vitamin C include citrus fruits, dark-green leafy vegetables and cantaloupe (which is also a good source of vitamin A).

Water. Drink plenty of water every day — at least 8 glasses — to hydrate your skin from the inside out. It's best to drink purified or bottled water — or tap water that has been run through a double-carbon filter.

Zinc. Because zinc allows stored vitamin A in the liver to be released into the bloodstream, it is very important for skin health. Either take a zinc supplement, or eat lots of zinc-rich pumpkin seeds.

solution and make a fresh batch.

DEW Centuries ago, Scottish and English women went out early in the morning to collect fresh dew from leaves and flowers to wash their faces. The dew, slightly sticky with mucilage from the plants, smoothed the skin. The women also believed that it erased blotches, smoothed out wrinkles and prevented the effects of aging.

FENNEL If you have oily skin, try cleaning it with fennel. Dirt tends to cling to oily skin, and this herb is very effective in removing it.

ROSEMARY European queens and ladies of the nobility used rosemary as a beautifying agent. To make a cleanser, they soaked rosemary leaves in white wine. Rosemary has a woody, pine-like aroma mixed with the sweetness of wildflowers. Rosemary oil also stimulates blood flow under the skin surface. And it contains diosmin, a flavonoid that strengthens fragile blood vessels.

SOAPWORT Since medieval times, Arabs, Chinese and Indians all used soapwort as a skin cleanser. Mix the juice of the plant with water to form a sudsy lather.

NATURAL TONERS

CUCUMBER Cucumbers have a cooling effect on the skin and eyelids. Cucumber juice makes a good toner. And in Europe and North America, massaging the face with fresh cucumber slices is a popular beauty treatment.

HYSSOP Boil 1 tablespoon of hyssop in 1 cup of water for 10 minutes and then strain. Refrigerate until cool and then use regularly as a toner to minimize oily skin.

LAVENDER This lovely flower makes a powerful astringent for oily complexions. Boil some lavender flowers (either fresh or dried) in a few cups of water. After the solution cools, use it to mist or wipe your face throughout the day.

LEMON To tone the skin of your throat, moisturize and then cover with a washcloth soaked in an infusion of hot water and lemon juice. Leave the cloth on for 2 minutes and then replace it with a cloth soaked in ice-cold water. Alternate the two applications 4 times and then apply a firming mask.

And to give your face a youthful glow, apply 1 part of lemon oil mixed with 2 parts of glycerin.

VINEGAR Dilute apple cider vinegar at least half and half with water and use for an astringent.

WATER Dunk your face right into a big bowl of ice water to lessen puffiness.

WITCH HAZEL This excellent natural astringent is a common ingredient in commercial skin-care products. To make your own toner, mix a few drops of witch hazel extract in water and splash it on your face.

YOGURT Yogurt applied directly to the skin helps maintain the proper acid balance (pH) that protects skin from germs and chemical toxins.

NATURAL MOISTURIZERS

ALDER BUCKTHORN Alder buckthorn grows in the damp marshes of Southeast England. Available from herbalists as a tincture or in a syrup, it can be used to make a lotion for dry skin. Steep 4 ounces of the twig bark in 1 quart of boiling water. Allow it to cool, and then apply directly or as a compress.

ALMONDS The aromatic oil of almonds is excellent for softening the hands and cuticles. Just rub it on.

ALOE Cleopatra, the legendary beauty, massaged fresh aloe gel into her skin every day. And Josephine, wife of the emperor Napoleon, reportedly used a lotion prepared from milk and aloe gel for her complexion. Today, aloe, a natural moisturizer and skin healer, is added to many commercial skin creams and lotions.

AVOCADO The high fat content of the avocado (rich in the very beneficial vitamin E) makes it an excellent moisturizer for the skin.

CALENDULA Recommended by herbalists all over the world, the softening oils found in the

---

A Recipe for Homemade Aftershave

To soften dry, damaged skin after shaving, make your own aftershave lotion using equal parts aloe vera juice (sold bottled at health food stores) and sage tea.

Special Face and Body Treatments

■ **Steam your pores clean with an herbal facial.** Simply boil a pot of water and add some bay, chamomile, comfrey, lemon balm, rosemary or thyme. Take the pot off the heat and lower your face into the steam. This works even better if you "tent" your head and the pot with a towel to prevent the steam from escaping.

■ **Enjoy a hot towel treatment.** Soak a small towel in hot water. Then lie down, place the towel over your face — and relax while the heat perks up your complexion.

■ **Have a massage.** The therapeutic value of massage — for the face as well as the body — has been undisputed for centuries. It stimulates blood flow and increases lymphatic drainage.

■ **Give yourself a herbal bath.** Ninon de Lenclos was a famous French beauty who discovered the beautifying powers of the herbal bath — what she called the "magic" water. She mixed a handful of dried lavender flowers, dried rosemary leaves, dried mint, chopped comfrey roots and thyme, and made an infusion in 1 quart of water. She added this infusion to her bath and then soaked in it for 15 minutes.

   The minerals from these herbs are absorbed through the skin, nourishing the cell structure. The mucilage in the plants also softens the skin.

petals of the calendula flower are especially effective on dry, hard, sore, chaffed or chapped skin. In fact, many commercial lotions contain calendula.

_____ **GELATIN** Use plain gelatin to soften rough, dry hands and feet. Follow the instructions on the box, but allow the gelatin to set only until it is semi-hard. Then massage it into the skin.

_____ **GLYCERIN** Any glycerin product helps retain moisture in the skin. So pick up some glycerin cream at your local health food store and apply it after you bathe to your hands, feet, legs and elbows.

_____ **HONEY** Because of its ability to trap and hold moisture, honey is an excellent moisturizer for rough, dry skin.

444

- **Pamper your skin with sea salt.** Just add ½ cup of sea salt to a tub of warm water — and enjoy.

- **Don't just bathe — luxuriate** in a tub of water moisturized with several drops of any essential oil. Pick your favorite scent, fill the tub with warm or hot water, and soak. Your skin will be softened by the emollients in the oils while you breathe in the therapeutic fragrance of wild flowers or herbs.

- **Soften your skin with comfrey.** Boil 1 ounce of comfrey leaves in 2 pints of water for about 20 minutes and then strain. Add immediately to your tub.

- **Try a buttermilk bath** — they've been popular in American rural communities since the days of the Western frontier.

- **Put a cup of oatmeal into some cheesecloth,** muslin or a tea ball and add it to your bathwater.

- **Treat yourself to a full-body wrap** at an upscale skin-care salon. You will emerge from your cocoon with your skin moisturized and nourished from head to toe.

JOJOBA From the deserts of the U.S. and Mexico comes the jojoba plant, which yields one of the best all-around natural oils for nourishing the skin. Jojoba contains vitamin E as well as other vitamins and minerals that make skin silky and soft.

MAYONNAISE Mayonnaise is one of the most popular European treatments for wrinkles caused by dry skin. The Europeans also use safflower oil, vitamin A oil, vitamin D oil, vitamin E oil and lanolin.

PAPAYA To smooth rough, dry hands, squeeze as much juice out of a fresh papaya as possible and then soak in the liquid for a few minutes.

POTATOES Potatoes are an excellent source of minerals which are good for the skin. To soften the skin — especially the hands — try this: Boil a potato and mash it with a little milk and a few drops of glycerin and rose water. Then rub the mixture into your hands.

ROSE WATER Make a rose water spritzer to keep your face moist during the day. First make the rose water by simmering petals in boiling water. Strain and cool. Then, in a small spray bottle, combine 2 teaspoons of the rose water with a cup of bottled or purified water.

SESAME OIL Following an herbal bath, women in the Far East like to rub scented vegetable oils — especially sesame oil — into their skin. The oil softens skin by preventing perspiration or other moisture from washing away natural oils.

SPEEDWELL The leaf of this plant is useful to treat patches of dry skin. Just take some fresh speedwell, bruise the leaves and rub directly on your skin.

Alpha-Hydroxy Acids (AHAs) — Nature's Wrinkle Removers

Whereas Retin-A was heralded in the 80s as a miracle anti-wrinkling agent, today the buzzword is AHA. This acid is naturally found in food products, primarily fruit. Like Retin-A, it smooths the skin — but without the unpleasant side effects of redness, irritation, burning or photosensitivity.

The most popular AHA is glycolic acid, although lactic acid provides good results as well. Both work by thinning the outer layers of the skin so wrinkles (especially crow's feet) become less obvious. They also plump the top layers of the skin, thereby making the face seem firmer.

If you're interested in trying AHAs, we recommend that you consult with a skin-care specialist first to determine if they're right for you.

WHEAT GERM OIL Use wheat germ oil — or cotton seed oil — to lubricate and moisturize your skin after cleansing.

NATURAL EXFOLIANTS AND SCRUBS

ALMONDS Finely crushed almonds are excellent for exfoliating the skin on the entire body.

BRAN For a healthy, rosy complexion, try using finely ground bran (or cornmeal) as a scrub to prevent blackheads and remove impurities from oily skin. Used daily, these grains will also soak up excess oil from your skin — without the chemical harshness of store-bought scrubs.

LOOFAH Rub a loofah over your wet skin while you're taking a shower or bath — and rub away dead cells that can make your skin look dull.

OATMEAL To gently scrub away excess dirt and make-up, make a paste made from a bit of honey and 2 teaspoons of oatmeal. Gently rub into your skin for a minute or two, and then rinse off.

PINEAPPLE The enzymes in this tasty fruit work well as an exfoliant for the hands. Simply extract the juice from a fresh pineapple and use it to rinse your hands thoroughly.

SEA SALT While you're taking a shower, massage sea salt on your body for an all-over silky softness without the expense of a commercial body scrub.

SEAWEED This gentle detoxifying, exfoliant wrap for the complexion has been passed down to us from the Orient: Take some brown or green seaweed (readily found in health food stores) and soak in water for at least 10 minutes. Then lie down and wrap your face with the wet seaweed (avoiding the delicate eye area). Leave it on for 15 minutes, remove and rinse well.

NATURAL FACE MASKS

AVOCADO Mash up half an avocado and smear it on your face. The oils in the avocado will plump and moisturize your skin. Then make a soothing eye treatment with the other half of the fruit. Slice, chill and place on your eyelids for about 10 minutes while you lie down and relax.

BANANA Use a mashed banana as a mask for dry skin.

BUTTERMILK For a homemade facial freshener, pat buttermilk on your face and then rinse it off with cold water.

EGG WHITES A mask of plain egg whites is an excellent astringent that's also good for firming skin on the face and throat. Just spread on (avoiding the eye area) and wait 15 minutes before rinsing. If you have oily skin, mix in a few drops of lemon juice.

HONEY Because of its humectant properties, honey is a great mask. It attracts moisture to the skin, so a liberal application of pure honey is perfect for dry skin. It also plumps wrinkles and makes skin look young and supple. Leave the honey on until your skin feels taut, and then rinse with warm water.

MANGO Women in the Sulawesi tribe of Indonesia make a face mask from the pulp of mango fruits. The pulp is massaged into the face and left to dry. Once dry, it is rinsed off, leaving the pores unclogged and the skin tight.

MUD Aztec, Mayan, Egyptian, Moroccan and Italian women have used mud as a firming mask, both for the face and the entire body. Today, pre-packaged face and body muds are widely available.

WHIPPED CREAM To prevent wrinkles, combine a little whipped cream with some raw grated potato or beetroot. Apply this mask to your face, let it dry and rinse off.

YOGURT Warm a little plain yogurt (the kind made with live cultures) and spread it over your face to help control oily skin. Or try this yogurt-based recipe: Place a small orange, sliced but not peeled, into a blender along with 1 teaspoon of lemon juice and a handful of rose petals. Blend until liquefied. Add ½ cup of yogurt and blend a few seconds more. Pat the mask on your face, leave it on for 15 to 20 minutes, then rinse with cool water.

NATURAL REMEDIES FOR SKIN IRRITATIONS

BUTTERMILK To help soothe an especially dry complexion, give your face a buttermilk bath. Just dip a washcloth into buttermilk and pat it on your face. Let air-dry, and then rinse.

CHAMOMILE To decrease the redness and irritation of dry skin, especially dry skin resulting from a windburn, steam your face with chamomile just before bedtime. This soothing remedy smells nice and earthy, and will rehydrate your dry complexion. Here's how to do it: Boil 8 chamomile tea bags in a quart of water and then place them in a bowl. Sit in a comfortable chair, bend your face over the bowl, and drape a towel over your head to make a tent. Breathe in the relaxing vapors while your skin is being healed.

EVENING PRIMROSE If you have oily skin, chances are you have other skin problems, ranging from an occasional pimple to a major case of acne. Evening primrose oil is your answer. Dab it on — right out of the capsule as soon as you feel a blemish coming on.

ST. JOHN'S WORT This multi-purpose herb is often recommended for topical use on the skin to heal minor cuts and abrasions. It can also heal the chapped, dry skin everyone can get in cold weather. Simply add the oil to your bathwater.

WARNING! If you want to look young as long as possible, stay away from alcohol and tobacco. Alcohol robs skin cells of valuable moisture, causing premature wrinkling. And there are more than 200 chemicals in cigarette smoke that damage all the cells in your body — including your skin cells — and cause them to age rapidly and die early.

SMOKING

Though researchers have proven over and over again that smoking contributes to cancer, heart disease and lung disease, it's a killer habit that's tough to break. Most smokers know how dangerous it is, yet when they try to quit — no matter how strong their motivation and willpower — they find that they are faced with one of the biggest challenges of their lives.

This is a powerful physical and psychological addiction, and you need all the support you can get to fight it. Medications and patches are helpful — but they can be quite expensive. And even if you decide to try this medical approach, you're still going to need help from some of the following natural alternatives if you want to give yourself the best chance of kicking the nictotine habit permanently.

BAYBERRY Try sucking on a bayberry (or wild cinnamon) leaf to help keep your smoking urges at bay.

BIRCH In the southeastern U.S., particularly in Appalachia, people who want to stop smoking chew on birch branches to help curb the oral fixation.

LICORICE Natives of the West Indies like to chew on licorice sticks or on sugar cane stalks. Inspired by this idea, one doctor we heard of recommends that his patients chew licorice sticks to break the smoking habit — and he has apparently been very successful. Smokers like having something to chew on or hold in their mouths, and a licorice stick is a safe substitute for a cigarette.

MARJORAM A Chinese herbal remedy to help curb the desire to light up a cigarette is to drink a tea made from marjoram or magnolia bark. These teas make the throat very dry — and that makes smoking unpleasant.

RADISH When a Chinese smoker wants to quit, he or she gets a little help from this traditional recipe: Mix grated fresh radish with 2 teaspoons of honey and drink it like a juice.

Helpful Hints

Here are some suggestions from Dr. Robert D. Willix to help you with your fight to quit smoking. Dr. Willix is the author of _Healthy at 100_ and the editor of the monthly newsletter, _Health & Longevity_.

■ **Breathe deep.** Try inhaling and exhaling as fully as possible. It will help you relax.

■ **Try to delay the urge.** Whether you light up or not, the urge to smoke will pass if you can just wait it out.

■ **Exercise.** You absolutely must exercise when you are trying to quit smoking. Aerobic exercise, especially, helps reduce stress — which is going to increase while you're trying to kick the habit. Also, exercising makes you feel better about yourself and your health as you work toward becoming smoke free. We recommend walking at a brisk pace or jogging 5 to 6 times a week for 20 to 30 minutes per session.

■ **Find non-smoking friends.** If you're trying to quit cigarettes, it's best not to hang around people who smoke or frequent places where smokers congregate.

■ **Join a support group.** Even if you have plenty of non-smoking friends, you may want to enlist a few new ones who are experiencing (or have experienced) the same withdrawal symptoms as you.

■ **Keep your hands busy.** Knit, sew, crochet, doodle, write letters, take up wood carving, try putting a puzzle together, work on your computer, use Chinese exercise balls — or do anything else you can think of to keep your hands occupied.

■ **Keep yourself busy.** Don't just sit or stand around. Staying occupied is important to help take your mind off of smoking.

SALT Another Chinese trick: Lick a little salt with the tip of your tongue whenever you feel the urge to smoke. This is said to break the habit within 1 month.

WATER The urge to smoke can sometimes be subsided just by taking a sip of water.

■ **Make a list.** Make a list of all the reasons you want to quit — and keep the list in your wallet or purse so you can refer to it any time you're tempted to light up. Your list will probably include at least some of the following:
- I want to quit because I'm short of breath.
- I want to quit because my smoking hurts my kids.
- I want to quit because I'm sick and tired of my breath and hair and clothes smelling like smoke.
- I want to quit because it's important for me to be in control of my own life.
- I want to quit to save $23.80 a week.

■ **Try taped motivational aids.** Cassette tapes that combine subliminal messages with straightforward messages of positive reinforcement are available at health food stores and bookstores, and through catalogs.

■ **Plan ahead.** If you're going to a place where you know many people will be smoking, take the time to give yourself plenty of positive reinforcement beforehand. Think of all the advantages to not smoking. Imagine how healthy you'll look, how good the food will taste, how much better your clothes and breath will smell, etc.

■ **Try visualization.** While trying to kick the habit, it really does help to think of your lungs as clean and clear, your breath sweeter smelling, your mouth better tasting, your teeth whiter, your appearance more youthful overall, and so on.

■ **Combine visualization with a deep breathing exercise** to help ease the stress of withdrawal. Here's how to do it: Picture in your mind something that makes you feel good or happy — then relax. Close your mouth and slowly inhale as deeply as possible. Remain relaxed and hold the breath for a count of four. Gently exhale, slowly, and empty your lungs completely. Repeat these steps 5 times.

Curiosity Box

In India, boiled oats have been used for many years to treat opium addiction. A welcome side effect of this treatment is that the addicts often lose interest in cigarettes as well as opium.

Interestingly, researchers in Scotland recently found that fresh oats really do diminish nicotine cravings. They believe it works because oats are high in alkaline and change the preference of your taste buds. Other high-alkaline foods that may make it easier for you to quit smoking are spinach, beet greens, raisins, figs, dried lima beans, dandelion greens and almonds.

Roll Your Own Herbal Cigarettes

Smoking began with the Indians. They smoked tobacco for ritual and spiritual purposes, not as an everyday habit. And because they added botanicals and flavored herbs to the tobacco in their pipes, they cut down on the nicotine content.

The more you add to tobacco, the less nicotine it has. And although you can buy herbal cigarettes in some natural food stores, here are a few roll-your-own fillers to try:

- Rosemary (used in tobacco mixtures for centuries in England)
- Beech tree leaves (smoked by Germans during WWI)
- Corn silk
- Tonka beans
- Myrica gale (used by Norwegians)
- Licorice
- Sage
- Marjoram

SORE THROAT

Although sore throats are common, their severity and causes vary widely. The pain can range from a mild scratchy feeling to a soreness so intense it inhibits swallowing and breathing. They can be caused by anything from a simple localized infection or irritation to a serious viral or bacterial disease. Most sore throats, however, are the result of the common cold, a mild allergy, or exposure to polluted, dry air.

For a sore throat accompanied by a fever, see your doctor. Mild sore throats, though, can be treated safely at home using these international remedies.

AGRIMONY In Europe, the agrimony plant is a favorite remedy for sore throats. It tones the membranes and helps keep mucous secretions fluid. French singers and public speakers use this agrimony gargle: 1 teaspoon of dried leaves, flowers and stems from the plant are infused in 1 quart of boiling water for 20 minutes. The flavor is like apricots, but licorice or honey is often added to improve the taste and to increase the soothing effect.

BLACKBERRY Louisiana, with its rich mix of native and immigrant cultures, has many folk remedies for sore throats. One is a gargle made from blackberries.

CAYENNE PEPPER In New Orleans, people treat a sore throat (and hoarseness) with cayenne pepper seeds. They soak the seeds in water and use the resulting liquid as a gargle.

CITRICIDAL Researchers worldwide are testing a substance called citricidal — an extract made from the seeds and pulp of citrus fruits — as a remedy for sore throats. The researchers theorize that citricidal may be able to kill a variety of disease-causing bacteria and viruses, including those that cause strep throat.

**ELDERBERRIES** Make a hot tea to soothe your inflamed throat by simmering elderberries and then straining the liquid from the fruit. Drink it as hot as you can take it, sweetened with honey, several times a day. For an added antiseptic effect, add ginger and cloves to the berry tea after it has come to a boil.

**GRAPEFRUIT JUICE** The Seminole Indians couldn't have told you why it worked, but for a sore throat, they squeezed the juice from a grapefruit, gargled it, and drank whatever was left over. Modern-day nutritionists, of course, will tell you that it is the vitamin C content of the fruit that helps relieve throat pain.

**HONEY** For centuries, Hungarians have used honey to treat sore throats. The best way to administer this sweet cure is to take 1 teaspoon of honey, place it on your tongue, and let it trickle down your throat. Similar treatments are common in Asia and Greece, and in Italy, opera singers have found that the honey is even more effective when it is mixed with lemon juice. An old-time American remedy for sore throats is a gargle made from a mixture of honey, salt and baking soda dissolved in water.

All of these honey cures do indeed bring relief, but that relief is not long-lasting. The honey acts as a hypertonic osmotic, which means that its presence causes fluid to be pulled out of the inflamed tissue, thus shrinking swelling and easing discomfort. Unfortunately, the symptoms return as soon as the honey is gone.

**OLIVES** The Chinese soothe sore throats by keeping pitted olives in their mouths throughout the day. This probably works because olives stimulate the secretion of saliva, which dilutes bacteria.

**POMEGRANATE** The pomegranate has been cultivated in Israel for more than 5,000 years, and over the centuries, the Israelis have found medicinal uses for many parts of this fruit. One example — a gargle made from boiling the rind in water to treat sore throats.

SAGE The Germans, the English and the French share a sore throat remedy that involves boiling sage leaves in water and vinegar. They allow the concoction to cool and then use it as a gargle.

Another German recipe for a sore throat is to steep 1 to 2 teaspoons of dried sage leaves in 1 cup of boiling water for 10 minutes. Use as a tea or gargle.

SALT The Pennsylvania Dutch treat sore throats with a gargle made of warm water and salt.

VIOLETS The Greeks gave this sore throat remedy to the Romans, who, in turn, gave it to the rest of Europe. Meanwhile, the Chinese discovered it on their own. What's the secret? Violets. Gargling violet tea is a many-fold treatment. It is slightly sedative, it has a mild topical anesthetic effect and the mucilage from the flowers coats the throat.

STOMACHACHE

Most ordinary stomachaches are caused by poor eating habits — eating too much, eating too fast and/or eating the wrong foods. For example, coffee, regular (not herbal) tea, carbonated drinks and alcoholic beverages (especially beer and wine, which have a high acid content) irritate the stomach lining. Mayonnaise, fried foods, overly salty foods and dairy products trigger digestive disorders in many people. And hard-to-digest foods like cabbage and beans can cause discomfort even in people with the hardiest of constitutions. So, if you are prone to stomachaches, common sense should tell you that you've got to make some changes.

Still, no matter how careful you are about your diet, you're going to have an occasional bout with bloating, aching, cramping and gas. And though the discomfort will almost always pass on its own, why suffer when there are so many simple home remedies to ease the pain?

ACIDOPHILUS Pick up some acidophilus capsules at your health food store. (The refrigerated or "live" cultures are best). Acidophilus helps restore "good" bacteria in the digestive system.

BANANA Bananas are gentle on your tummy and easy to digest — a tried-and-true remedy for stomachaches.

BASIL Boil a bit of sweet basil to make a stomach-soothing tea.

CARAWAY SEED A brew of caraway seed can help ease any stomach problems — especially those accompanied by nausea or hiccuping. Simply boil 2 teaspoons of caraway seeds with 1 teaspoon of cinnamon and 1 teaspoon of dried ginger. Cool slightly, and sip slowly.

CHAMOMILE Drinking a strong brew of chamomile tea (a natural calmative) several times a day can alleviate even the most serious stomachaches and cramps.

CHIVES A Chinese remedy for upset stomach calls for 1 glass of cow's milk mixed with half a glass of fresh chive juice and 3 teaspoons of fresh ginger juice. This medicinal "milkshake" is heated before drinking.

CINNAMON The Chinese also treat stomach pains by dissolving 1 teaspoon of ground cinnamon in a cup of warm water. They cover the cup for 15 minutes, and then drink the liquid like tea.

DANDELION An old German remedy for upset stomachs is dandelion tea.

FENNEL The Greeks find that adding fennel to recipes often helps squelch stomach upset.

GINGER Ginger is a very effective stomach soother. Take it in the form of gelatin capsules, available at most health food stores — or try some of the following Chinese folk remedies:
- Make ginger tea by mixing ½ teaspoon of dried ginger in a cup of tea.

- Use lots of ginger in your cooking.

- Pulverize 2 teaspoons of litchi or licorice and boil in a small amount of water with 1 teaspoon of fresh ginger.

HONEY The British make a soothing drink that calls for ¼ cup of honey in 1 cup of warm water.

KUMQUATS The Chinese make a tea out the juice of the kumquat to treat stomachache. They boil 10 dried kumquats in 6 cups of water, and drink the liquid 3 times a day.

PAPAYA This popular tropical fruit not only tastes great, it helps improve digestion. Islanders eat it whenever their stomachs are acting up.

___**PEPPERMINT** Peppermint (a natural antispasmotic) yields a volatile oil that the British use as a medicine to alleviate stomachache. When added to tea, it regulates the flow of bile to aid digestion.

Try combining peppermint, chamomile and lemon balm in hot water. (Kids like it with a little apple juice mixed in too.)

___**PERSIMMON** Eat fresh persimmon to aid your ailing digestive tract.

___**RICE** To treat an acid stomach, The Philadelphia College of Pharmacy and Science recommends eating ½ cup of cooked rice, a complex carbohydrate that binds up excess acid. This all-natural antacid is extremely easy to digest.

STRAINS AND SPRAINS

Even mild muscle injuries may not require a trip to the doctor, but they can be quite painful. A strain occurs when the muscle tissue is stretched or torn. A sprain is more serious, involving damage to the ligaments and joints. Sprains are often accompanied by tenderness and swelling in the area surrounding the immediate impact — and they may bruise in vivid shades of black and blue. Both types of injuries are most likely to occur when the muscles are weak and unable to absorb the impact of a sudden movement or jarring jolt.

The best way to prevent strains and sprains is to exercise regularly. The stronger the surrounding muscles, the less likely you are to injure your ligaments and joints. However, once you have been injured, stop exercising that muscle group immediately. If you continue, you will only exacerbate the damage.

With or without professional care, a muscle injury can take days, weeks or even months to fully heal. But with the help of the following natural remedies, you can speed up the healing — and be more comfortable in the process.

ARNICA Used externally, a compress made with diluted tincture of arnica is great for sore muscles or sprains, because this herb is a natural anti-inflammatory and analgesic. Arnica ointment is also widely used in both Europe and North America to relieve pain and inflammation. Two substances in arnica, helenalin and dihydrohelenalin, are what give it its unique properties.

BANANA If you have a sprain, you may want to pick up a few extra bananas. After eating the fruit with your morning cereal, save the skin and apply it to your injury. Banana peels not only help alleviate the pain, they can even minimize the black and blue bruising. Try it this way: Run some very cold water over a piece of cloth and then wring thoroughly. Put the banana peel over the wounded area, cover with the cold cloth and secure with gauze tape.

BAY Oil of bay — which is made by pressing oil from the berries and leaves of the plant — is reputed by many to ease sprains. Add a few drops to your bath and soak your pain away.

CABBAGE Put cabbage leaves directly on your injury. Secure with gauze and tape, or bind with a cloth made out of a soft material like flannel, terry, fleece or muslin.

CAYENNE PEPPER A liniment made with cayenne pepper is a good external treatment for muscle injuries. Capsaicin, the active chemical in these peppers, relieves pain when applied to the skin. Capsaicin affects the sensory nerves and stimulates blood flow to the area, which reduces inflammation.

COMFREY Bruised comfrey leaves can speed up the healing process. The recommended method is to boil about 8 ounces of comfrey in a small amount of water for about 5 minutes. Once the preparation has cooled to the touch, put the whole thing — leaves and all — in a soft cloth and apply to your injury.

For larger or more serious sprains, it's best to wrap the wounded area with a poultice made only with the comfrey liquid. Simply boil the leaves (a couple of ounces should be enough for each application) in ¾ of a pint of water for 20 minutes. Strain and use the water to saturate a large, soft cloth. Leave on your injury until the poultice cools. Then remove and replace with a fresh one.

HYSSOP This ancient remedy was used by the American Indians for many purposes, one being the healing of sprains. Modern-day healers tell us to rub the leaves until you get the juice out of them, and then apply directly to the sprain.

ICE Ice will help decrease swelling. Apply it for the first 24 hours after the injury.

OATMEAL Combine equal parts of oatmeal and comfrey, and boil the two together for about 5 minutes. Once the mixture has cooled, squeeze out as much of the excess liquid as possible and stuff it into a soft cloth. Put this poultice directly on your sprain and leave it there until it cools.

POTATOES According to American folklore, raw potato juice or hot potato water can soothe a sprain. Simply add the juice to your bath (or foot bath) and soak.

SALT The iodine in unrefined salt, such as sea salt, is soothing when applied to a sprain as a hot compress. Sea salt can be purchased at your grocery store or health food store.

THYME For swellings and sprains, steep 1 teaspoon of thyme in 1 pint of boiling water for 10 to 15 minutes. Then add to your bathwater and soak in it.

WITCH HAZEL Saturate a cloth with distilled witch hazel and apply it to your injury.

WORMWOOD Make an infusion by steeping 2 teaspoons of wormwood leaves or tops in 1 cup of water. Soak a cloth in this infusion and apply the compress to your sprain.
CAUTION: *Use wormwood externally only. It's poisonous if ingested.*

STRESS

In today's fast-paced world, just about everyone is affected by stress — at home and on the job. The symptoms are many and varied, and can include fatigue or insomnia, depression, headache, back or neck pain, irritability or edginess, and weight loss or gain. Less common, but potentially more serious manifestations of stress include heart palpitations, shortness of breath, diarrhea, nausea, panic attacks, inability to concentrate, agoraphobia (chronic fear), excessive smoking or drinking, drug use — and even serious physical illness like heart disease, asthma, emphysema and ulcers.

Since there is no way to completely eliminate stress from our lives, it's very important to learn how to defuse its potentially damaging effects on our bodies and minds. The good news is there are many lessons to be learned — from people all around the world — to help manage and control stress without resorting to expensive professional help or dangerous pharmaceuticals.

ANISE Anise tea is said to be helpful in treating headaches and stomachaches commonly associated with stress.

BORAGE Though raw borage flowers can act as a stimulant, people in Wales use this plant to encourage relaxation. In fact, they refer to it as the "herb of gladness." They soak borage in sherry and water, boil the mixture, and then drink it in the early evening or before bedtime. They also occasionally add borage to cocktails, just as you might put olives in a martini.

Native Americans made a borage tea by steeping 1 heaping teaspoon of dried borage in a cup of boiled water for 10 minutes, and then straining. It can also be made by boiling fresh leaves and stems in water. Try it — it tastes like cucumber.

CATNIP Cats may be on to something when they happily chew on catnip leaves. The aromatic oils in this plant, which contain similar compounds to those found in the naturally soothing valerian root, seem to send them into ecstasy.

Helpful Hints

■ **Eat a healthy diet.** Keeping your physical machine primed is a wonderful preventive measure to take against stress.

■ **Avoid sugar.** Refined white sugar compounds stress by making you jittery and ruining your sleep. If you must use a sweetener, opt for fructose (fruit sugar) or turbinado (raw sugar). They're much safer than the chemically processed alternative.

■ **Use soothing herbs.** A host of spices including fennel, ginger, cumin, cloves and spearmint have been said to promote a feeling of well-being when consumed in the daily diet.

Use herbs in the bath, too — especially valerian, chamomile, parsley and sweet flag. In ancient Greece and Rome, this was a popular way to relieve stress and anxiety. The most effective way to prepare an herbal bath is to wrap the dried herbs in a cheesecloth, and hang it from the water faucet.

■ **Eat plenty of complex carbohydrates.** Because they promote the release of serotonin (a neurotransmitter produced in the brain that has natural sedative properties), carbohydrates help counteract the effects of stress on your body.

Instead of eating more bread (which is loaded with yeast and can cause candida problems), eat lots of vegetables, potatoes, brown rice, grains, cereals and spinach pastas. Some experts argue that "carbs" don't work as well when mixed with meat protein, so whenever possible, try for a straight carbohydrate meal that includes a non-meat protein like garbanzo beans, lentils or tofu.

■ **Exercise.** Regular exercise is important to maintain physical and mental health — especially when you're going through a period of increased stress or anxiety. The reason: Exercise releases endorphins (chemicals that give you a natural "high") in your brain. If you don't want to join a

Because catnip is a natural tranquilizer, it can be used by humans as a stress-reducer and as a sleeping aid. Make catnip tea by pouring boiling water over dried catnip and letting it steep. Use a tea ball or strain thoroughly before drinking.

---

gym and aerobicise your tension away, a brisk walk around the block every day will do the trick.

■ **Treat yourself to a massage.** A good massage — maybe using a few drops of jasmine oil mixed into a cup of vegetable oil — can loosen up tense muscles and relax the body. Albanians believe that a massage also frees the mind and enhances creativity. They alternately massage the neck and shoulders, and then apply hot compresses.

■ **Find a creative outlet.** Throughout the U.S., art therapy is used to ease nervous tension. By drawing, sculpting or painting the images that are troubling them, patients get some degree of relief from stress disorders.

Actually, any hobby that can help you escape from the pressures of the moment is a good remedy for stress.

■ **Decorate your home or office with yellow.** Dr. Alexander Schauss' studies at the American Institute for Biosocial Research indicate that the color yellow has an energizing effect and can even lift your spirits — perhaps because it is the color of sunshine.

■ **Relax with the sounds of nature.** Many new age artists are producing albums filled with the peaceful sounds of waterfalls, rain and ocean waves. So pop one in your CD player, put on some headphones to eliminate outside noise and kick back. For reasons researchers don't yet understand, music is aesthetically pleasing to the psyche and thereby therapeutic in any stressful situation.

■ **Be positive.** Whenever you have to face a potentially upsetting situation, think of all the possible outcomes — from the best to the worst — and expect the best.

CELERY A traditional Chinese remedy for stress is fresh celery juice mixed with honey. The Chinese believe this has a mild sedative effect. You might also want to try eating lots of fresh celery and flavoring food with dried celery seeds and leaves.

CHAMOMILE The Germans and the English swear by chamomile tea for its strong relaxing effect. Try it sweetened with a little honey.

The English relax with chamomile in a different way. They add a large sachet of chamomile flowers to their bathwater. You can get the same effect by steeping a handful of the dried herb in hot water for 15 minutes before adding it to your tub.

CHERRIES Though the fructose in fruit is a natural sugar, which can rev you up instead of calm you down, scientists in Germany have recently found that cherries contain minute amounts of a sedative chemical.

COWSLIP The cowslip is a flower that grows in the meadows and pastures of England, and in other parts of Europe, Siberia, western Asia and northern Africa. The blossoms are mixed with sugar, honey, water and lemon juice to make a beverage that acts as a mild sedative that can help you fall asleep.

The Alexander Technique

Frederick Alexander, a retired Shakespearean recitalist from Australia, developed an interesting way to reduce stress. Apparently, Alexander had vocal problems that ruined his career. And when he tried to figure out what had caused these problems, he determined that he had been misusing his body while speaking and acting. He believed that this was true for many people — that they unconsciously tensed up their bodies at work and while performing everyday tasks. So, he developed "The Alexander Technique," a sequence of simple movements that teach people to change bad habits that create tension and stress. Students learn to sit, bend, talk and walk in ways that promote optimum functioning of their bodies.

For a list of certified teachers in your area, contact the American Center for the Alexander Technique at the Abraham Goodman House, 129 W. 67th St., New York, NY 10023, (212) 799-0468.

CRAMP BARK Cramp bark is a muscle and nerve relaxant that is commonly taken as a tea. Prepare the tea by steeping a teaspoon of the herb in a cup of boiled water for about 7 minutes. Strain and drink. **CAUTION:** *The berries of the cramp bark tree are poisonous.*

GINSENG Popular throughout the Orient, Siberian ginseng is reportedly able to help people resist the effects of stress. For more about the many benefits of ginseng, turn to page 64.

LAVENDER Because lavender has sedative properties, it is good for calming anxiety and tension. Try a relaxing massage with lavender oil to ease stress.

LEMON Advocates of aromatherapy will tell you that scents can have a powerful effect on your state of mind — which is the reason the Japanese

---

NERVE-CALMING TEA

Valerian tea is rather neglected as a homemade remedy because the roots smell so strong during preparation. The flavor is also quite "singular," so use valerian in a mixture with other pleasant-tasting herbs, as in the following recipe:

> 8 tsps. valerian root
> 6 tsps. hops
> 3 tsps. peppermint leaves
> 3 tsps. hibiscus flowers

It is best to soak these herbs overnight in lukewarm water, heat up to drinking temperature in the morning, and then strain them off. The results are excellent. One of the most remarkable things about valerian is that it is calming, yet does not inhibit concentration and awareness.

Valerian seems to totally fascinate and hypnotize cats, so store it carefully if there are felines about the house.

Reprinted from "The Family Herbal" by Barbara and Peter Theiss, published by Healing Arts Press, an imprint of Inner Traditions International, Rochester, VT.

Relax With Yoga

Yoga is a form of meditation derived from a 4,000-year-old Indian tradition. It literally means "union," and works on several levels to bring the body and the mind into balance. Yoga releases energy, while calming tense muscles and ridding your mind of anxious thoughts.

The moon asana (described below) is an especially calming posture that you might want to try. **CAUTION:** *Don't do this if you have high blood pressure.*

- Kneel on a flat surface and sit on your heels.
- Grasp your right wrist with your left hand behind your back.
- Inhale, and as you exhale, bend forward slowly from the hips until your forehead is on the ground, or as close to the ground as you can get it. (If your forehead doesn't reach the ground, rest it on a folded towel.)
- Let go of your wrist and allow your arms to rest on the floor on each side of you.
- Hold this position for a moment or two.
- Then, as you slowly inhale, lift yourself back up until you are once again upright in a kneeling position.

Turn to page 6 for more information about yoga.

use lemon oil with an aroma lamp when they want to ease psychological or emotional stress.

And lemon is a main ingredient in this popular Gypsy remedy for stress that is safer and more effective than over-the-counter tranquilizers. They drink a juice made from lemons, oranges, honey and hot water.

LEMON BALM Arabs are fond of the scent of lemon balm and use it as a perfumed oil to treat nervousness, fatigue (or even exhaustion), tension and depression.

Lemon balm tea promotes relaxation when taken at bedtime — and when taken in the morning, it's refreshing and invigorating.

LETTUCE A substance in lettuce, called lactucarium, is a calming agent — one more good reason to eat plenty of fresh, green salads.

MAGNESIUM Since magnesium has natural sedative properties, you can calm jittery nerves and relax tight muscles simply by adding 2 to 3 cups of Epsom salts to your bath. Soak for at least 20 minutes to get all the anti-stress benefits you'll need to face another day.

MILKWORT Another popular Chinese remedy for tension is a tea made with chopped milkwort root mixed with licorice.

MINT In some countries with hot climates, bunches of fresh mint are placed around the house to freshen the air and provide a relaxing feeling of coolness. This herb is an excellent aromatic that improves with age.

OATS Oats provide many nutrients that help our bodies tolerate tension. They are essential for maintaining a properly functioning nervous system, and have been found to be helpful in alleviating depression, fatigue, lethargy, weakness and even exhaustion.

ONIONS Onions have long been praised in holistic circles for their general healing properties — and because they contain quercetin, studies indicate that they may also induce relaxation.

PASSIONFLOWER Passionflower contains alkaloids that are both tranquilizing and non-addicting. And because this herb has no known toxicity in small doses, it is a popular ingredient in several sedative/hypnotic drug mixtures in Europe that are used to treat anxiety and tension. Try ½ teaspoon of the passionflower in 1 cup of boiling water.

PERIWINKLE The Madagascar periwinkle has been esteemed for its medicinal properties since the days of the Roman Empire. Because it is a natural sedative, periwinkle tea is used to treat nervous conditions.

ROSEMARY Rosemary tea has been consumed for centuries by Arab, Chinese and European people to ease stress. Thanks to its high calcium content, rosemary seems to calm the nerves when taken as a tea. It also acts like aspirin to help subdue stress-related headaches. An added bonus: Rosemary doesn't upset the stomach the way aspirin can.

SAGE Reputed to be beneficial for the nervous tension associated with menopause, sage also eases common, everyday anxiety. Use sage to flavor poultry recipes or make it into a soothing tea. You can even burn fresh sage like incense.

SERPENTWOOD Mahatma Gandhi, the Hindu nationalist and spiritual leader who kept his cool in the face of major civil turmoil in India, regularly drank a tea made from serpentwood. This herb has been used as a "soother of the mind" in India for over 4,000 years. The root was regularly chewed by the holy men of that country who sought tranquillity in order to meditate.

ST. JOHN'S WORT St. John's wort was originally used in Europe to ward off witches and heal deep sword cuts — and it is now used as a natural

---

Progressive Relaxation

According to Dr. Robert D. Willix in his newsletter "Health & Longevity," progressive muscle relaxation is a very effective — and easy-to-learn — stress-management technique. Simply follow these 6 steps to melt away all the tension from your body:

- ■ **Sit down.** (If you lie down, you run the risk of falling asleep.) Then close your eyes and do nothing for a minute or two.
- ■ **Open your eyes for 10 to 30 seconds,** and then close them and do nothing for another minute or two.
- ■ **Open your eyes for 10 to 30 seconds.**
- ■ **Close your eyes and concentrate on your scalp.** Take a deep breath through your nose and, as you exhale through your nose, consciously relax the muscles of your scalp. (You may find it helpful to first tense those muscles and then relax them.)
- ■ **Work your way down your body,** relaxing your face muscles, neck, shoulders, upper and lower back, arms, hands, fingers, diaphragm, abdomen, pelvis, thighs, legs, feet and toes. Give yourself as long as 15 minutes to do this.
- ■ **When you're finished, take 10 deep breaths** — and focus on a pleasant image in your head.

antidepressant. One to two droppers of the fluid extract — mixed with water, and taken 3 times daily on an empty stomach — is the usual treatment.

THYME Thyme has antispasmodic properties and can relax muscles. As far back as the 15th century in Europe, thyme tea at bedtime was used to treat people who were nervous and suffered from nightmares.

WOOD BETONY If you suffer from tension headaches or migraines, herbalists recommend wood betony tea. In addition to alleviating fatigue and anxiety, this herb is a powerful relaxer for the nervous system.

Bach Flower Remedies

Bach flower remedies have been used for years to relieve emotional problems and other causes of stress. Dr. Edward Bach, a renowned British scientist, developed 38 different natural herbal recipes made from the petals and heads of flowers preserved in unflavored brandy. (The liquid is dropped under the tongue 4 times a day.)

For more information, contact the Flower Essence Society at Box 1769, Nevada City, CA 95959, (916) 265-9163.

SUNBURN

In years past, we thought of sunburn as a hazard only for fair-skinned people. But today, we know that we all need to protect ourselves from over-exposure to the sun in order to avoid long-term skin damage — and the possibility of cancer.

Fortunately, there are many products on the market that offer protection from the sun's dangerous UVB rays. So, whether you're sunbathing, gardening, picnicking or skiing, be sure that every bare inch of your body is thoroughly covered with a sunscreen — preferably one with an SPF of 10 or higher. If you're sunning for the first time of the season or have very fair skin, use one with an SPF of 15 or even 20.

If you wind up with a serious sunburn — one where the skin is not only red, but severely swollen and blistered — you may need professional attention. And if your sunburn is accompanied by chills, fever, nausea or vomiting, you may have sunstroke, and you need immediate emergency care. However, for most minor sunburn, the following natural remedies will suffice to speed your recovery and minimize your discomfort.

ALOE Bottled aloe vera juice is great for relieving the soreness that accompanies a sunburn — and, unlike aloe vera directly from the plant, it's not at all messy. To make a cooling spritzer, mix ¼ cup aloe vera juice in a spray bottle with 1 teaspoon of vitamin E oil and 10 drops essential oil of lavender. Spray the affected area often.

CALENDULA Mix a tincture of calendula with a bit of olive oil (preferably virgin olive oil) and dab on the seared skin. Or bathe the skin with a calendula infusion.

CHAMOMILE The calmative properties of chamomile are relaxing and refreshing when used to bathe a sunburn.

CUCUMBER Either use a juicer to extract the liquid from a cucumber, or carefully squeeze out as much as you can by hand. Soak a cloth in the juice and place directly on the burn.

HONEY Combine equal parts of honey and buttermilk, and apply to your burn.

LAVENDER Essential oil of lavender is reputed to heal sun-scarred skin. Add a few drops to your cool bathwater.

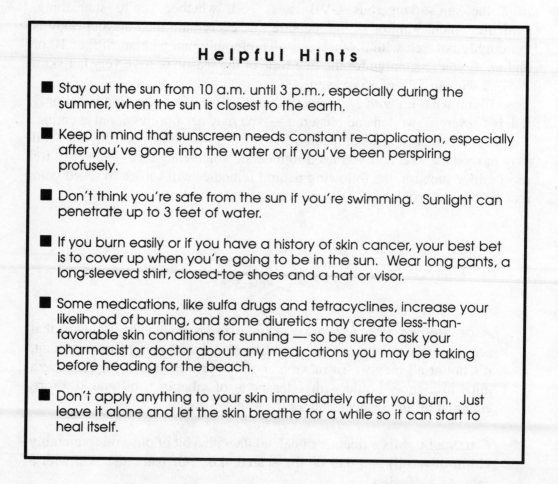

Helpful Hints

■ Stay out the sun from 10 a.m. until 3 p.m., especially during the summer, when the sun is closest to the earth.

■ Keep in mind that sunscreen needs constant re-application, especially after you've gone into the water or if you've been perspiring profusely.

■ Don't think you're safe from the sun if you're swimming. Sunlight can penetrate up to 3 feet of water.

■ If you burn easily or if you have a history of skin cancer, your best bet is to cover up when you're going to be in the sun. Wear long pants, a long-sleeved shirt, closed-toe shoes and a hat or visor.

■ Some medications, like sulfa drugs and tetracyclines, increase your likelihood of burning, and some diuretics may create less-than-favorable skin conditions for sunning — so be sure to ask your pharmacist or doctor about any medications you may be taking before heading for the beach.

■ Don't apply anything to your skin immediately after you burn. Just leave it alone and let the skin breathe for a while so it can start to heal itself.

NETTLE Used in a diluted form, ointment or tincture of nettle — even cold nettle tea — provides sunburn relief.

PEPPERMINT To cool your sunburn, try this wonderfully aromatic herb. Either make some peppermint tea or use a cup of lukewarm water mixed with 2 drops of peppermint oil. Let the infusion chill, and then wash the burned area gently and repeatedly with it.

POTATOES A mixture of pureed potatoes and carrots helps soothe burns when applied directly on the damaged skin.

ST. JOHN'S WORT This multi-purpose herb — in oil or ointment form — can reduce the inflammation of a sunburn.

STRAWBERRY After washing, soothe your sunburned skin by rubbing it with a cut strawberry.

TEA In Taiwan, tea is the favored way to ease sunburn pain. Cold tea compresses or baths quickly remove the sting of tender, sunburned skin.

WATER Take a washcloth soaked in cold, but not frigid, water and place over the burn. Then re-saturate the compress with fresh, chilled water every 15 minutes or so.

YOGURT To ease the burning of well-done skin, apply chilled, fresh, plain yogurt made with live cultures.

TEETHING

Even the most tranquil baby can become a terror when teething — with good reason. The pain can be non-stop and excruciating. The first sign that baby is starting to go through the teething process is usually excessive drooling and restlessness. The gums become red and swollen, possibly even blistered where the new tooth is coming in. And most children become cranky and/or clingy, sometimes refusing to eat or sleep. These symptoms are often accompanied by fever, a cold, diarrhea, rashes on the face, or ear, nose and throat infections.

Painkillers are not the answer. Teething biscuits and frozen teething rings work to some extent, but babies also need plenty of TLC — and help from the following natural ways to curb the pain and soothe the irritability.

APPLE Unsulphered dried apple rings are a tasty alternative to conventional teething rings.

CARROT Mothers in Scotland have found that a frozen carrot makes a good natural teething aid. Chewing offers some relief, and the cold eases swelling and tenderness. As the carrot is chewed it dissolves in baby's mouth.

CHAMOMILE French mothers combine chamomile oil, which is soothing as well as calming. They gently rub the oil directly on the baby's gums.

CLOVES Aromatherapists say that a natural teething solution can be found in essential oil of clove. Dilute a few drops in a tablespoon of olive oil and rub onto baby's gums. This can be done up to 4 times a day.

GARLIC The Europeans use garlic for adult toothaches — and as a treatment for teething babies. Apply a bit of garlic oil directly onto the gums. The antibacterial properties of garlic will minimize the possibility of an infection that could lead to complications.

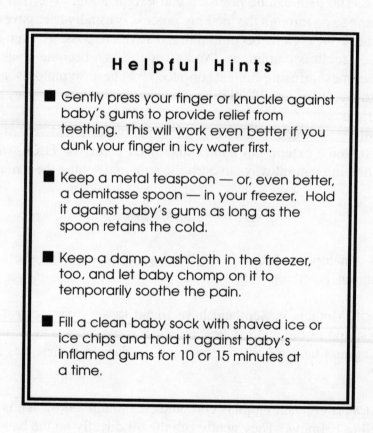

Helpful Hints

■ Gently press your finger or knuckle against baby's gums to provide relief from teething. This will work even better if you dunk your finger in icy water first.

■ Keep a metal teaspoon — or, even better, a demitasse spoon — in your freezer. Hold it against baby's gums as long as the spoon retains the cold.

■ Keep a damp washcloth in the freezer, too, and let baby chomp on it to temporarily soothe the pain.

■ Fill a clean baby sock with shaved ice or ice chips and hold it against baby's inflamed gums for 10 or 15 minutes at a time.

TOOTHACHE

Toothaches are almost always caused by a large cavity or some other destruction to the tooth itself — and require professional attention. See your dentist as soon as possible. You can cause more damage and spread infection by ignoring the pain.

If your toothache is the result of a blow to the head or face, you need emergency care — even if that means going to the nearest hospital. The same goes for a toothache that is accompanied by a fever or chills, swelling of the face, headache or eye ache, stiffness in the neck, bleeding, loss of a tooth or any other unusual symptom. (If you've had a tooth knocked out, wrap it in a wet towel and take it with you. In many cases, it can be replaced.)

However, for minor toothaches, we have ways to help you deal with the discomfort until you can get to the dentist.

CLOVE A simple home remedy for toothaches that's been used for centuries by Europeans calls for bruised leaves of clove to be placed on the affected tooth. This apparently works because a mild antiseptic is contained in the leaves.

Oil of cloves, a strong antiseptic, can be used on a plug of cotton to pack a cavity until you can get to a dentist. Or, just dab a bit of the oil on the aching tooth for temporary relief.

ECHINACEA Echinacea is a good anesthetic for toothaches. Make echinacea tea and use it as a mouthwash.

FIG A German with a toothache will cook a dried fig in milk and apply it to the painful area.

GARLIC Many Europeans use garlic as a toothache remedy. Chew on a clove, or hold it against the tooth. The antibacterial properties of garlic are well-known.

GINGER In Germany, ginger is sold as a remedy for toothache.

GOLDENSEAL Goldenseal is a favorite North American Indian medicine — used to treat sore gums, canker sores, cold sores and toothaches. To relieve pain from a toothache, use a cotton-tipped swab to place the powder directly on the affected area. You can also gargle with goldenseal powder mixed with tincture of myrrh and water. Goldenseal is a very strong antiseptic, disinfectant and astringent.

Curiosity Box

Throughout history, the rich and famous have suffered from dental problems. King Louis XIV angrily revoked religious freedom in France while in the throes of a major dental infection. England's Queen Elizabeth I had to be convinced by her entire court that having a tooth pulled was painful, but endurable. (To help convince her, a bishop had one of his own good teeth pulled while she watched.) And George Washington, who wore wooden dentures, had such problems with his teeth and gums that he was plagued for most of his later life with the inability to chew.

CAUTION: *Goldenseal should not be used during pregnancy. It stimulates the uterus to contract.*

HOPS Dried and taken as an infusion, hops help soothe the pain of toothaches.

MARIGOLD Not just a pretty posy, the marigold was used by English country people as a remedy for toothache. The juice of the marigold petals mixed with vinegar was rubbed on gums and teeth to relieve pain. In addition to acting as an antibacterial agent, marigold contains mucilage to coat and soothe the affected area.

OREGANO Oil from the oregano plant, a favorite flavoring spice in

Italian cuisine, was used by medieval Europeans for toothaches. They massaged the tooth and gums with the oil. Oregano contains thymol, which is a natural antiseptic.

PEPPERMINT To ease toothache or other mouth pain, the Chinese make a tea by boiling 1 teaspoon of fresh peppermint in 1 cup of water and adding a little salt. Peppermint is an antiseptic and contains menthol, which relieves pain when applied to skin surfaces.

PERIWINKLE To stop a toothache, chew on periwinkle, an herb that grows wild in Europe and is cultivated in the U.S. It is known for its astringent and sedative properties.

WINTERGREEN The Quebec Indians knew that fresh wintergreen leaves would relieve aching teeth. Oil of wintergreen contains salicylate, natural aspirin.

YARROW This herb can be made into an infusion and taken to calm aching teeth. Yarrow is another herb that contains natural aspirin compounds. For instructions on how to make an infusion, turn to page 82.

Helpful Hints

■ To ease a toothache or bring down the swelling after extensive dental work, try heat or ice. Some people find relief by applying a heating pad or hot towel to their face. Others are more successful when they use an ice pack or a towel soaked in ice water.

■ If you're bleeding after oral surgery or after having a tooth pulled, a cool tea bag can help. Use it to apply mild pressure to the wounded area for at least 15 minutes.

TOOTH CARE

A tooth is made up of calcium phosphate. It is constantly supplied with nutrients and blood to help keep it alive and to fight decay. The exterior of each tooth is protected by enamel, which is one of the strongest materials in the human body. It has to be strong, because your teeth can apply more than 200 pounds of biting power per square inch.

But tooth enamel isn't impenetrable. Acid, which forms when bacteria in the mouth process sugars in food, can pierce the enamel and eat away at the tooth, creating cavities (also called caries). If detected early, the decayed material can be removed and the resulting hole can be filled. But, if allowed to progress, the bacteria will eat their way to the root of the tooth, producing a toothache and eventually requiring painful root canal surgery or loss of the tooth. Regular, preventive dental care not only protects your teeth from decay, it also keeps a yellowing substance called "plaque" from forming and building up on your teeth when proteins and bacteria interact with your saliva.

So, to maintain good dental health and to prevent future problems as you age, make sure you schedule regular visits to your dentist — and choose natural alternatives to the overpriced oral hygiene products hyped in the mass-market media.

BAKING SODA The best product for cleaning and polishing your teeth is in your kitchen cabinet. Baking soda has just the right consistency for a dentifrice — not too scratchy to remove the enamel, but with enough scouring action to remove plaque. It also neutralizes the acids in your mouth that can eat into tooth enamel.

Use the baking soda together with hydrogen peroxide, and you have an unbeatable combination. The peroxide has an effervescence that

Inflamed Gums

Sore, red, tender or bleeding gums may be the result of poor oral hygiene, heredity or serious gum disease. The best way to prevent gum irritation is to brush both your teeth and gums, twice a day — and floss daily. If your gums are already irritated or infected, floss and brush (with a soft-bristled toothbrush) gently, but thoroughly. You'll aggravate the condition if you scrub, rub or scrape. You can also help heal your aching gums, without medication, by using the following all-natural remedies:

Agrimony. The apricot-flavored herb called agrimony can be soothing for sore gums. It is used regularly by Europeans — especially by singers and speakers who use their voices for a living. Just boil some of the plant (flowers, stems and leaves can all be used) in water, add a bit of honey to sweeten and drink like tea.

Goldenseal. Goldenseal has long been used in North America as a folk remedy for discomfort in the mouth. This herb is antibacterial, which is important since bacteria is often the root of gum disease. Also, it has an astringent effect, which reduces the swelling of inflamed gum tissue.
To brew up some goldenseal tea, just add 1 teaspoon of the powdered herb to 1 cup of boiling water and then steep for about 10 minutes, covered. Add some honey and then use the tea as a rinse, not a drink.

Hydrogen peroxide. The foaming in your mouth when you gargle or rinse with hydrogen peroxide comes from the solution's attack on bacteria in your mouth. So use peroxide daily to fight gum infection.

Sage. Tannins in this herb are helpful to minimize gum tenderness.

Salt. A teaspoon of salt in a glass of hot water is a very effective treatment for painful gums. Gargle and rinse with this solution hourly until the irritation subsides.

Vervain. Make a mouthwash out of vervain to help relieve the pain of inflamed gums by steeping 2 teaspoons of the herb in 1 cup of boiling water, covered.

Vitamin C. Just as it is helpful in preventing bruises, vitamin C is also beneficial for weak, bleeding gums.

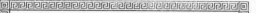

can float away particles from between your teeth — and it has bacteriostatic properties. A highly effective way to maintain dental hygiene is to first soak your toothbrush in hydrogen peroxide, and then dip it in baking soda before brushing.

BERGAMOT OIL Bergamot oil, which smells good enough to be used as a perfume ingredient, is used in Italy to treat a variety of ailments. Bergamot contains thymol, which has antiseptic action. It can be used as a mouthwash and to help cure mouth infections.

CHEDDAR CHEESE Studies show that dairy products help prevent cavities when consumed at the end of a meal. In Canada, researchers have shown that cheddar cheese can reduce the ability of table sugar to cause cavities by 56 percent. It has also been shown to neutralize plaque and minimize damaging acids in the mouth. Cheddar cheese contains concentrated amounts of the minerals calcium, phosphate and casein. Other aged cheeses that may be useful as cavity-fighters include Monterey jack and Swiss.

Curiosity Box

In centuries past, people went to extremes to preserve their teeth. Until the 18th century, many Europeans had their teeth scraped with an iron file and then dabbed with a solution of corrosive nitric acid. For a while, their teeth were dazzlingly white. However, this practice completely eroded natural tooth enamel, causing massive tooth decay among European nobles. Because such dental decay was so common in princely circles, other extreme measures were resorted to in order to replace the missing teeth.

As far back as 800 B.C. in Etruscans (an ancient part of central Italy), dentures were made by extracting teeth from the recently deceased. Renaissance Europe had a similar practice, except that the donors were still living — the poor sometimes sold their healthy teeth for a nego-tiated fee. And some stories tell of extractions made during historical battles — not only on dead soldiers, but also on the wounded. Thousands of teeth were pulled from soldiers felled during Napoleon's battle at Waterloo. And in the U.S., nearly as many dentures were provided by soldiers killed during the Civil War.

CHERRIES According to studies at Forsyth Dental Research Center, black cherry juice is a potent antibacterial agent when used to fight tooth decay.

GREEN TEA Chinese green tea may be nature's best anti-cavity mouthwash. The tea is rich in fluoride, which protects against tooth decay.

RASPBERRIES In the rolling hills and fields of the English countryside, farmers swear that the best way to keep teeth clean is by eating something sweet — but not just any sweet will do the trick. What these farmers recommend is the wild raspberry.

SAGE Many Arabs, American Indians and Far Eastern Indians rub their teeth with sage leaves to cleanse them.

STRAWBERRIES The Swedes clean their teeth with a fresh strawberry. The strawberry is cut in half, and each half is rubbed over the teeth and gums. Strawberries whiten teeth and remove plaque as well.

THYME The leading property of thyme is an antibacterial oil called thymol, which can be found in many store-bought mouthwashes. Make your own mouthwash by steeping 2 teaspoons of thyme (or sage) in a covered cup of boiling water. Strain, allow to cool, and then use as a rinse.

TWIGS For thousands of years, villagers in India have been chewing fresh twigs of the Neem tree to keep their teeth clean. And in the Middle East, the Miswak, or Peelu tree, is sought after as a very effective natural toothbrush. These trees are prized for their naturally astringent, purifying and tooth-whitening properties. Today, there are many toothpastes available commercially that contain these ingredients.

WHEY In Norway, farmers chew on solid whey to prevent cavities, to keep their teeth white and to prevent gum disease. Whey is one of the dairy by-products of cheese. Norwegians also use whey in its liquid form as a gargle.

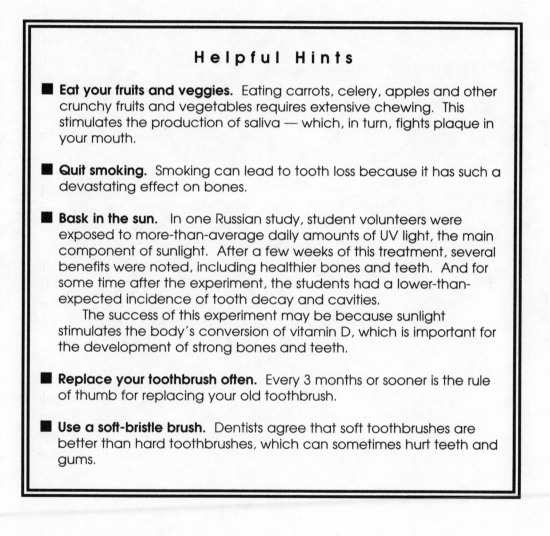

Helpful Hints

■ **Eat your fruits and veggies.** Eating carrots, celery, apples and other crunchy fruits and vegetables requires extensive chewing. This stimulates the production of saliva — which, in turn, fights plaque in your mouth.

■ **Quit smoking.** Smoking can lead to tooth loss because it has such a devastating effect on bones.

■ **Bask in the sun.** In one Russian study, student volunteers were exposed to more-than-average daily amounts of UV light, the main component of sunlight. After a few weeks of this treatment, several benefits were noted, including healthier bones and teeth. And for some time after the experiment, the students had a lower-than-expected incidence of tooth decay and cavities.

   The success of this experiment may be because sunlight stimulates the body's conversion of vitamin D, which is important for the development of strong bones and teeth.

■ **Replace your toothbrush often.** Every 3 months or sooner is the rule of thumb for replacing your old toothbrush.

■ **Use a soft-bristle brush.** Dentists agree that soft toothbrushes are better than hard toothbrushes, which can sometimes hurt teeth and gums.

ULCERS

An ulcer is a hole that has formed either in the lining of the stomach (a gastric ulcer) or in the small intestine (a duodenal ulcer). Though scientists don't know exactly what causes ulcers, research points the finger at a number of probable culprits — a diet heavy with spicy or fried foods, too much alcohol, smoking, stress and possibly even a newly discovered bacteria.

Ulcers may improve on their own, but, if left untreated, can lead to serious complications that might require surgery. The smartest way to treat them is to prevent them. Still, if you have already developed an ulcer, we can offer some help.

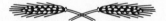

ALFALFA In rural areas of the United States, alfalfa is used to ease stomach ulcer pain. Alfalfa is an excellent source of vitamin K, which helps blood clot and can prevent hemorrhages.

Use fresh alfalfa leaves like lettuce by adding them to your sandwich or tossing them into a fresh salad. Dried, crushed alfalfa leaves can be used to brew a tea. Try flavoring it with honey, orange or lemon peel and a little mint.

COMFREY The British, French and Greeks use comfrey to treat just about every digestive complaint. Comfrey tea is said to be especially effective for soothing gastric ulcers.

FIGS Fresh or dried, figs contain significant amounts of the enzyme ficin. And in laboratory tests, ficin has shown it can kill the bacteria that has recently been associated with ulcers.

HONEY Fresh honey soothes ulcers and aids digestion. It has been used in Europe and Asia to relieve stomach inflammation for hundreds of years. Try a teaspoon by itself, or dissolve it in a cup of hot tea.

LICORICE The Greeks use licorice for all sorts of stomach ailments. It's readily available, it tastes good, and it contains carbenoxolone, which has been shown to protect the stomach lining from natural gastric acid.

TUMERIC Used by East Indians as a spice as well as a dietary aid, tumeric is believed to increase the production of bile which breaks down fats and protects the lining of the stomach. Try dissolving a teaspoon of the herb in warm milk to soothe ulcers.

URINARY TRACT INFECTIONS

Urinary tract infections are relatively common in both men and women. They are usually caused by bacteria in the bladder. Though annoying, uncomfortable and, sometimes, embarrassing, these infections are easily treatable. The most common symptom is frequent, painful urination. Don't ignore it. If left untreated, a urinary tract infection can become chronic and spread to the kidneys where it can cause serious damage.

Because this malady is so widespread, it's not surprising that so many home remedies have been developed to treat it.

BARLEY A brew of barley can help keep the urinary tract functioning. Simmer 1½ ounces of barley in 2 pints of water, covered, for 30 minutes, flavoring it with a bit of lemon during the last 10 minutes of cooking. Strain and drink.

BLUEBERRIES Many types of berries contain a substance that seems to prevent bacteria from adhering to the urinary tract lining. A cup of blueberries a day is a tasty, nutritious way to fight off bladder infections.

COMFREY A herbal remedy for urinary tract infections calls for 1 ounce each of comfrey root, yellow-dock root, yarrow root and dandelion root, plus 2 ounces of licorice root. Put the herbs in a tea ball and steep in boiling water. Take a tablespoon 3 or 4 times a day.

CRANBERRIES The Pequot Indians of New England were the first to recognize the value of cranberries to prevent urinary tract infections. Today, many doctors around the world prescribe this healthful and reliable remedy. The Indians ate the berries, however the juice is more convenient — and just as effective.

NASTURTIUM The Germans use the nasturtium flower to treat urinary tract and bladder infections. The plant is believed to have antibiotic properties.

PARSLEY The men of Holland believe they can prevent prostate problems by drinking parsley tea. Parsley is a good source of vitamin A, and because it is a diuretic, it promotes urination which helps prevent bladder infections.

RASPBERRIES An old English remedy for urinary tract infections and ovarian cysts advises women to douche with a mixture of red raspberry tea, black currant and witch hazel leaves, and a little powdered myrrh. These herbal ingredients are anti-fungal, antiseptic and good for the circulation.

SANDALWOOD Sandalwood is prized in Pakistan for its sweet scent — and for its ability to ease urinary tract infections. A few drops of sandalwood oil added to a warm bath helps soothe the external irritation that often accompanies this condition. Or, boil a heaping teaspoon of sandalwood in a cup of water and drink twice a day.

SAW PALMETTO The saw palmetto tree produces a berry that is believed to be an effective treatment for urinary tract infections. Make a decoction by putting ½ to 1 teaspoon of berries in a cup of water. Boil for 5 minutes. Drink 2 cups per day.

UVA-UREI The uva-urei shrub, a.k.a. bearberry or Indian tobacco, is a hardy member of the evergreen family that is used by Native Americans to treat kidney and bladder inflammation, and to treat the back pain associated with kidney problems. It is available in leaf, powder or capsule form.

VARICOSE VEINS

Varicose veins are unsightly and painful, appearing as a network of redish-blue or blue lines radiating along the calf or thigh. The discoloration is caused by blood (which is blue until exposed to the air) backing up and enlarging a vein when there isn't enough pressure to maintain an even flow to the heart. Seen more frequently in women than in men, they are usually caused by spending long periods of time standing or sitting. They also occur when continuous pressure is put on the vein (in pregnancy, for example).

Varicose veins are a sign that your legs need more exercise. Exercise strengthens the large leg muscles that support the veins and maintain adequate pressure. There are also a number of popular folk remedies that can help.

BLACKSTRAP MOLASSES In South Africa, sugar-cane farmers swear by blackstrap molasses to ease circulatory problems, including varicose veins.

HORSE CHESTNUT The French treat varicose veins with horse-chestnut tea, which they say shrinks the veins to normal size. The horse-chestnut leaves contain tannins and flavonoids, which strengthen vein walls.

MELILOT Melilot contains anti-inflammatory and anticoagulating comarins, which take pressure off the veins. Most people prefer to take melilot as a tea.

NETTLE Herbs that contain silica, such as horsetail and nettle, help build strong connective tissue that supports the veins. Take in capsule form or drink as a tea.

VINEGAR The English, Scots and Germans treat varicose veins with an apple-cider vinegar lotion. They massage their legs with it to shrink the veins and relieve related cramping and muscle tiredness. To try it, add 1 teaspoon of apple-cider vinegar to 1 teaspoon of your regular body lotion.

You can also soak a cheesecloth bandage in vinegar and wrap the bandage around your varicose veins. Then lie down for at least an hour with your legs elevated. Repeat twice a day.

YARROW Teas and poultices made from yarrow, hawthorn, rue and St. John's wort are recommended by herbalists to treat varicose veins because of the flavonoids (especially rutin) in these herbs.

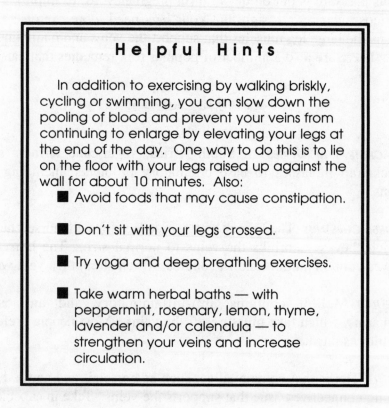

Helpful Hints

In addition to exercising by walking briskly, cycling or swimming, you can slow down the pooling of blood and prevent your veins from continuing to enlarge by elevating your legs at the end of the day. One way to do this is to lie on the floor with your legs raised up against the wall for about 10 minutes. Also:

■ Avoid foods that may cause constipation.

■ Don't sit with your legs crossed.

■ Try yoga and deep breathing exercises.

■ Take warm herbal baths — with peppermint, rosemary, lemon, thyme, lavender and/or calendula — to strengthen your veins and increase circulation.

VISION PROBLEMS

Eyes are amazingly complex structures, served by a complex circuitry of nerves requiring more space in the brain than any other part of the body. To work properly, the eyes must be nourished — especially by vitamin A, which modern researchers have proven to be critical for healthy eyes and good vision. Exposure to light is also important. The retina, the part of the eye that actually sees, requires a minimum of 2 to 3 hours of natural light every day.

A person with average vision is capable of distinguishing among millions of different colors and degrees of light and shadow. About one-tenth the size of a 35mm camera, eyes are infinitely more versatile, constantly focusing, adjusting, absorbing, processing, sorting and interpreting thousands of images. We probably take more pictures with our eyes in a few minutes than most photographers take in a lifetime with their cameras. Though, like a camera, our eyes wear out with age.

Despite the natural aging process, several cultures have found ways to preserve good eyesight and eye muscle function — secrets that you can take advantage of.

BILBERRY During World War II, pilots swore that eating bilberry jam improved their night vision. Bilberries, also called European blueberries, are used in Germany to make Heiderbeersekt (sparkling) and Heidelbeerwein (non-sparking) wines. The berries can be eaten raw or cooked.

BITTER GOURD A traditional Chinese recipe for good eyesight is the regular consumption of bitter gourd seeds, which are packed with vitamins and minerals.

BLACK CURRANT Black currants are very high in vitamin C and contain flavonoids. Both of these nutrients protect blood vessels and improve eyesight.

CARROT Your mother was right — carrots do improve your eyesight. They are an excellent source of vitamin A, and eaten regularly are believed to prevent night blindness.

COLLARD GREENS This leafy green vegetable is full of vitamins, minerals and phytochemical compounds that are effective in maintaining eyesight and eye health. Research shows that a weekly ½ cup serving of collard greens cuts the risk of eye disease by one-third. Collard greens are best when they are steamed like spinach.

EYEBRIGHT In the Highlands of Scotland and cold climes of Iceland, eyebright is thought to be a powerful sight enhancer. It is brewed into a tea and taken daily to keep vision sharp.

EXERCISE!

William Horatio Bates, an early 20th century American optometrist, developed a number of exercises designed to strengthen eye muscles. Although his methods met with opposition in the United States and Great Britain, they were well received in Germany and used by their armed forces. His eye exercise manual, published in 1919, is called *Better Eyesight Without Glasses.*

And in China, children do eye exercises in school every morning. By focusing on near and then far objects, you, too, can give your eyes a workout to help maintain their ability to focus quickly and accurately.

FENNEL Since Ancient Greek times, fennel tea has been thought to improve vision. Herbalists recommend drinking it to maintain good eyesight or using it as an eyewash to soothe irritation.

PUMPKIN SEEDS High in zinc, pumpkin seeds are food staples in China and India, where they are believed to play an important role in maintaining eyesight.

SUNFLOWER SEEDS Grown throughout the world and considered a tasty snack by children and adults, sunflower seeds are high in zinc and other vital nutrients. Like pumpkin seeds, they are believed to slow the natural deterioration of eyesight that accompanies aging.

VIOLET PETALS The British claim that eating violet petals and leaves significantly improves vision. This makes a lot of sense, since violets contain a significant amount of vitamin A.

Turn to page 243 for more information about eye care, eye irritation and sties.

VOMITING

One of the more unpleasant reactions the human body is capable of is vomiting, the forced expulsion of food or bile up from the stomach and out of the mouth. One of your body's ways of getting rid of toxins, it can be caused by illness, by something you ate or drank, or by a negative reaction to medication.

See your doctor immediately if vomiting lasts more than 24 hours, if it is violent and uncontrollable, or if it contains blood. However, for occasional vomiting brought on by food poisoning, too much alcohol or the flu, try one of these old, but reliable remedies.

CARAWAY One Chinese treatment calls for boiling 2 teaspoons of caraway seeds with 1 teaspoon of cinnamon and 1 teaspoon of dried ginger. Drink it hot and as often as needed to soothe the stomach and quell the nausea.

CHIVES Mix 2 teaspoons of fresh chive juice into 8 ounces of milk. Add 1 teaspoon fresh ginger and heat till warm. Drink before meals to reduce vomiting.

COCONUT The Chinese like coconut milk to stop vomiting and replace the essential nutrients lost through dehydration. They recommend drinking a glass of fresh coconut milk with an ounce of sugar and a dash of salt 3 times a day for 3 days.

GINGER Ginger tea is a popular Chinese remedy for nausea and vomiting. One recipe calls for adding dried orange peel to the brew.

HONEY For dry heaves, try mixing 1 teaspoon of honey in a small cup of ginger juice. Sip it slowly.

PEPPERMINT Good tasting and good for you, peppermint tea helps soothe the stomach and fight off nausea and vomiting. Peppermint's healing power comes from its high menthol content. Steep 1 teaspoon of dried leaves in a cup of hot water or buy one of the many commercially packaged peppermint teas.

PINEAPPLE This tropical fruit is used by most island cultures to curtail vomiting and nausea. Eat four slices of fresh pineapple or drink a glass of pineapple juice whenever symptoms occur.

For more remedies, refer to motion sickness on page 371, nausea on page 387 and morning sickness on page 413.

WARTS

In Mark Twain's novel Tom Sawyer, Tom and his buddy Huck Finn visit a graveyard at midnight with a dead cat in an effort to get rid of a wart. Despite the fact that most warts (with the exception of plantar warts and venereal warts) are painless and harmless, people have resorted to such drastic and ridiculous wart remedies for centuries.

Warts can be caused by any one of the papovaviruses. They can be contracted on any part of the body, be it skin or mucous membrane. They occur most frequently in children and usually disappear on their own after a few months. But, as harmless as they are, warts can be unsightly — especially when they grow in prominent places, such as on the hands or face.

Although warts are never cancerous, they are contagious. Warts can quickly spread not only all over your body, but they can travel onto someone else too. Therefore, you should never, ever scratch or pick at warts.

Painful warts — plantar warts (which grow on the foot and can be excruciating when located at a point of pressure) and venereal warts — should be treated by a physician. It's not necessary to see a doctor for any other type of wart. If you do, he'll attempt to remove it — quickly, but painfully — using acid to burn it off, nitrogen to freeze it off, an incision to cut it off or even electric shock (all at considerable expense to you).

If you're not ready to submit to any of these tortures —and if you're not willing to wait for the wart to disappear on its own — consider one of the following alternatives.

ALOE Fresh juice right from the aloe usually helps with warts. First you need to file down the affected area and then apply the gel. Do this every day until the wart disappears.

APPLE CIDER VINEGAR A Canadian remedy for wart removal calls for soaking a cotton ball in some apple cider vinegar and placing it under a band-aid. They do this every night for at least 2 weeks. Eventually the wart should blacken and fall off on its own.

BANANA The healing mucilage found inside a banana peel has been known to help warts go away. To try this, tape the inside peel on the wart and leave overnight until it disappears. Reportedly this technique works well with planters' warts, which usually must be removed through more painful procedures.

CASTOR OIL The Brahman physicians of India treat warts with castor oil and garlic. Castor oil contains a large quantity of vitamin A, which is known to be effective in treating skin ailments in general. And raw garlic irritates the skin just enough to cause the offending virus to be attacked and destroyed by the body's immune system.

You can also try taping a slice of garlic to the wart — but be sure to first protect the surrounding skin with petroleum jelly.

COD LIVER OIL A popular old wives' tale is to apply cod liver oil to a wart to get it to disappear

DANDELION Consider this wart remedy, popular among the sheepherders of Australia. They simply break a dandelion stem in half and drip the milky white sap on the wart. Sap applications should be repeated over several days. In a week or 2, the wart should turn dark and fall off.

FIGS The Romans prepared a sap from fresh fig leaves, which they used to remove warts.

HOT BATHS For plantar warts, which are heat-sensitive, you can try a hot bath. As with aloe, you must file down the wart first, to expose the softer skin underneath. Then, soak in a steaming tub (jacuzzi's work well). You'll need to do this every day, for at least 15 minutes, for a couple of weeks.

LEMON Try soaking some lemon slices in apple cider vinegar and a bit of salt for 2 weeks. Then, rub the lemon slices on the wart daily for several weeks until it removes the wart.

POTATO The Pennsylvania Dutch removed warts by rubbing the white part of half of a raw potato on the wart. According to folklore, the piece of potato was buried after use, or the cure was not effective.

VITAMIN A As with other skin problems, often taking vitamin A orally or applying it topically will heal the condition. If you are having a problem with warts, try upping your daily intake of vitamin A. Supplements are fine but there's less of a chance of toxicity if you take it in its natural form of beta-carotene, which is readily available in many foods. See the chart of food sources for beta-carotene on page 50.

VITAMIN E Apply vitamin E oil right from the capsule to your wart a couple of times a day. This old and easy remedy is probably the most successful method for getting rid of warts.

WEIGHT CONTROL

Americans are almost addicted to dieting. We spend millions of dollars trying to lose weight, trim down and redesign our bodies. And there's a good reason for it — the majority of us really are overweight!

We eat too much and we eat the wrong foods. The basic diet of this country is overloaded with ingredients that keep us struggling to keep the weight down. In fact, the typical American diet contains more than double the recommended amounts of fat and protein, and less than half the recommended amount of carbohydrates. Is it any wonder that so many of us spend our lives trying one "quick fix" diet after another, only to gain back the pounds and inches over and over again?

The truth is, it's not that difficult to maintain your body weight at a healthy and attractive level without starving yourself or depriving yourself of the foods you love. Other cultures all over the world have proven that it's possible. So all you need to do is tap into that traditional reservoir of knowledge — and supplement it with everything modern science has learned about the important connection between good health and nutrition.

- **Stop going on crash diets.** They offer only temporary results, and can even be harmful. Make a commitment to yourself to maintain a healthy diet as a regular part of your lifestyle on a permanent basis. If you eat the proper foods in adequate quantities — and exercise regularly — you'll not only lose weight, you'll have a healthier body, a stronger heart, improved self esteem and a happier life.

- **Stop counting calories.** Instead, start counting percentages and the calories will take care of themselves. Your daily diet should contain 60 percent to 70 percent carbohydrates, 15 percent to 20 percent

---

EXERCISE!

A healthy diet must be accompanied by regular exercise. To maximize weight loss, exercise 30 minutes every day. Then, once you've achieved your ideal weight, you can reduce that to 3 sessions a week.

When you exercise, you help your body use the energy from the food you've eaten, and keep it from storing the fat in your diet. In addition to burning calories, exercise also helps to build muscle tone and maintain a healthy cardiovascular system. But if working out at the gym isn't your cup of tea, there are some alternate ways to get a good workout:

- If possible, walk or ride your bicycle to work.
- Take the stairs instead of the elevator.
- Park your car at the far end of the shopping center parking lot — and walk to the stores.
- If you ride the bus, get off a few blocks before your stop and walk the rest of the way.
- Take vacations which involve hiking, swimming and other physical activities.

---

protein, and 15 percent to 20 percent fat.

- **Eat at least 3 meals a day**, including a good breakfast. Some cultures believe that the main meal of the day should be eaten between noon and 2 p.m., with a light evening meal and no food after 8 p.m. If this doesn't work for you, eat your meals at hours that fit in with your schedule.

- **Include the following in your daily diet**: 3 to 5 whole fruits, 3 to 4 servings of different cooked vegetables, 3 slices of whole grain bread, at least 1 serving of rice, potatoes or pasta, and 8 to 10 glasses of water.

- **Eliminate or reduce** the butter, margarine and sour cream that you eat.

■ **Have red meat no more than 3 times a week**, and keep your portions down to 3 to 4 ounces. Replace the red meat in your diet with veal, pork, skinned chicken and fish. Fresh ocean fish and free-range chicken are best. Keep in mind that while fish is a good food for cutting calories, shellfish has a higher fat content and should be eaten in moderation.

Beans, rice, grains, seeds and nuts (except for peanuts) are also good replacement sources for animal protein.

■ **Eat cheese no more than 3 times per week**, choosing those made from skim milk, such as feta, farmer's or mozzarella.

■ **Limit your intake** of sugar, alcohol, caffeine and artificial sweeteners.

■ **Instead of focusing on what you can't eat**, try to eat more of the foods you should eat.

■ **Go ahead, cheat a little!** Some experts say you've got to cheat occasionally if you're going to make good nutrition a lifelong habit. After all, it's easier to give up sirloin steak or chocolate cake if you know that you can still have it now and then. So every so often (but not too often), treat yourself to something that you really love to eat. If you're like many people who stay on a healthy diet, you may even lose your taste for the rich desserts and other fattening foods.

■ **Read those labels** — they're loaded with important information. Many people are buying "low fat" foods these days only to find that they're not really cutting their fat intake substantially. The label may say "low fat," but that means nothing if most of the calories in the product are derived from fat. Experts disagree on the exact percentage to aim for, but it's safe to say that the fewer fat calories there are in a particular item, the better it is to include in your diet. For example, if two different salad dressings each have 100 calories per serving, but dressing A has 80 calories from fat and dressing B has only 20 calories from fat, you should obviously choose dressing B.

■ **Take your time.** Remember, your goal is to change your eating habits for life, so it's best to make those changes gradually. A

International Weight Control Tricks

■ The typical Chinese diet is ideal for weight control because it is made up of so many easy-to-digest, nutritious foods that are high in fiber and water. Though high-fiber foods pass quickly through your system (which is probably where the idea came from that "an hour after you eat Chinese food, you're hungry again"), they are also very low in fat and calories. That means you can eat plenty of water chestnuts, bamboo shoots, Chinese cabbage and bean sprouts and not gain weight.

■ Bulgur is one of the staples of the middle Eastern diet. This highly nutritious form of wheat is a good source of protein, niacin and iron — and it's fat and sodium free.
Bulgur is sold in three forms: coarse, medium and fine. Coarse is best for stuffings, and fine makes a great salad. It's also good when added to bread dough and batters. When you buy it at the grocery store, it has already been parboiled, dried and cracked. So all you need to do to cook it is pour boiling water over the grains, then drain off the liquid. To keep bulgur fresh, store it in a tightly covered glass jar in your refrigerator.

■ Italians love to eat. Still, they manage to maintain generally trim figures. And, yes, they have a few secrets that explain how they are able to manage this. For one thing, they eat lots of pasta, which is low in fat and high in beneficial complex carbohydrates. They also eat lots of garlic, which protects their hearts and blood vessels. A lesser-known Italian diet trick is fennel seed tea. They credit this drink with an amazing ability to suppress the appetite.

■ The Mongol people drink green tea to lose weight and stay slim. Tea really does help to eliminate fat in the body. In fact, if you save the leaves after making tea, and rub them on your hands, you will feel the grease-removing effect.

sure way to return to your bad eating habits is to make too many drastic changes all at once. That's why crash diets fail.

■ In times of extreme cold, the body's metabolism slows down to nearly nothing in an effort to preserve valuable energy. And in mild cold, the body tries to pad itself with insulating fat, so you may actually feel hungrier than usual. That may be the reason why, in chilly Great Britain, research has shown that a warm drink can reduce hunger by raising body temperature. The warmth also makes you feel better, making it more likely that you'll move around and burn calories.

But be careful. A hot cup of coffee or tea probably won't do the trick unless it's decaffeinated. Caffeine is notorious as an appetite stimulant — which is the exact opposite of what you are looking for.

■ Even though caffeine is an appetite stimulant, the Chinese have learned to use it by combining it with the powdered leaves of the ma huang plant when they need a little help to lose weight. The caffeine increases the metabolism, burning fat faster and creating more energy to move and exercise. The ma huang also increases the metabolism a bit — and it decreases the urge to eat.

■ Kelp and other forms of seaweed have been used worldwide for centuries as diet aids. In Ireland, for example, a type of seaweed called carrageen is said to stimulate the metabolism — probably because it contains iodine, a metabolic booster.

■ Next time you're hungry, try this Chinese acupressure technique that's said to decrease the appetite: Squeeze your earlobes for 1 minute.

YEAST INFECTIONS

A vaginal yeast infection is considered to be a woman's disease, even though men may unknowingly act as carriers. Symptoms include redness, mild to severe itching, irritation, swelling, rawness, and a white discharge, often accompanied by painful intercourse, burning urination and/or an unpleasant odor.

This common malady (caused by the overgrowth in the vagina of a fungus called candida or monilia) is reported to affect 50 percent of all women at some point in their lives. More serious yeast infections like candidiasis (an infection of some other part of the body) or systemic candidiasis (an infection that has invaded the entire system) are more difficult to diagnose, because they tend to be signaled by a series of vague, intermittent symptoms like clumsiness, forgetfulness, mood swings, body aches, inability to concentrate, hay fever, dizziness, insomnia, mild gastrointestinal discomfort, frequent urination, acne, headaches, sugar and starch or yeast cravings, earaches, cold hands and feet, anxiety, irritability, hives, lethargy and menstrual irregularities.

Actually, yeast colonies are a natural part of our systems. They live in our digestive tracts, and are harmless as long as they are in balance with other bodily flora. They become a problem (in the vagina and in other parts of the body) only when the immune system is weakened, and the fungus is allowed to grow out of control. This can be due to a number of factors, including poor nutrition, exposure to chemical irritants, hormonal changes (such as menstruation and pregnancy), diabetes and the long-term use of antibiotics.

A yeast infection usually doesn't clear up by itself. It almost always needs to be treated with antifungal medication. At the same time, the body's natural defense mechanisms must be beefed up to keep the infection from returning again and again. Here, then, are our recommendations to keep you as comfortable as possible while you are under treatment — and to help protect you from recurring infection.

ACIDOLPHILUS To encourage the growth of good flora in your system, take acidophilus. Look for live lactobacillus acidophilus cultures in capsule form (refrigerated) at your health food store — or take it in powder form (1 or 2 teaspoons per day).

Acidophilus capsules can also be inserted directly into the vagina. Push them in as far as you can without discomfort — right before bed, for optimal results.

CINNAMON A natural antifungal, cinnamon has been known to keep yeast in check throughout the ages and is widely used for treating candida in China today. Drink cinnamon tea to help control the yeast level in your body.

CRANBERRY JUICE Start drinking this highly acidic juice at the first sign of vaginitis. Buy yours at your health food store to avoid brands loaded with sugar. And try mixing it with sparkling water and some fresh squeezed lemon juice for a tasty, fizzy remedy.

GARLIC Eat lots of garlic every day. Garlic's natural antifungal properties are said to help fight off a candida infection without resorting to costly drugs.

GOLDENSEAL Not only will this herb help build up your natural immune system when taken orally, it can relieve the agony of a vaginal yeast infection when used as a douche.

IRON Iron deficiency, in addition to causing a form of anemia, is also responsible for contributing to vaginitis.

MILLET Whole grains and vegetables help the body clear itself of toxins in the digestive tract. But be careful — oatmeal and wheat products are not recommended for those with candidiasis. Instead, try whole grains like millet and spelt.

ONION Like garlic, onions have more than just flavoring capabilities. They help boost the immune system and help ward off yeast infections.

_____ **WATER** Eight 8-ounce glasses of water is the minimum you should be drinking, especially if you have a candida problem. The more you urinate, the easier it is for your body to flush out impurities.

_____ **YARROW** Another natural remedy for candida is yarrow. Yarrow tea is used by many European women — as a drink or as a douche — to clear vaginal infections.

Dietary Bad Guys

While you're treating a yeast flare-up, it is helpful to eat foods like freshly squeezed fruit juices, beans and grains. They have a high acid content, which is exactly the opposite of what yeast need to thrive. And stay away from the following:

■ **Sugary foods.** Refined, white sugar is the biggest culprit of all in promoting yeast overgrowth, but even raw sugar, honey or molasses are not recommended. If you must eat sweets, settle for fruits or other naturally sweetened foods like carrots.

Also, be careful with dried fruits, which have an extremely high sugar content, salad dressings, ketchup and barbecue sauce, sodas, and commercially prepared fruit juices.

■ **Yeast.** Foods that contain yeast or mold contribute to a candida condition. That includes pizza dough, most breads, pickled vegetables, smoked meats, aged cheeses, fermented foods and drinks, and alcoholic beverages.

Alcohol is especially bad because it's not only full of yeast from fermentation, it's full of sugar.

■ **Dairy products.** Dairy products create phlegm — a perfect breeding ground for yeast. Furthermore, the hormones in dairy products may be responsible for some systemic imbalances.

If you're worried about your calcium intake, take a supplement.

Helpful Hints

■ **Minimize stress.** The more agitated or anxious you get, the harder your body has to work to help you heal. Lowering stress is the best thing you can do to boost your immune system.

■ **Keep cool and dry.** Moisture and heat create a breeding ground for candida.

■ **Wipe yourself well after eliminating**, wiping from front to back to avoid spreading yeast to the genital area.

■ **Don't douche.** Douching robs the vagina of the friendly bacteria that fight off yeast.
   If you must douche, do it infrequently and (because commercial preparations often contain chemical irritants) use the age-old homemade formula of 1 tablespoon of vinegar to 1 quart of water.

■ **Change your birth control.** If you have recurring vaginitis and you take birth control pills, you may want to switch to another method, because birth control pills alter your body's delicate hormonal balance.

■ **Use condoms.** Besides protecting you from sexually transmitted diseases (STDs) and pregnancy, condoms minimize the irritation sometimes caused by spermicides or your partner's semen.

■ **Urinate after sex.** This will wash away any irritating invaders lurking near the opening of your bladder after intercourse.

■ **Avoid deodorant tampons or sanitary napkins.** Although these are not reported to cause yeast infections, they could irritate the genital area or aggravate an existing condition.

■ **Don't sit all day.** Although it's difficult for some people to unchain themselves from their desks, force yourself to take breaks that require you to get up and move around. And be sure the area you're working in is cool, dry and well-ventilated.

■ **Shower — don't bathe — every day,** using an unscented, non-deodorant soap. And dry yourself with a clean towel after each shower to minimize yeast infections.

■ **Try a soothing salt soak.** To help treat a vaginal yeast infection, fill your tub to waist level with comfortably warm water, and then add about ½ cup of natural sea salt (you can get this at supermarkets as well as at health food stores). Sit in the water until it cools, preferably with your legs spread apart as much as possible.

   For even better results, put a ½ cup of vinegar into the bath water along with the salt. Yeast flourishes in an alkaline environment, so by doing this and helping restore the acidity in your vagina, you can lower your yeast count.

■ **Stick to white, unscented toilet paper.** Not only is it better for you, it's better for the environment.

■ **Skip the pantyhose.** If you must wear stockings for your job, wear thigh-highs with elastic bands or pantyhose with a cotton crouch (especially in the summer, or if you live in a hot, humid climate).

■ **Wear loose clothing made of natural fibers.** If you're troubled by vaginitis, don't wear tight underwear, pants, or shorts. Baggy jeans or slacks and skirts are a better choice for you. Buy natural fibers that "breathe." Unlike synthetics, cotton, linen and silk don't trap moisture next to your skin.

■ **Wear white cotton panties** — and don't wear any panties when you sleep. Cotton absorbs moisture. And although the dyes in colored panties won't necessarily cause an infection, they could aggravate a candida condition.

■ **Change out of wet clothes ASAP.** Damp bathing suits, sweaty aerobics gear, etc., help create the moist conditions that encourage a candida outbreak.

YOGURT Yogurt is an important part of the diet in virtually all Middle Eastern countries and in the Balkan mountains. And modern scientific studies have shown that the active bacteria cultures in yogurt effectively prevent yeast infections. We're not talking, here, about the processed, pasteurized yogurt commonly found in Western supermarkets. To be effective, the yogurt must be made from raw, unprocessed milk and have live cultures in it.

Plain yogurt can not only be eaten to prevent yeast overgrowth, it can also provide relief from the itching of vaginal infections. At bedtime, insert yogurt directly into your vagina with a store-bought applicator. Or smear some on your genitals and then put on a clean pair of cotton panties.

NOTE: You can make your own yogurt right at home by buying acidophilus milk and letting it sour a bit.

ZINC This vitamin has been known to help boost the immune system and actually speed natural healing.

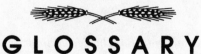

G L O S S A R Y

Agrimony

Agrimonia eupatoria (also known as Burr, Cockleburr, Hairyvein, Marigold, Sticklewort)

Description: A deep green perennial herb that is a member of the Rose family. This slightly aromatic herb is native to Europe and is now commonly found in Asia, Canada and the U.S. The plant has medicinal value. The seeds, plant (in cut, powdered or capsulated form) and an extract can be purchased.
Application: Heartburn, inflamed gums, migraine, sore throat
Available at: Herb stores, mail-order catalogs

Alder Buckthorn

Rhamnus frangula (also known as Buckthorn, Dogwood)

Description: A dense shrub or small tree that grows rapidly. The bark is used medicinally and can be purchased whole or in cut, powdered, capsulated or extract form.
Application: Skin care
Available at: Herb stores, mail-order catalogs

Alfalfa

Medicago sativa (also known as Buffalo Herb, Purple Medic, Sweet Lucerne)

Description: A deep-rooted, perennial plant that is rich in vitamins, minerals and trace elements. The leaves have medicinal value. Seeds, leaves (whole or in cut or powdered form), capsules or extracts can be purchased. Alfa-mint tea is also available.

Application: Appetite stimulant, arthritis, backache, colitis, gout, hangover, headache, irritable bowel syndrome, rheumatism, ulcers

Available at: Grocery stores, health food stores, herb stores, mail-order catalogs, nurseries

Allspice

Pimento officinalis (also known as Clove Pepper, Jamaica Pepper, Pimento)

Description: The dried berry of the pimento, an evergreen tree that grows to 40 feet high, in the West Indies, South and Central America, and Mexico. This aromatic herb has a flavor that resembles a blend of cinnamon, pepper, clove and juniper. Eugenol is the active healing ingredient, and it works as a carminative, removing gas from the upper intestines. In combination with cloves, it is also helpful in cases of diarrhea. The berries are collected when mature, but not yet ripe.

Application: Diarrhea, flatulence, indigestion, menstrual cramps

Available at: Grocery stores, health food stores, herb stores, mail-order catalogs

Aloe

Aloe vera (also known as Barbados Aloe, Curacao Aloe)

Description: A perennial plant that is a member of the Lily family and looks like a cactus. It originates from tropical Africa and is now found worldwide. The leaves have medicinal value. Plants and powders can be purchased.

Application: Acne, burns, constipation, insect bites, menopause, menstrual cramps, skin care, sunburn, warts

Available at: Grocery stores, health food stores, herb stores, mail-order catalogs, nurseries

Amaranth

Amaranthus hypochondriacus (also known as Lady Bleeding, Pilewort, Prince's Feather, Red Cockcomb)

Description: An annual herb that is high in protein and cultivated mainly in the central U.S. The leaves have medicinal value. Seeds, leaves (in cut or powdered form) and capsules can be purchased.
Application: Menstrual cramps
Available at: Herb stores, mail-order catalogs

Angelica

Angelica archangelica (also known as European Angelica, Garden Angelica)

Description: A perennial, aromatic flowering herb that is a member of the Carrot family and has a taste similar to licorice. The rootstock, root and seeds have medicinal value. Seeds (whole or in powdered or capsulated form) and roots (in cut, powdered, capsulated or extract form) can be purchased.
Application: Acne, common cold, headache, heartburn, menstrual irregularity
Available at: Health food stores, herb stores, mail-order catalogs, nurseries

Anise

Pimpinella anisium (also known as Anisum, Sweet Cumin)

Description: An annual plant that is an aromatic member of the Carrot family and has a flavor similar to licorice. The seeds and leaves have medicinal value. Seeds (whole or in powdered or capsulated form) can be purchased.
Application: Bad breath, cough, flatulence, insomnia, stress
Available at: Grocery stores, health food stores, mail-order catalogs

Arnica

Arnica montana (also known as Leopardsbane, Mountain Tobacco, Wolfsbane)

Description: An aromatic, perennial plant found in mountainous regions of Canada, the northern U.S. and Europe. The flowers and rootstock have medicinal value. The plant, seeds, flowers (whole or in cut or powdered form) and extracts can be purchased.

Application: Bruises, muscle ache, sprain

Available at: Health food stores, mail-order catalogs

Arrowroot

Maranta arundinacea (also known as Bermuda Arrowroot, Maranta, St. Vincent Arrowroot)

Description: A native of South America and the West Indies that is cultivated in parts of the southern U.S. The root is a valuable source of carbohydrates that can be made into a nutritive drink, especially for infants and convalescents. It has a softening effect on the mucus membranes of the body and is used where there is inflammation and irritation. The root is available in powdered form and can be boiled in milk and water.

Application: Urinary tract infection

Available at: Health food stores, herb stores, mail-order catalogs

Barley

Hordeum vulgare

Description: An annual plant whose grain is rich in vitamin B and vitamin E and is also a good source of dietary fiber.
Application: Constipation, heart disease, high blood pressure, kidney stones, urinary tract infection
Available at: Grocery stores, health food stores, nurseries

Basil

Ocimum basilicium (also known as Common Basil, St. Josephwort, Sweet Basil)

Description: An annual plant that is a member of the Mint family. It is aromatic and contains pungent oils such as thymol and camphor. The herb is used medicinally and can be purchased whole or in cut, powdered or capsulated form.
Application: Bad breath, congestion, shingles
Available at: Grocery stores, health food stores, herb stores, mail-order catalogs, nurseries

Bay

Laurus nobilis (also known as Bay Laurel, Sweet Bay)

Description: An evergreen bush or tree that yields aromatic leaves and small, black berries. The leaves and berries have medicinal value. The leaves (whole or in cut, powdered or capsulated form) and the berries (in cut, powdered or capsulated form) can be purchased.
Application: Sprain
Available at: Herb stores, mail-order catalogs, nurseries

Bee Propolis

Description: A waxy, resin-like substance excreted by bees to protect their hives. Contains pollen, amino acids, vitamins and trace minerals.
Application: Migraine
Available at: Bee farms, health food stores, mail-order catalogs

Bergamot

Monarda didyma (also known as Beebalm, Mountain Balm, Oswego Tea)

Description: A citrus fruit with a rind that yields an essential oil.
Application: Tooth care
Available at: Health food stores, mail-order catalogs

Betony

Stachys officinalis (also known as Lousewort)

Description: A perennial plant that is ornamental. The flowering herb has medicinal value. Seeds and leaves (in cut, powdered or capsulated form) can be purchased.
Application: Cuts
Available at: Herb stores, mail-order catalogs

Bilberry

Vaccinium myrtillus (also known as Blueberry, Burren Myrtle, European Blueberry, Huckleberry, Hurtleberry, Whinberry, Whortleberry, Wineberry)

Description: A shrubby perennial whose berries are closely related to the cranberry. The leaves and berries have medicinal value. The leaves (whole or in cut, powdered or capsulated form) can be purchased.
Application: Vision
Available at: Grocery stores, health food stores, mail-order catalogs

Birch Bark

Alba, Betula lenta (also known as Canoe Birch, Paper Birch, White Birch)

Description: The bark from a family of hardy trees with a silvery or whitish trunk. The bark yields salicin, which is natural aspirin.
Application: Backache, headache, smoking (quitting)
Available at: Health food stores, herb stores, mail-order catalogs

Bitterroot

Apocynum cannabinum (also known as American Hemp, Hemp Dogbane)

Description: Native to the U.S., this perennial herb has branching stems that reach 3 to 5 feet in height. The stems, leaves and root produce a bitter, milky white sap. The root has medicinal value.
Application: Diabetes
Available at: Herb stores, mail-order catalogs

Black Cohosh

Cimicifuga racemose (also known as Bugbane, Snakeroot, Squaw Root)

Description: A perennial plant that grows from 3 to 8 feet in height. It is topped with an array of white flowers. Native to the U.S., the roots and rhizome have medicinal value. It is available in powder form.
Application: Menstrual cramps, osteoporosis
Available at: Herb stores, mail-order catalogs

Borage

Borago officinalis (also known as Bugloss, Burrage)

Description: An annual plant that is self-seeding and in ancient times was thought to evoke courage. The herb and flowers have medicinal value. Seeds, flowers (in cut, powdered or capsulated form) cut leaves, dried herb and an extract can be purchased.
Application: Chicken pox, depression, eczema, fatigue, fever, stress
Available at: Herb stores, mail-order catalogs, nurseries

Bulgur

(also known as Cracked Wheat)

Description: Similar to whole wheat, with the bran and germ of the grain retained. It is an excellent source of protein and carbohydrates.
Application: Dieting
Available at: Grocery stores, health food stores, mail-order catalogs

Burdock

Arctium lappa (also known as Bardana, Hardock, Lappa, Thorny Burr)

Description: A biennial plant whose flowers clump together to form a burr, which will cling onto anything that brushes up against it. The root, seed and leaves are used medicinally. The root (in cut, powdered, capsulated or extract form) and the seeds (whole or in extract form) can be purchased.

Application: Baldness, bruises, burns, cancer prevention, cradle cap, eczema

Available at: Herb stores, mail-order catalogs

Calendula

Calendula officinalis (also known as Marigold)

Description: An annual composite flowering plant that is native to the Mediterranean and Egypt. It grows about 2-feet high and produces yellow, orange or maroon flowers which have medicinal value.

Application: Antiseptic, bruises, cuts, sedative, skin toner, toothache

Available at: Health food stores, herb stores, nurseries

Camphor

Cinnamomum camphora (also known as Gum Camphor, Laurel Camphor)

Description: Camphor is obtained from large trees in Taiwan. The chipped wood undergoes a process of steam distillation. The distillate is rich in camphor oil, which is separated and then heated to evaporation to obtain pure oil.

Application: Bruises, inflammation

Available at: Heath food stores, herb stores, mail-order catalogs

Caraway

Carum carvi

Description: A biennial or perennial plant whose seeds are aromatic and can be found in rye bread. The seeds are used medicinally and can be purchased whole or in powdered or capsulated form.

Application: Appetite stimulant, flatulence, menstrual cramps, vomiting

Available at: Herb stores, mail-order catalogs

Cardamom

Elettaria cardamomum

Description: A perennial plant that is an aromatic spice native to East India. The seeds are used medicinally and can be purchased along with the plant.

Application: Bad breath

Available at: Grocery stores, herb stores, mail-order catalogs

Catnip

Nepeta cataria (also known as Catmint, Catnip, Catwort, Field Balm)

Description: A perennial herb that is a member of the Mint family and grows wild in Europe, North America and temperate Asia. It is gray-green in color, has a mounded shape, a characteristic square stem, and highly scented heart-shaped leaves that cats are attracted to. The leaves contain volatile oil.

Application: Colic, flatulence, fever, insomnia, menopause, menstrual cramps, stress

Available at: Health food stores, herb stores, mail-order catalogs

Cayene Pepper

Capsicum frutescens (also known as Bird Pepper, Capsicum, Chili Pepper)

Description: A shrubby perennial plant that is native to Africa and India. It grows in most tropical and subtropical countries and is cultivated in parts of Mexico and South America. The fruit is the medicinal part of the plant. It is a pepper pod with many seeds and a leathery skin in various shades of red and yellow.

Application: Circulation, colitis, fatigue, hangover, heartburn, shingles, sore throat

Available at: Grocery stores, health food stores

Celery Seed

Apium graveolens (also known as Garden Celery, Wild Celery)

Description: The seed of the celery plant, which is a biennial herb and member of the Carrot family. It is widely cultivated but also grows wild in the salty soils of North and South America, Europe and Africa. The fruit, which is a small ribbed ovate seed, is used medicinally.

Application: Arthritis

Available at: Grocery stores, health food stores

Chamomile

Chamaemelum nobile (also known as Camomile, Ground Apple, Roman Camomile); Matricaria chamomilla (also known as German Chamomile, Wild Chamomile)

Description: These two annual species are closely related. Roman Chamomile is a low growing compact herb and much less common than German Chamomile, which is taller and more rangy in habit. Both plants have daisy-like flowers that give off a deliciously fresh apple-like smell when crushed. Both grow wild in meadows, along roadsides and abandoned places, but are also widely cultivated in gardens. The flowers are used medicinally.

Application: Acne, bronchitis, calluses, eye care, gall bladder stones, haircare, heartburn, insomnia, menstrual cramps, muscle ache, muscle cramp, skin care, stomachache, stress, sunburn, teething

Available at: Grocery stores, health food stores, mail-order catalogs, nurseries

Chickweed

Stellaria media (also known as Mouse-Ear Satin Flower, Rongue Grass Winterweed)

Description: An annual herb with white flowers that grows to 15 inches tall. It is native to Europe and grows in temperate zones of North America. The plant and leaves have medicinal value. Young leaves, which are rich in vitamin C, are often added to salads.

Application: Chicken pox, eczema

Available at: Herb stores, mail-order catalogs, nurseries

Chinese Green Tea

Description: A non-fermented drink made from green tea leaves.

Application: Cancer prevention, tooth care

Available at: Health food stores, mail-order catalogs, Oriental markets

Chinese Parsley

See Coriander.

Chinese Tiger Balm

Description: A healing ointment which contains aromatic oils of camphor, menthol, peppermint and clove, and an East Indian oil called cajeput that increases blood flow to surface skin.
Application: Backache, muscle ache, muscle cramp, rheumatism
Available at: Health food stores, mail-order catalogs, Oriental markets

Chive

Allium schoenoprasum

Description: A perennial bulbous plant and a member of the Onion family. It is native to Sweden, Greece and the Alps, but is widely cultivated all over the world. Like the onion, it has hollow green leaves and a flowering stem that shoots up from the bulb. The leaves have medicinal uses, and the oil has the medicinal properties of allium, which works as an antiseptic.
Application: Bruises, vomiting
Available at: Grocery stores, health food stores, herb stores, mail-order catalogs, nurseries.

Cholchine

Colchicum autumnale (also known as Autumn Crocus)

Description: A perennial herb with a flowering head resembling a crocus. It thrives in the woodlands and mountainous regions of Europe, Canada and the U.S. Alkaloid is derived from the seeds and roots.
Application: Gout
Available at: Herb stores, mail-order catalogs, nurseries

Chrysanthemum

See Feverfew.

Citricidal
Description: An extract made from the seeds and pulp of citrus fruits.
Application: Diarrhea, sore throat
Available at: Health food stores

Clover (Sweet)
Melilotus officinalis (also known as Sweet Lucerene, Yellow Melilot, Yellow Sweet Clover)
Description: A member of the Pea family, sweet clover is a biennial herb that grows throughout Europe and most of North America. It is cultivated as animal fodder. It has a very distinctive vanilla smell. The leaves have medicinal value.
Application: Kidney stones, toothache
Available at: Herb stores, mail-order catalogs, nurseries

Clove
Caryophyllus aromaticus
Description: Unopened, aromatic flower bud of a woody, evergreen tree native to the tropics.
Application: Bad breath, diarrhea, teething
Available at: Grocery stores, health food stores, herb stores, mail-order catalogs

Coltsfoot
Tussilago farfara (also known as British Tobacco, Coughwort)
Description: A perennial herb that contains mucilage and is rich in zinc, calcium and potassium. It grows in damp places in the U.S., Europe and the East Indies. The creeping rhizome sends up scaly flower stems, which are topped by large yellow flowers, and leaves that stand on long stalks above the ground. Both flowers and leaves are used medicinally.
Application: Eczema
Available at: Herb stores, mail-order catalogs

Comfrey

Symphytum officinale (also known as Healing Herb, Knitback, Slippery Root)

Description: A member of the Borage family, with its large broad leaves and purple blooms. It is a common perennial plant found in moist places in the U.S., Europe and Asia. The rhizome is fleshy, whitish on the inside, black on the outside, and contains a glutinous juice. The medicinal part is the rootstock.

Application: Athlete's foot, bruises, chicken pox, cough, cuts, eczema, gall bladder stones, skin care, sprain, ulcers, vaginal dryness

Available at: Herb stores, mail-order catalogs

Common Ash

Fraxinus excelsior (also known as Bird's Tongue, European Ash)

Description: A large, European tree whose bark, leaves and seeds are all used medicinally. The bark is available whole or in cut or powdered form.

Application: Gout, rheumatism

Available at: Herb stores, mail-order catalogs

Coriander

Coriandrum sativum

Description: One of the twin herbs that come from the same annual plant, widely grown in North and South America, Europe and the Mediterranean. Coriander refers to the seeds, while it's twin, Chinese Parsley, refers to the leaves. The brownish — almost spherical — seeds have a spicy aroma when they ripen.

Application: Bad breath, colic, diabetes, heartburn

Available at: Herb stores, mail-order catalogs

Cowslip

Caltha palustris (also known as Marsh Marigold, Meadow Bouts)

Description: A perennial herb that can be found in the Northeastern U.S. near streams, ponds and marshes. The stem grows 1 to 2 feet tall and bears one or more dark-green, kidney-shaped leaves with rounded teeth along the margin. Bright yellow flowers are seen during April and May.

Application: Headache, insomnia, stress

Available at: Herb stores, mail-order catalogs

Cramp Bark

Viburnum opulus (also known as Guelder Rose, High Bush Cranberry)

Description: An ornamental shrub from the Honeysuckle family that has white flowers and red berries.

Application: Menstrual cramps, muscle cramp, stress

Available at: Health food stores, herb stores, mail-order catalogs

Cypress

Cypressaceae

Description: A swamp growing tree found in Florida and Louisiana. Its oil has medicinal value.

Application: Cellulite

Available at: Health food stores, mail-order catalogs

Damiana

Turnera diffusa (also known as Turnera)

Description: A shrub native to Mexico and a member of the Turneraceae family. The leaves are touted as a powerful aphrodisiac and a sexual tonic for both men and women. They contain a complex volatile oil which is responsible for the characteristic bitter, fig-like taste and odor. The leaves may be smoked like tobacco or drunk as a tea.
Application: Aphrodisiac, depression, fatigue, frigidity, impotence
Available at: Health food stores, herb stores, mail-order catalogs

Dandelion

Taraxacum officinale

Description: Perhaps the world's most famous weed, found in lawns, pastures, fields and gardens. The dandelion's bright yellow flowers grow on succulent stems. The hollow stem contains a milky substance that oozes when broken. All parts of the plant are used for healing. The leaves are rich in vitamin A and calcium.
Application: Appetite stimulant, arthritis, boils, constipation, corns, diabetes, stomachache, warts
Available at: Grocery stores, health food stores, herb stores, mail-order catalogs

Devil's Claw

Harpagophytum procumbens (also known as Grapple Plant, Wood Spider)

Description: A native South African plant that is a member of the Pedaliaceae family. The herb is edible and has peculiar fruits that are claw-like pods. It is common in the southwestern states and in Mexico. The part used is the secondary storage roots, which has anti-inflammatory, analgesic and anti-rheumatic effects.
Application: Arthritis, backache, fever, rheumatism
Available at: Herb stores, mail-order catalogs

Dill

Anethum graveolens

Description: A native herb of the Mediterranean that is a hardy annual member of the Umbellifer family. Dill produces yellow umbrella-like flowers in clusters. After flowering, a crescent-shaped seed is developed. Both leaves (Dillweed) and seeds have medicinal uses.

Application: Appetite stimulant, colic, flatulence

Available at: Grocery stores, herb stores, mail-order catalogs

Dogwood

Cornus florida (also known as Boxwood, Cornelia Tree, Florida Cornel)

Description: A native American tree that grows to 40 feet tall and is found in the eastern and central U.S. The rough brown bark is dried and used for medicinal purposes. It is sometimes used as a substitute for Peruvian Bark.

Application: Fever

Available at: Herb stores, mail-order catalogs

Dong Quai

Angelica polymorpha (also known as Dang Gui, Tang Kuei, Tang Kwei)

Description: The root of a native Chinese plant that is a member of the Apiaceae family. It tastes like celery and is used for its laxative, antispasmodic, blood purifying and tonic properties. Some of the purported properties can be accounted for by the presence of seven different coumarin derivatives.

Application: Menopause, menstrual cramps

Available at: Health food stores, herb stores, mail-order catalogs

Echinacea

Echinacea angustifolia (also known as Coneflower, Sampson Root)

Description: A native American plant that is a herbaceous perennial from the Composite family and grows wild in the central plains. It bears beautiful flowers resembling those of the Black-Eyed Susan, with prominent cone-shaped discs, and color ranges from purple to white. The root is the medicinal part.

Application: Acne, boils, chronic fatigue syndrome, cold sores, common cold, cuts, earache, flu, infertility, insect bites, toothache

Available at: Health food stores, herb stores, mail-order catalogs, nurseries

Elderberry

Sambucus canadensis (also known as Black Elder, Common Elder, Sweet Elder)

Description: A native American shrub that grows wild in the central and eastern U.S. It grows 5 to 12 feet high, and produces white wheel-shaped flowers in large terminal clusters from May to July, that are followed by dark purplish-blue berries. The berries have culinary uses, and the leaves and flowers have medicinal uses.

Application: Cough

Available at: Herb stores, mail-order catalogs

Elderflower

Sambucus canadenisis, Sambucus nigra, Sambucus racemosa (also known as Bourtree, European Elder, Pipe Tree)

Description: A member of the Honeysuckle family, this tree-shrub is found throughout Europe and North America. Used for hundreds of years in folk and herbal medicines, the bark, roots and flowers have medicinal value, though the raw plant is toxic.

Application: Eye care

Available at: Herb stores, mail-order catalogs, nurseries

Elecampane

Inula helenium (also known as Wild Sunflower)

Description: A beautiful perennial herb with a thick fleshy root that has a camphor-like fragrance and bright yellow flowers that look like Sunflowers. It grows wild in Europe and Asia, and in North America from Nova Scotia to North Carolina. The fibrous root is the part of the plant used for healing, and it is considered good only in the second year of growth. It is known for its bitterness and pungency.

Application: Shingles

Available at: Health food stores, herb stores, mail-order catalogs

Ephedra

Ephedra sinica (also known as Ma Huang)

Description: A jointed, almost leafless shrub, that resembles stunted pine trees. It is rich in ephedrine and pseudoephedrine and can be found growing in the southwestern U.S.

Application: Allergies, asthma

Available at: Herb stores, mail-order catalogs

Eucalyptus

Eucalyptus globulus (also known as Australian Fever and Blue-Gum)

Description: A native of Australia and Tasmania, and one of the tallest trees in the world. It is known for its shimmering, long, narrow, blue-green leaves and a strong camphoraceous fragrance. In the U.S., it grows in the Pacific Southwest. The aromatic oil which is present in mature leaves is primarily composed of Eucalyptol, which is considered a healing substance.

Application: Allergies, asthma, bronchitis, cold sores, cough, croup, fever, rheumatism

Available at: Grocery stores, health food stores, mail-order catalogs

Evening Primrose

Oenothera biennis (also known as Evening Star, Night Willow, Scabish)

Description: A biennial herb that grows from 3 to 6 feet in height in meadows and along roadsides. It has a hairy stem and very thin leaves. The stem and the oil have medicinal value.

Application: Eczema, menopause

Available at: Health food stores, herb stores, mail-order catalogs

Evergreen

Sedum purpurem (also known as Frog Plan, Live-Forever, Orpine)

Description: A fleshy perennial with stalkless leaves and a tuberous rhizome. Native to Eurasia, it grows wild throughout most of North America. The leaves have medicinal value.

Application: Urinary tract infection

Available at: Herb stores, mail-order catalogs, nurseries

Eyebright

Euphrasia officinalis

Description: An elegant annual that is found predominantly in the meadows and dry pastures of England, some grassy areas of western Asia, and is only rarely domesticated in North America. Flowering occurs between July and September, and all parts of the plant except the root are used for healing. The herb is gathered when the plant is in full flower and dried in a cool dark place.

Application: Vision

Available at: Health food stores, herb stores, mail-order catalogs

Fennel
Foeniculum vulgare

Description: A beautiful perennial plant (and a relative of dill) that is native to the Mediterranean region and is widely cultivated in the U.S. and Europe. Its bright yellow flowers are produced as flat-topped clusters from July to October, and are followed by aromatic seeds that are rich in vitamins and minerals. Both root and seed are used for healing.

Application: Asthma, bad breath, colic, dieting, eye care, flatulence, skincare, stomachache, vision

Available at: Grocery stores, health food stores, herb stores, mail-order catalogs

Fenugreek
Trigonella foenum-graecum

Description: An annual leguminous plant that is cultivated for its medicinal and culinary uses. Its healing secret lies in its aromatic seeds, which contain mucilage, calcium and other minerals. It is native to western Asia and the Mediterranean, but is naturalized in North America.

Application: Allergies, aphrodisiac, bad breath, body odor, boils, breast cancer prevention, colitis, congestion, frigidity, impotence, menopause

Available at: Health food stores, herb stores, mail order catalogs

Feverfew
Chrysanthemum parthenium (also known as Chrysanthemum, Featherfew)

Description: A cultivated perennial herb and member of the Daisy family that is cultivated in North America but is native to southern Europe. It is often mistaken with chamomile because of its dome-shaped floral receptacle. Feverfew has only recently become available in health food stores in the U.S.

Application: Arthritis, backache, insect repellent, menstrual cramps, migraine

Available at: Herb stores, mail-order catalogs

Feverwort

Eupatorium perfoliatum (also known as Boneset, Crosswort, Indian Sage)

Description: A prairie growing herb that reaches 5 inches in height and produces wrinkled leaves and whitish flowers. A staple of American frontier medicine, the leaves and flowers have medicinal value.

Application: Fever

Available at: Herb stores, mail-order catalogs

Fo-Ti-Tieng

Description: A product that has a registered trademark and should not be confused with the herb (*fo-ti* or *he-shou-wu*). Fo-Ti-Tieng is a mixture of herbs, mainly the stem and leaves of a diminutive variety of Gotu Kola (*Cantella asiatica*). The other components are the root of Indian physic and small amounts of kolanuts.

Application: Aging

Available at: Herb stores, mail-order catalogs

Garlic

Allium sativum (also known as Clove Garlic)

Description: A bulbous member of the Lily family, made up of 4 to 15 bulblets or cloves. Origin is uncertain but it may be indigenous to southern Siberia. The bulb is the medicinal part, but it has to be crushed or chopped to activate the medically active compounds. Two of these sulfur-containing compounds are allicin (which is responsible for garlic's strong odor) and ajone. Allicin has antibiotic properties, and ajone has anticoagulant properties.

Application: Arthritis, athlete's foot, cancer prevention, common cold, cough, earache, flu, gall bladder stones, genital herpes, heart disease, high blood pressure, high cholesterol, insect repellent, irritable bowel syndrome, teething, toothache, yeast infection

Available at: Grocery stores, health food stores, herb stores, mail-order catalogs

Geranium

Geranium maculatum (also known as Cranesbill, Crowfoot, Dovefoot, Shameface, Wild Geranium)

Description: A perennial herb, that has greyish-green leaves and grows to 2 feet tall. Native to North America, it grows wild from Maine to Manitoba and can be found as far south as Georgia and as far west as Kansas. The rhizome and root have medicinal value.

Application: Body odor, genital herpes

Available at: Health food stores, herbal stores, mail-order catalogs, nurseries

Ginger

Zingiber officinalis (also known as African Ginger)

Description: An exotic tropical plant and a native of China that is a perennial with a highly aromatic rootstock. It is cultivated in tropical countries, especially Jamaica. The rootstock is the medicinal part and it is thick, fibrous and knotty with a buff color. It is rich in essential oils, gingerols and zingerones.

Application: Arthritis, asthma, backache, bad breath, baldness, burns, circulation, common cold, constipation, fever, flatulence, headache, heartburn, heart disease, hiccups, high blood pressure, irritable bowel syndrome, laryngitis, menstrual cramps, migraine, motion sickness, muscle ache, muscle cramp, rheumatism, stomachache, toothache, vomiting

Available at: Grocery stores, health food stores, herb stores, mail-order catalogs, nurseries, Oriental markets

Ginkgo

Ginkgo biloba (also known as Maiden Hair Tree)

Description: A native of the Far East and the oldest living tree species on earth, Ginkgo's fan-shaped leaves have medicinal uses. The active compounds are flavonoid, glycoside and ginkgolides, and its preparations have been extensively tested in people. It plays a big part in traditional Chinese medicine. It is available as a concentrated extract of the plant.

Application: Aging, impotence, memory loss

Available at: Health food stores, herb stores, nurseries

Ginseng

Panax schin-seng (also known as Chinese Ginseng, Wonder-of-the-World)

Description: A small perennial plant with an aromatic root, that is native to Asia. The native American variety (*P. quinquefolius*) is very similar in appearance and has essentially the same constituents. The medicinal part is the root, which is rich in saponins.

Application: Aging, fatigue, high cholesterol, impotence, jet lag, menopause, stress

Available at: Health food stores, herb stores, mail-order catalogs, Oriental markets

Goldenrod

Solidago virgaurea (also known as European Goldenrod)

Description: A perennial herb that grows wild in Europe and Asia. It is a common herb that embraces a genus with over 130 species. One variety is native to North America and can be found in open fields and along roadsides. The short rootstock produces a slender stem with serrated leaves and yellow flowers that appear from July to October. The flowering tops and leaves have medicinal uses.

Application: Arthritis, gout, insect bites

Available at: Herb stores, mail-order catalogs

Goldenseal

Hydratis canadensis (also known as Ground Raspberry, Indian Dye, Indian Paint, Orange Root, Poor Man's Ginseng, Yellow Root)

Description: A small perennial plant that is a native American wildflower. It is cultivated, but is relatively rare and expensive. The thick, knotty, yellow rootstock is the medicinal part, as it contains two alkaloid compounds, berberine and hydrastine. These compounds have an array of effects on the human body. The plant bears a red fruit resembling raspberry and can be found in the rich soils of river deltas.

Application: Canker sores, cold sores, eye care, inflamed gums, menopause, shingles, toothache, yeast infection

Available at: Herb stores, mail-order catalogs

Gotu Kola

Hydrocotyl asiatica (also known as Bramhi, Herb of Enlightenment)

Description: A creeping marsh-loving plant that is native to India, China and the South Pacific, but isn't well-known outside of its native range. It grows in mountainous tropical regions and is rich in flavonoids and terpenes. These active ingredients offer anti-inflammatory and antibacterial effects. It is available as capsules and extract preparations.

Application: Aging, burns, cuts, fatigue

Available at: Herb stores, mail-order catalogs

Grindelia

Grindelia robusta (also known as Gum Plant, Gum Weed)

Description: A bushy perennial plant that is native to the coastal areas of California. Several stems grow together and produce leathery leaves. Two to 5 yellow flower heads appear from August to September. The medicinal parts are the leaves and the flowering tops.

Application: Insect bites

Available at: Herb stores, mail-order catalogs

Hairyvein

See Agrimony.

Hawthorne

Crataegus oxyacantha (also known as English Hawthorne, Thorn Apple Tree)

Description: A small, spiny tree of the Rose family that has pink or white blossoms and brightly colored fruits. It grows as a shrub or a tree in Europe and is a common plant in the English countryside. The plant is rich in flavonoids and can be purchased as an extract. The flowers and fruits have medicinal uses.

Application: High blood pressure, high cholesterol

Available at: Herb stores, mail-order catalogs

Honey

Description: The saccharine secretion deposited by the bee in the honeycomb. The bee collects the nectar from various flowers and stores it in its crop. It is acted upon by secretions from glands in the bee's head and thorax, which converts it from sucrose to simple sugars. On returning to the hive, the bee regurgitates the honey into the wax comb.

Application: Acne, aging, allergies, aphrodisiac, burns, eye care, fatigue, flatulence, insomnia, muscle cramp, ulcers

Available at: Grocery stores, health food stores, herb stores

Hops

Humulus lupulus

Description: A fibrous vine of the Mulberry family that provides the main flavoring agent in beer. It is a perennial climbing plant that may grow up to 20 feet long. Hops grows wild in many parts of the world, but is cultivated in the U.S. The scaly cone-like fruit is the medicinal part. It is rich in lupulin and estrogen-like compounds.

Application: Aphrodisiac, impotence, toothache

Available at: Herb stores, mail-order catalogs

Horse Chestnut

Aesculus hippocastanum

Description: A large ornamental tree that is native to Asia and south eastern Europe. It is rich in a number of compounds collectively called aescin, that gives it astringent properties. The fruit is the part used for healing, and it is available in extract form. It is a prickly green capsule which contains 1 to 6 shiny brown seeds.

Application: Varicose veins

Available at: Herb stores, mail-order catalogs, nurseries

Huckleberry

Vaccinium myrtilloides (also known as Sourtop Blueberry)

Description: A low-growing shrub with short stalks that produce pasty blue berries from July through September. A member of the Heath family, it prefers sandy or peaty acid soil. The leaves and berries have medicinal value.

Application: Diabetes

Available at: Herb stores, mail-order catalogs, nurseries

Hyssop

Hyssopus officinalis

Description: A member of the Mint family that is a bushy evergreen herb indigenous to southern Europe. It is a traditional herb used since Biblical times because it has astringent properties. The plant has square stems, opposite lance-shaped leaves, and bluish-purple flowers that grow from June to October. The leaves contain hyssopsin and tannin.

Application: Asthma, cough, congestion, croup, diarrhea, skin care, sprain

Available at: Herb stores, mail-order catalogs

Irish Moss

Chandrus crispus (also known as Carrageen)

Description: A curly red, purple or yellow-green seaweed that grows along the rocky coast of Ireland and other cold coastal regions. The entire plant has medicinal value.

Application: Bronchitis

Available at: Health food stores, mail-order catalogs

Ivy

Hedera helix (also known as English Ivy, True Ivy)

Description: A popular ornamental plant, that is cultivated world wide. It has a woody stem and glossy, dark-green leaves and is a member of the Ginseng family. The exudate, leaves and berries have medicinal value.

Application: Calluses, corns

Available at: Herb stores, mail-order catalogs

Jasmine
Jasminum officinalis

Description: A vine-like member of the Olive family that is indigenous to warm places of the eastern hemisphere. It is cultivated in the U.S. for its extremely fragrant flowers that are used commercially and medicinally.
Application: Aphrodisiac
Available at: Herb stores, mail-order catalogs, nurseries

Jojoba
Simmondsia chinensis (also known as Goat's Nut)

Description: An evergreen shrub of the Buxaceae family that is abundant in Mexico and the southwestern U.S. Jojoba oil is obtained from the peanut-sized seeds of the Jojoba plant.
Application: Skin care
Available at: Grocery stores, health food stores, herb stores, mail-order catalogs

Juniper
Juniperus communis

Description: An evergreen shrub found in dry rocky places of Europe, Asia and North America. It grows 2 to 6 feet high and has brown bark, needle-shaped leaves, and yellow or green flowers from April to June. The fruit is a berry-like cone which is green the first year and ripens to a dark purple the second year. The berries, which can be eaten fresh but are most commonly made into a concentrated oil, are used for healing.
Application: Cellulite
Available at: Herb stores, mail-order catalogs, nurseries

Kelp

Fucus vesiculosus (also known as Kelpware, Seaweed, Sea Oak)

Description: A nutritionally rich plant that grows in the sea along coasts and border inlets of the North Atlantic and North Pacific Oceans. It is brown and has large, flat, leaf-like fronds. An ash or powder which is rich in iodine is obtained by burning the plant. Kelp is also rich in silicon, which is important in treating conditions of the skin and hair.

Application: Baldness, cancer prevention, dieting, fatigue, hair care, heartburn, skin care

Available at: Health food stores, mail-order catalogs

Lavender

Lavendula vera

Description: A Mediterranean shrub that is a bushy perennial with woody stems and small opposite gray-green leaves. Highly aromatic flowers appear in the mid-summer and range in color from pale lavender to deep purple. The flower is the medicinal part. It is cultivated in the U.S. for its volatile oils.

Application: Acne, aphrodisiac, body odor, bruises, burns, cold sores, cradle cap, cuts, depression, frigidity, head lice, impotence, insect bites, insect repellent, migraine, muscle ache, skin care, stress, sunburn

Available at: Health food stores, herb stores, mail-order catalogs, nurseries

Leek

Allium porrum

Description: A cultivated perennial that is a type of onion and member of the Lily family. Its round stem grows from a bulging bulb and is surrounded at the bottom by a sheath of linear leaves. The stem is topped by white or red flowers during June and July. Leeks have similar properties to garlic.

Application: Burns

Available at: Grocery stores

Lemon Balm

Melissa officinalis (also known as Balm Root, Mediterranean Melissa, Sweet Balm)

Description: A perennial member of the Mint family that is one of the most fragrant herbs and has a long history of medicinal use. The leaves release a pleasant lemony fragrance when crushed. It has a characteristic square stem and ovate-toothed leaves. The entire herb is used for healing because it is rich in volatile oil and polyphenols.

Application: Acne, cold sores, depression, eczema, genital herpes, headache, heartburn, high blood pressure, menopause, menstrual cramps, shingles, skin care, stress

Available at: Health food stores, herb stores, mail-order catalogs, nurseries

Licorice

Glycyrrhiza glabra (also known as Licorice Root, Sweet Licorice, Sweet Wood)

Description: A graceful shrub with woody stems and spreading, pinnate leaves, that belongs to the Legume family. The sweet-flavored root has many branching rootlets and is rich in mucilage, a substance that soothes and protects. When used for healing purposes, the roots are first dried.

Application: Aphrodisiac, blisters, ulcers

Available at: Health food stores, herb stores, mail-order catalogs

GLOSSARY • L

M

Magnolia

Magnolia glauca (also known as Beaver Tree, Indian Bark, Sweet Magnoila)

Description: An evergreen tree that bears large distinctive cream-colored flowers from May to August and is found in the Atlantic and Gulf Coast states. The smooth ash-colored bark is the medicinal part, and it can be substituted for Peruvian Bark.

Application: Aphrodisiac, impotence

Available at: Health food stores, herb stores, mail-order catalogs, nurseries

Ma Huang

See Ephedra.

Marigold

See Calendula.

Marjoram

Origanum vulgare (also known as Mountain Mint, Wild Marjoram)

Description: A tender perennial herb of the Mint family that is indigenous to Portugal and North Africa, naturalized in most Mediterranean countries, and cultivated in the U.S. It has a creeping woodstock, square downy stems, small ovate leaves and purple two-lipped flowers that grow in clusters from July to October. It is closely related to Oregano and is sometimes substituted for it.

Application: Heartburn, smoking (quitting)

Available at: Grocery stores, herb stores, mail-order catalogs, nurseries

Meadowsweet

Filipendula ulmaria maxim (also known as Bridewort, Queen-of-the-Meadow)

Description: A stout perennial herb that reaches 6 feet in height. Found in marshes and wet lands, meadowsweet grows wild from Newfoundland south to Virginia and west to Ohio. The rhizome, leaves and root all have medicinal value.

Application: Cradle cap

Available at: Herb stores, mail-order catalogs, nurseries

Mediterranean Melissa

See Lemon Balm.

Melilot

Melilotus (also known as Sweet Clover)

Description: A common name for about 20 species of fragrant, annual or biennial herbaceous plants in the Pea family. When crushed or dried, they give off a fragrance similar to that of coumarin.

Application: Varicose veins

Available at: Health food stores, herb stores, mail-order catalogs

Milk Thistle

Silybum marianum

Description: A tall spiny plant native to the Mediterranean, which has large purple flowers and white-veined leaves that produce a milky sap. The medicinal parts are the leaves and seeds. The leaves have a bitter taste, and the seeds contain a complex compound called Silymarin.

Application: Gall bladder stones

Available at: Herb stores, mail-order catalogs, nurseries

Milkwort

Polygala amara (also known as Bitter Milkwort, Snake Root)

Description: A European perennial that grows in meadows and may refer to any herb or shrub of the genus Polygala. It has a simple stem, 4 to 6 feet tall, a rosette of basil leaves, and terminal blue, red or white flowers that appear from April to June. The entire plant has medicinal uses.

Application: Depression, stress

Available at: Herb stores, mail-order catalogs

Motherwort

Leoneirus cardeaca (also known as Lion's Ear, Lion's Tail, Throwwort)

Description: A perennial herb that has tiny pink, white or purple flowers from June through September. The Chinese believe that this member of the Mint family prolongs life. It is shaggy looking and grows to 5 inches tall. Native to Europe, it grows from Nova Scotia south to Texas and South Carolina. The tops and leaves have medicinal value.

Application: Menopause

Available at: Health food stores, herb stores, mail-order catalogs, nurseries

Mugwort

Artemisia vulgaris (also known as Sailor's Tobacco)

Description: A soft green plant with greenish-yellow flower heads that grow in spikes. It is an ornamental perennial plant found in temperate regions of North and South America, along roadsides, waste places and bushy areas. The rootstock and the herb both have medicinal uses.

Application: Asthma, earaches

Available at: Herb stores, mail-order catalogs

Mustard Seed

Brassica hirta (also known as White Mustard)

Description: A member of the aromatic Mustard family and a close relative of broccoli and cabbage. The mustards are distinguished by their strong smell and yellow four-petaled flowers that appear to form a rounded cross. Mustard grows anywhere. The seeds, which are the medicinal part of the plant, are quite hardy and can remain viable for years.

Application: Heartburn, hiccups, high cholesterol

Available at: Herb stores, mail-order catalogs, nurseries

Nasturtium

Tropaedum majus (also known as Indian Cress, Watercress)

Description: A low-growing, bushy annual, native to South America. It has saucer-shaped leaves, and large red, orange or yellow flowers that bloom from June to October. It is a peppery tasting herb that is high in tannin. The flowers, seeds and leaves have medicinal uses.

Application: Congestion, flu, tooth care, urinary tract infection

Available at: Grocery stores, herb stores, mail-order catalogs, nurseries

Nettle

Urtica dioica (also known as Stinging Nettle)

Description: A thorny perennial plant with bristly hairs covering its dark green, heart-shaped leaves. These hairs are actually hollow tubes filled with an irritating substance, which can produce an itchy burning rash if touched. Nettle is found in the temperate regions of Europe, Asia, South Africa and the Andes. It contains an array of vitamins and minerals, large amounts of chlorophyll and histamine. The dried herb has medicinal value.

Application: Allergies, arthritis, dandruff, eye care, kidney stones, sunburn, varicose veins

Available at: Herb stores, mail-order catalogs

Oak Bark (White)

Quercus alba (also known as Stone Oak, Tanner's Oak)

Description: A member of the Beech tree family that grows to 15 feet and is native to North America. It is distinguished by its light grey bark which gives off a reddish cast. The bark, which is usually purchased in powder form, has medicinal value.
Application: Laryngitis
Available at: Health food stores, herb stores

Oats

Avena sativa (also known as Common Oats, Panicle Oats)

Description: A cultivated cereal grass that grows all over the world in the temperate zones. The seed, which is about one-half inch in length, has nutritional and healing properties. Oats are a soothing mucilaginous medicine.
Application: Source of fiber
Available at: Grocery stores, health food stores, herb stores, mail-order catalogs, nurseries

Onion

Allium cepa

Description: A perennial plant that grows from an edible bulb that is a member of the Lily family. It is native to Asia but is grown all over the world. The erect stem carries a number of small flowers that are white, pink or purple. As a medicine, onion contains smaller doses of garlic's antibacterial and antifungal components. The bulb is the medicinal part.
Application: Asthma, baldness, boils, bronchitis, burns
Available at: Grocery stores, herb stores, mail-order catalogs, nurseries, Oriental markets

Oregano

Origanum valgare

Description: A bushy perennial plant of the Mint family with erect square stems. This pungent herb is native to the Mediterranean and Central Asia, but is widely naturalized and cultivated in the U.S. and Europe. It is a culinary herb with medicinal properties. The essential components are thymol and cavacol.

Application: Head lice, toothache

Available at: Grocery stores, health food stores, herb stores, mail-order catalogs, nurseries

Parsley

Petroselinum crispum

Description: A sweet, annual herb of the Carrot family that has tender, bushy, bright-green leaf clusters. Parsley grows wild from Sardinia east to Lebanon and is cultivated throughout the temperate zones. It is rich in vitamins A and C, minerals and chlorophyll. The entire plant, including the root, has medicinal uses.

Application: Bad breath, kidney stones, urinary tract infection

Available at: Grocery stores, herb stores, mail-order catalogs, nurseries

Passionflower

Passiflora incarnata

Description: A native from Florida west to Texas and north to Illinois, characterized by a colorful showy bloom with coiling tendrils. The flowers are purple or brilliant pink, and the fruit is a sweet edible berry called grandella. An extract that is derived from the leaves, flowers and fruity tops has a narcotic and sedative effect.

Application: Depression, menopause, stress

Available at: Herb stores, mail-order catalogs, nurseries

Pennyroyal

Hedeoma pulegioides (also known as American Pennyroyal)

Description: A variety of mint with very fragrant leaves, much sharper than spearmint or peppermint. This common wildflower grows in the Eastern U.S. in dry fields. Pennyroyal should not be used internally.

Application: Insect repellent

Available at: Herb stores, mail-order catalogs

Peppermint

Mentha piperita

Description: A perennial mint with dark green leaves and small pink flowers. It is a hybrid of other mint species but more medically potent than the others. The active ingredient that gives it healing properties is menthol, a potent aromatic chemical in the plant's volatile oil. The healing part is the leaf, which may be purchased whole, in tea bags or as a distilled oil concentrate.

Application: Bad breath, earache, fatigue, flatulence, flu, headache, heartburn, hiccups, jet lag, menopause, stomachache, stress, sunburn, toothache, vomiting

Available at: Grocery stores, health food stores, herb stores, mail-order catalogs, nurseries

Periwinkle

Vinca major (also known as Greater Periwinkle, Lesser Periwinkle, Vinca minor)

Description: A creeping plant that grows wild in Great Britain and Europe. A pale blue flower grows on a long stalk from each stem joint during March and April. The herb has sedative and astringent properties.

Application: Stress, toothache

Available at: Health food stores, herb stores, mail-order catalogs

Peru Balsam

Myroxylon balsamum

Description: A Peruvian tree that is native to the Pacific coast of El Salvador. It exudes a thick resin that has a bitter taste and smells like vanilla. It is available as an oil.

Application: Asthma, bronchitis, cough

Available at: Health food stores, mail-order catalogs, nurseries

Pilewort

Hieracifolia erechtites (also known as Fireweed)

Description: A native North American annual found in woods and waste places. It is a coarse, hairy plant characterized by whitish brush-shaped flower heads and a disagreeable odor and taste. It has astringent properties and the entire plant is used for healing.
Application: Hemorrhoids
Available at: Herb stores, mail-order catalogs

Plantain

Plantago major (also known as Snakeweed, White Man's Foot)

Description: A perennial weed that grows wild in the U.S. along roadsides, in lawns and places with poor soil. The tiny mucilaginous seeds and the juice from the plant have medicinal uses. The leaves are broad and ovate, and the flower stalks are topped with long slender spikes of tiny yellow-green flowers.
Application: Bruises
Available at: Health food stores, mail-order catalogs, nurseries

Psyllium

Plantago ovata/plantago psyllium (also known as Flea Seed, Fleawort)

Description: Psyllium is found in Europe, North America and western Asia. It grows to 15 inches tall and has narrow leaves that grow in opposite pairs. The seeds, which can be purchased as a powder, have medicinal value.
Application: Cuts
Available at: Health food stores, herb stores

Quince

Cydonia oblonga (also known as Cydonium, Quince seed)

Description: A hardy shrub that has slender branches and white or light pink flowers. Its yellow pear-shaped fruits are globular and somewhat hairy before maturity. The ripe, nutritious, edible fruits are gathered in the autumn. The seeds are removed, crushed and dried for their astringent properties.

Application: Arthritis, rheumatism

Available at: Grocery stores, nurseries

Raspberry
Rubus idaeus

Description: A perennial shrub reaching 3 to 6 feet in height with prickly cane-like stalks. Small white flowers appear May through July followed by red fruits from June through October. It grows throughout the northern regions of the U.S. High concentration of tannins provide a number of medicinal uses. The leaves are usually brewed into tea.

Application: Menstrual cramps, nausea, pregnancy

Available at: Grocery stores, health food stores, herb stores, mail-order catalogs

Rose Hips
Rosa canina (also known as Dog Rose)

Description: The bright scarlet or deep red pear-shaped fruits found at the base of the rose flower. This member of the Rose family is a rich source of vitamin C. Extracts from the dried fruit are incorporated into a number of natural vitamin preparations.

Application: Fever, skin care

Available at: Health food stores, herb stores, mail-order catalogs, nurseries

Rosemary
Rosmarinus officinalis

Description: A woody evergreen shrub with an intense piney scent, native to southern France. This member of the Mint family has small, narrow, dark-green leaves which are almost needle-like. Tiny pale blue flowers appear in summer. The leaves and flowers are the parts used for healing purposes and they are harvested in their second year when they are rich in a volatile oil containing camphor.

Application: Circulation, cradle cap, hair care, headache, heartburn, jet lag, memory loss, rheumatism, skin care, stress

Available at: Grocery stores, health food stores, mail-order catalogs, nurseries

Royal Jelly

Description: A white, milky, highly nutritious, viscous secretion from the pharyngeal glands of the worker bee. Bee larvae and future queens are nourished by it. It is said to be beneficial when used externally because it is rich in proteins, B vitamins and predominantly pantothenic acid.

Application: Aging

Available at: Health food stores, mail-order catalogs

Saffron

Crocus sativus (also known as Spanish Saffron)

Description: A widely cultivated perennial plant found in many places, but particularly in the Mediterranean regions and Iran. It has no true stem, so the flower rises directly from the earth. The fragrant, lavender, white or purple flowers have long reddish-purple stigmas which are used for flavoring and coloring.

Application: Backache

Available at: Grocery stores, health food stores, herb stores, mail-order catalogs, nurseries

Sage

Salvia officinalis (also known as Garden Sage, Sagebrush)

Description: A shrubby perennial with square, woody or wiry stems that are covered with hairs. The velvety grayish-green leaves appear to be wrinkled and puckered. This native of the Mediterranean is widely cultivated in the U.S. for its culinary, ornamental and medicinal values. The leaves have antiseptic properties, and its oil contain camphor and cineol.

Application: Athlete's foot, bad breath, body odor, canker sores, cellulite, cold sores, diarrhea, fever, inflamed gums, laryngitis, menopause, menstrual irregularity, sore throat, stress, tooth care

Available at: Grocery stores, health food stores, mail-order catalogs, nurseries

Sandalwood

Santalum album

Description: A small parasitic tree that produces an aromatic oil and is native to India. The stem grows 20 to 30 feet high, and its heavy, straight-grained wood varies in color from yellow to orange when mature. The medicinal properties of sandalwood reside in the oil, which is extracted from the wood with alcohol and water. The oil has antiseptic, disinfectant, diuretic and astringent properties.

Application: Urinary tract infections

Available at: Herb stores, mail-order catalogs, Oriental markets

Sassafras

Sassafras officinalis (also known as Ague Tree, Cinnamon Wood)

Description: The dried outer bark of the root of a tree that can be found in Virginia, Kentucky, Tennessee and Kansas. This member of the Laurel family can grow to be 100 feet high and bears ovate leaves and greenish-yellow flowers. An oil extract with an agreeable spicy odor is obtained by distilling the oil from the chips of the root and tree stump.

Application: Common cold, cuts, eye care, fever

Available at: Grocery stores, herb stores, mail-order catalogs

Savory

Satureja hortensis (also known as Bear Herb, Summer Savory)

Description: An annual plant that is a member of the Mint family. The entire plant is strongly aromatic and has a spicy flavor that is widely used in cooking. Savory has a branching root that produces hairy stems and soft, hairless, linear leaves that are grayish in color. Dried leaves are available commercially.

Application: Diabetes

Available at: Grocery stores, health food stores, mail-order catalogs, nurseries

Saw Palmetto

Serenoa serrulata (also known as Sabal)

Description: A shrubby fan palm plant that grows along the coast from South Carolina to Florida. The berries of this plant, fresh or dried, have therapeutic value and have an effect on glandular tissue. They are olive-like, dark purple, and grow in bunches that ripen from October to December.

Application: Aphrodisiac, impotence, urinary tract infection

Available at: Herb stores, mail-order catalogs, nurseries

Senna

Cassia angustifolia (also known as Cassia)

Description: A legume that is native to the upper Nile areas of Egypt, India and the Mediterranean regions. It has whitish stems and bears yellowish-green flowers. The fruit is an oblong pod that encloses 6 to 7 heart-shaped seeds. The leaves are small, grayish-green and shaped like the head of a lance. The pods and the leaves have an irritating effect on the muscles of the colon, and the taste is unpleasant.

Application: Constipation

Available at: Health food stores, mail-order catalogs

Serpentwood

Rauvolfia serpentina

Description: A small tropical tree or shrub that contains a milky white sap. It grows in the moist forests of India, Indonesia, Burma and Ceylon. The root is the source of the drug Reserpine, which is widely used as a tranquilizer.

Application: Stress

Available at: Health food stores, mail-order catalogs

Slippery Elm

Ulmus rubra (also known as Indian Elm, Moose Elm, Sweet Elm)

Description: A native of the northern and central U.S. that grows in moist woods and attains a height of 50 to 60 feet. The bark of the tree is thick, tough and dark brown. The inner bark is pinkish-white and contains mucilage, which is the tree's healing ingredient.

Application: Burns, colic

Available at: Grocery stores, herb stores, mail-order catalogs

Soapwort

Saponaria officinalis (also known as Bouncing Bet, Soap Root)

Description: A hardy perennial with a single erect stem bearing ovate pointed leaves that yield a soapy lather when bruised. Soapwort is a native of western Asia that has become naturalized in North America. The branching rootstock is rich in saponin. The juice is extracted from the root and leaves and used for healing.

Application: Skin care

Available at: Health food stores, mail-order catalogs

Soybean

Glycine max

Description: A member of the Legume family that is native to Asian temperate regions. Like other legumes, soybeans are high in anti-cancer protease inhibitors. Soybean is also valued for its high protein content and for the fact that it raises the good HDL cholesterol content in the body and lowers the destructive LDL cholesterol levels. It is a tall and strong growing bean. The oil and soy flour are used.

Application: High cholesterol

Available at: Grocery stores, health food stores

Speedwell

Veronica officinalis (also known as Gypsyweed, Veronica)

Description: A low growing perennial with flowering stalks reaching 16 inches in height. A member of the Snapdragon family, it has small blue, lavender or white flowers that appear May through July. The leaves have medicinal value.

Application: Skin care

Available at: Health food stores, herb stores, mail-order catalogs

Spikenard

Aralia racemosa (also known as Indian Root, Life-of-Man)

Description: A handsome perennial plant that is a member of the Ginseng family. The aromatic rootstock is pleasant tasting and fleshy and is used for healing purposes. Tiny green flowers appear in summer that later develop into dark purple berries.

Application: Arthritis, rheumatism

Available at: Herb stores, mail-order catalogs

Star Anise

Illicium anisatum

Description: A small tree that is native to China, Japan and Korea and is also grown in the southeastern states of the U.S. It has a star-shaped fruit, aromatic leaves and stem, and solitary auxiliary flowers that are white, pink or purple. The seeds have a strong flavor and odor similar to aniseed.

Application: Bad breath, fatigue

Available at: Health food stores, mail-order catalogs, Oriental markets

Stinging Nettle

See Nettle.

St. John's wort

Hypericum perforatum (also known as Amber, Goat Weed)

Description: A hardy perennial shrub that smells like turpentine or balsam. Native to Europe and naturalized in North America, St. John's wort produces flat-topped cymes of bright yellow flowers, whose petals are dotted with black along the margins. Its woody, branched root produces rounded stems that bear linear leaves. The leaves are covered with oil glands that look like holes. The medicinal ingredients in the herb are volatile oil, resin, tannin and dye.

Application: Depression, menopause, shingles, skin care, stress, sunburn

Available at: Herb stores, mail-order catalogs

Thyme

Thymus vulgaris (also known as Common Thyme, Garden Thyme)

Description: A perennial shrub, native to southern Europe and the western Mediterranean regions, that grows to be about 15 inches tall. The leaves are strongly aromatic because they contain the essential oil thymol. Thymol has antispasmodic and carminative properties, making it good for gastrointestinal complaints.

Application: Congestion, cough, croup, flatulence, head lice, heartburn, insomnia, laryngitis, sprain, stress, tooth care

Available at: Grocery stores, health food stores, mail-order catalogs, nurseries

Tumeric

Curcuma longa

Description: A tropical, aromatic, perennial herb that is a member of the Ginger family. It has enjoyed long use for its health benefits and as a culinary herb. The active chemical in turmeric is curcumin, which is also the major ingredient in Indian curry. The rhizome (underground stem) is the part used for healing. It is also a powerful antioxidant.

Application: Ulcers

Available at: Grocery stores, herb stores, mail-order catalogs

Uva Urei

Arctostaphylos uva urei (also known as Bearberry)

Description: A small evergreen shrub that is found wild in the northern U.S. and Europe. A single fibrous main root sends out several buried stems from which branching stems grow. The leaves are oval, entire and rounded at the apex. The flowers are white or pink and grow in terminal clusters. Uva urei is available in dried herb or capsulated form.

Application: Urinary tract infection

Available at: Health food stores, herb stores, mail-order catalogs

Valerian

Valeriana officinalis (also known as Phu)

Description: A tall herbaceous perennial herb with a hollow stem, bearing dark-green opposite leaves and pink-tinged flowers. The vertical rhizome with many attached rootlets is harvested in the second year of growth. Studies indicate that the active ingredient in the pungent root, called valepotriates, acts as a tranquilizer. It is available in the form of tinctures, capsules, teas and liquid extracts.
Application: Insomnia, menstrual cramps
Available at: Herb stores, mail-order catalogs

Vervain

Verbena officinalis (also known as Herb-of-the-Cross)

Description: A perennial that is native to Europe and is naturalized in North America and temperate regions. It is a spiky looking plant with purplish-white flowers and leaves that are opposite, oblong and deeply divided. The entire herb is reported to have broad healing properties.
Application: Depression, impotence, inflamed gums
Available at: Herb stores, mail-order catalogs

Violet

Viola odorata (also known as Sweet Violet, Viola)

Description: A low growing perennial herb that grows from a short rootstock and is a native to Europe, Asia and North Africa. It is leafy and stemless, producing purple, blue, yellow, white or variegated flowers in the second year of growth. Flowers are fragrant and solitary. The leaves and flowers have antiseptic and expectorant properties, but the flower by itself is healthful because it contains an abundance of vitamins A and C. An aspirin-like substance is also obtained from the plant.
Application: Headache, sore throat, vision
Available at: Herb stores, mail-order catalogs, nurseries

Wheatgrass

Triticum aestivum

Description: An annual cereal grass that is cultivated for its nutritional value. It is a richly concentrated source of vitamin E, important B-complex vitamins and an assortment of other nutrients. The major health benefit of wheat is its high fiber content.
Application: Cancer prevention
Available at: Health food stores, nurseries

Willow

Salix alba (also known as White Willow)

Description: A deciduous tree that grows in moist places in the temperate regions of the Northern Hemisphere. One of its active ingredients is salicin, a source of natural aspirin. This gives the herb its pain relieving and fever fighting properties. The rough, grey bark is the medicinal part.
Application: Arthritis, headache
Available at: Health food stores, mail-order catalogs, nurseries

Wintergreen

Gaultheria procumbens (also known as Canada Tree, Hillberry, Spice Berry)

Description: A native North American evergreen shrub that makes an attractive ground cover in woods from Canada to Georgia. Its creeping stems send up erect branches and bear alternate, oval leaves. Leaves are about 2 inches long, leathery, glossy on the top and paler beneath. The medicinal value in the aromatic leaves resides in the oil of winter green which is obtained by steam distillation. The oil's active constituent is methyl salicylate, a close relative of aspirin.
Application: Arthritis, tooth care
Available at: Health food stores, mail-order catalogs, nurseries

Witch Hazel

Hamamelis virginiana (also known as Hazel Nut, Tobacco Wood)

Description: An indigenous shrub throughout most of North America except in the western U.S. It grows in moist woodlands and may grow to be 12 feet high, with crooked stems and forking branches that are covered with a scaly brown bark. The leaves are round and grow alternately on the stems. The leaves, twigs and bark contain tannic acid, which is the principal active ingredient in witch hazel. A distillation of the extract is mixed with alcohol or water and is widely available as an astringent.

Application: Acne, body odor, eye care, genital herpes, hemorrhoids, insect bites, muscle cramp, skin care, sprain

Available at: Grocery stores, health food stores, herb stores, mail-order catalogs

Wormwood

Artemisia absinthium (also known as Green Ginger, Madderwort, Quing Hao)

Description: A perennial shrub-like plant with silky grey-green leaves and tiny yellow flowers that bloom July through September. The leaves and flower tops are the most often used parts of this member of the Rose family.

Application: Sprain

Available at: Health food stores, mail-order catalogs, nurseries

Yarrow

Achillea millefolium (also known as Milfoil, Soldier's Woodwort)

Description: A hardy, fragrant, perennial flowering plant that grows from 1 to 3 feet tall and is easily recognized when in bloom by its disc-shaped clusters of tiny, white, daisy-like florets. Yarrow originated in Europe and Asia but it is naturalized in temperate regions of North America. The leaves, flowers and stem are used for healing purposes. The plant has astringent properties and contains salicylic acid derivatives.

Application: Fever, high blood pressure, incontinence, toothache, varicose veins, yeast infection

Available at: Health food stores, herb stores, mail-order catalogs

Yucca

Yucca glauca (also known as Soapweed)

Description: A semi-desert, hardy plant that grows in the warmer parts of North America. The plant has stiff sword-shaped leaves known to contain large quantities of saponins. These are plant chemicals that produce froth and foam when mixed with water. The saponins act as the precursors to cortisone synthesis, and are the basis for its medicinal uses.

Application: Backache, dandruff, rheumatism

Available at: Herb stores, mail-order catalogs, nurseries

BIBLIOGRAPHY

Ackerman, Diane. "Aphrodisiacs; Foods to Love By," *Cosmopolitan*, October 1994.

Aesoph, Laurie M., N.D. "Three Ways to Increase Fertility for Men and Women," *Delicious!*, May/June 1993.

Aguilar, Nona. *Totally Natural Beauty*. New York, NY: Rawson Associates Publishers, 1977.

Aikman, Lonnelle. *Nature's Healing Arts: From Folk to Medicine to Modern Drugs*. Washington, DC: The National Geographic Society, 1977.

Balch, James F., M.D., and Phyllis A. Balch, C.N.C. *Prescription for Nutritional Healing*. Garden City Park, NY: Avery Publishing Group, Inc., 1990.

Berger, Amy H. "Get Rid of That Tired Feeling," *First Magazine*, December 1994.

Bianchini, Francesco, and Francesco Corbetta. *The Complete Book of Fruits and Vegetables*. New York, NY: Crown Publishers, 1976.

Bieler, Henry G., M.D. *Food Is Your Best Medicine*. New York, NY: Ballantine Books, 1965.

Bodanis, David. *The Body Book: A Fantastic Voyage to the World Within*. Japan: Dai Nippon Printing Company, 1984.

Bogusz, Stanley. "Foot Odor Elimination," *Concious Choice*, March/April 1995.

Bolyard, Judith L. *Medicinal Plants and Home Remedies of Appalachia*. Springfield, IL: Charles C. Thomas, 1981.

Boston Women's Health Book Collective. *The New Our Bodies, Ourselves*. New York, NY: Simon & Schuster, 1992.

"Botanical Extract Stops Diarrhea, Strep Throat, Gingivitis, Candidiasis, and More," *New Paradigm Digest*, Summer/Fall 1992.

Boyer, Pamela. "Strength Training for Troubled Nails," *Prevention*, April 1993.

Brace, Edward R. *A Popular Guide to Medical Language*. New York, NY: Van Nostrand Reinhold Company, 1983.

Braly, James, M.D. "Can Depression Make You Sick?" *Delicious!*, March 1993.

Bricklin, Mark. *The Practical Encyclopedia of Natural Healing*. Emmaus, PA: Rodale Press, 1983.

Brown, Dr. O. Phillips. *The Complete Herbalist*. North Hollywood, CA: Newcastle Publishers, 1993.

Brown, Royden. *The Bee Pollen Bible*. Phoenix, AZ: Plains Corporation, 1989.

Buchman, Dian Dincin. *Dian Dincin Buchman's Herbal Medicine*. New York, NY: Gramercy Publishing, 1979.

Burton Goldberg Group. *Alternative Medicine: The Definitive Guide*. Puyallup, Washington: Future Medicine Publishing, Inc., 1993.

Califano, Julia. "Looking Great When You're Tired," *McCalls*, March 1995.

Carlson, Delbert G., D.V.M., and James Griffin, M.D. *Dog Owners' Home Veterinary Handbook*. New York, NY: Howell Book House, 1992.

Carper, Jean. *The Food Pharmacy*. New York, NY: Bantam, 1988.

Carper, Jean. *Food — Your Miracle Medicine*. New York, NY: Harper Perennial, 1993.

Carroll, David. *The Complete Book of Natural Medicines*. New York, NY: Summit Books, 1980.

Carse, Mary, M.N.I.M.H. *The Herbs of the Hearth: A Self Teaching Guide to Healing Remedies*. Hinesburg, VT: Upper Access Publishers, 1989.

Chopra, Deepak, M.D. *Ageless Body, Timeless Mind*. New York, NY: Harmoney Books, 1993.

Clark, Amy Rosenbaum. "Self Care for Spring," *Vegetarian Times*, May 1994.

Clark, J. B. "Alternative Medicine Is Catching On," *Kiplinger's Personal Finance Magazine*, January 1993.

Clark, Linda, M.A. *A Handbook of Natural Remedies for Common Ailments*. New York, NY: Pocket Books, 1976.

Clark, Linda. *Get Well Naturally*. Old Greenwich, NY: The Devin-Adair Co., 1974.

Clayman, Charles B., M.D. *The Encyclopedia of Medicine*. New York, NY: Random House, 1989.

Coffin, Margaret M. *Death in Early America*. New York: Elsevier/Nelson, 1976.

Committee on Diet and Health, Food, and Nutrition Board, Commission on Life Sciences National Research Council. *Diet and Health: Implications for Reducing Chronic Disease Risk*. Washington, DC: National Academy Press, 1989.

Coon, Nelson. *Using Plants for Healing*. Emmaus, PA: Rodale Press, 1979.

Cowley, Geoffrey, with Mary Hager, Karen Springen, Jeane Gordon, and Joshua Cooper Ramo. "Vitamin Revolution," *Newsweek*, June 7, 1993.

Crerand, Joanne. "Home Remedy: Insomnia," *Natural Health*, March/April 1992.

Cummings, S., and D. Ullman. *Everybody's Guide to Homeopathic Medicines*. New York, NY: G.P. Putnam's Sons, 1991.

Dadd, Debra Lynn. *Nontoxic, Natural, & Earthwise*. Los Angeles, CA: Jeremy P. Tarcher, 1990.

Darrach, Brad. "The War on Aging," *Life*, October 1992.

Dausch, J. G., and D. W. Nixon. "Garlic: A Review of Its Relationship to Malignant Disease," *Preventive Medicine*, 1990, Vol. 19.

Diamond, H. and M. Diamond. *Living Health*. New York, NY: Warner Books, 1987.

Dolan, Edward F. *Folk Medicine Cures and Curiosities*. New York, NY: Ivy Books, 1993.

Douglas, Dr. William Campbell. "The Stinking Rose," *Second Opinion*, May 1992.

Drury, Neville, and Susan Drury. *The Illustrated Dictionary of Natural Health*. New York: Sterling Publishing Company, Inc., 1989.

Duffy, Gail. *The Countryside Cookbook: Recipes and Remedies*. New York, NY: Van Nostrand Reinhold, 1982.

Duke, James A., Ph.D. *CRC Handbook of Medicinal Herbs*. Boca Raton, FL: CRC Press, 1985.

Duke, James A., Ph.D. *Culinary Herbs: A Potpourri*. New York, NY: Trado-Medic Books, 1985.

Dunphy, Paul. "Acupuncture Promotes Fertility," *East West Natural Health*, March/April 1992.

Eller, Daryn. "Get the Glow," *Real Beauty*, September/October 1994.

Evelyn, Nancy. *The Herbal Medicine Chest*. Freedom, CA: The Crossing Press, 1986.

Ezzell, Carol. "Celery Studies Yield Blood Pressure Boon," *Science News*, May 9, 1992.

Finkel, Maurice, B.S., M.S., M.Ed., Ed.D., N.D. *Fresh Hope With New Cancer Treatments*. Englewood Cliffs, NJ: Prentice-Hall, 1984.

Fischer-Rizzi, Susanne. *Complete Aromatherapy Handbook*. New York, NY: Sterling Publishing, 1990.

Foster, Steven, and Yue Chongxi. *Herbal Emissaries: Bringing Chinese Herbs to the West*. Rochester, VT: Healing Arts Press, 1992.

"The French Paradox," *60 Minutes*, CBS News, November 17, 1991.

Furnell, Dennis. *Health From the Hedgerow*. London, England: B.T. Batsford Ltd., 1985.

Gallagher, John. *Good Health With Vitamins and Minerals*. New York, NY: Simon and Schuster, 1990.

Gardner, Joy. *Healing Yourself During Pregnancy*. Freedom, CA: The Crossing Press, 1987.

Geelhoed, Dr. Glenn W., M.D., M.P.H., FACS, ed. *International Health Secrets*. Baltimore, MD: Agora, 1993.

Geller, Robert M., M.D., and Kathy Matthews. *Natural Prescriptions*. New York, NY: Carol Southern Books, 1994.

Gillyatt, Peta. "Cultural Revolution," *Harvard Health Letter*, October 1994.

Gittleman, Ann Louise. "Seven Steps to Sturdy Bones," *Your Health*, March 1994.

Gordon, L. *A Country Herbal*. New York, NY: Mayflower Books, 1980.

Goulart, F. S. "Honey: Energy From the Hive (Nutritional Properties of Bee Pollen, Royal Jelly, Propolis, and Honey)," *Total Health*. October 1991.

Green, James. *The Male Herbal*. Freedom, CA: The Crossing Press, 1991.

Greenwood, D. "Honey for Superficial Wounds and Ulcers," *The Lancet*, January 9, 1993.

Grossman, Richard. *The Other Medicines*. Garden City, NY: Doubleday & Company, 1985.

Guiness, Alma E., Editor. *The Reader's Digest Family Guide to Natural Medicine*. Pleasantville, NY: The Reader's Digest Association, Inc., 1993.

Hamburg, Joan F. "Can Home Remedies Work?" *Parade Magazine*, July 1994.

Harris, B. C. *Ginseng: What It Is ... What It Can Do for You*. New Canaan, CT: Keats Publishing Inc., 1978.

Harris, Lloyd John. *The Official Garlic Lovers Handbook*. Berkley, CA: Aris Books, Harris Publishing Company, 1986.

Hauri, Peter J., Ph.D., and Linde Sherley, M.S., Ph.D. "Can't Sleep? Tired? Tense?" *Redbook*, May 1990.

Hausman, Patricia, and Judith Benn Hurley. *The Healing Foods: The Ultimate Authority on the Curative Power of Nutrition.* Emmaus, PA: Rodale Press, 1989.

Heinerman, John. *The Complete Book of Spices.* CT: Keats Publishing, 1983.

Hendler, Sheldon Saul. *The Doctors' Vitamin and Mineral Encyclopedia.* New York, NY: Simon and Schuster, 1990.

Herbert, Victor, Editor. *The Mount Sinai School of Medicine Complete Book of Nutrition.* New York, NY: Saint Martin's Press, 1990.

Hermann, Matthias. *Herbs and Medicinal Flowers.* New York, NY: Galahad Books, 1973.

Hewitt, James. *Teach Yourself Yoga.* Chicago, IL: NTC Publishing, 1993.

Hobbs, Christopher. "Let Go — Relax Naturally With Valerian and California Poppy," *Delicious!*, March 1992.

"A Honey of a Cure," *The Edell Health Letter*, August 1993.

Hsu, H-Y. *How to Treat Yourself With Chinese Herbs.* Long Beach, CA: Oriental Healing Arts Institute, and New Canaan, CT: Keats Publishing Inc., 1993.

Hurley, Judith Benn. *The Good Herb.* New York, NY: William Morrow and Co., 1995.

Hutchens, Alma R. *Indian Herbology of North America.* Boston, MA: Shambhala, 1991.

Hutt, Judy. "Nature's Pharmacy: Top Five Herbs for Women," *Delicious!*, May/June 1993.

Hylton, William H., and Claire Kowalchik, eds. *Rodale's Illustrated Encyclopedia of Herbs*. Emmaus, PA: Rodale Press, 1987.

Inglis, Brian, and Ruth West. *The Alternative Health Guide*. New York, NY: Alfred A. Knopf, 1983.

Israel, Richard. *The Natural Pharmacy Product Guide*. Garden City Park, NY: Avery Publishing Group, 1991.

Isyengar, B.K.S. *The Tree of Yoga*. Boston, MA: Shambhala Publications, 1988.

Jain, M. K., and R. Apitz-Castro. "Garlic: Molecular Basis of the Putative 'Vampire- Repellant' Action and Other Matters Related to Heart and Blood," *TIBS*, July 1987.

Jaret, Peter. "Foods That Fight Cancer," *Health Magazine*, March/April 1995.

Jensen, Bernard, Ph.D., D.C. "Natural Breast-feeding," *Delicious!*, May/June 1993.

Kaptchuk and Croucer. *The Healing Arts*. New York, NY: Summit Books, 1987.

Kastner, Mark, L.Ac., Dipl.Ac., and Hugh Burroughs. *Alternative Healing*. La Mesa, CA: Halcyon Publishing, 1993.

Kent, Saul. *Your Personal Life Extension Program*. New York, NY: William Morrow and Company, 1985.

Keys, John D. *Chinese Herbs*. Tokyo, Japan: Charles E. Tuttle Company, 1976.

Kingston, Jeremy. *Healing Without Medicine*. London, England: Aldus Books Ltd., 1976.

Kordel, Lelord. *Natural Folk Remedies*. New York, NY: Manor Books, 1976.

Kowalchik, Claire, and William H. Hylton, eds. *Rodale's Illustrated Encyclopedia of Herbs*. Emmaus, PA: Rodale Press, 1987.

Krakovitz, Rob. *High Energy: How to Overcome Fatigue and Maintain Your Peak Vitality*. Los Angeles, CA: Jeremy P. Tarcher, 1986.

Krampf, Leslie. "Choosing a Natural Deoderant," *Delicious!*, July 1994.

Krampf, Leslie. "Ooh! Baby Skin," *Delicious!*, September 1994.

Langer, Stephen. "Garlic: The New Cancer-Fighting Candidate," *Better Nutrition for Today's Living*, June 1991.

Lee, Paul. "Arnica Montana," *Total Health*, 1990.

Lee, William H., and L. Lee. *The Book of Practical Aromatherapy*. New Canaan, CT: Keats Publishing Inc., 1992.

Lee, William H., Ph.D. *Essential Oils That Build Natural Defenses*. 1991.

Leigh, S. "Aromatherapy: Making Good Scents," *Mothering*, Spring 1991.

Lin, Robert I-San. "Protection Against Occlusive Cardiovascular and Circulatory Diseases (Garlic & Health, Part 1)," *Total Health*, February 1993.

Lockie, A., and N. Geddes. *The Woman's Guide to Homeopathy*. New York: St. Martin's Press, 1994.

Lu, Henry C. *Chinese System of Food Cures*. New York, NY: Sterling Publishing Co., Inc., 1986.

Lucas, Richard M. *Herbal Health Secrets From Europe and Around the World*. New York, NY: Parker Publishing Company, 1983.

Lust, John. *The Herb Book*. New York, NY: Bantam Books, Inc., 1974.

Mabey, Richard, ed. *The New Age Herbalist*. New York, NY: Collier Books, Macmillan Publishing Company, 1988.

Maleskey, Gale. "Halting Herpes," *Prevention*, December 1988.

Manniche, Lise. *An Ancient Egyptian Herbal*. Austin, TX: University of Texas Press, 1989.

Marcin, Marietta Marshall. *The Complete Book of Herbal Teas*. New York, NY: Congdon & Weed, 1983.

Marieb, Elaine N. *Human Anatomy and Physiology*. CA: Benjamin Cummings Publishing Co., Inc., 1992.

Mars, Brigitte. "Natural Remedies for Childhood Ailments," *Delicious!*, September 1991.

Mayell, Mark. *Natural Health First Aid Guide*. New York, NY: Pocket Books, 1994.

McCaleb, Rob. "Ginseng: Energy Booster," *Better Nutrition for Today's Living*, January 1992.

McCaleb, Rob. "Ginseng: Mental Booster," *Better Nutrition for Today's Living*, July 1993.

McClure, Vimala. *The Vegetarian Alternative*. Willow Springs, MO: Nucleus Publications.

McIntyre, Anne. *The Complete Woman's Herbal*. New York, NY: Henry Holt, Co., 1995.

McVicar, Nancy. "The Hot New Pain Reliever: Jalapeno Juice," *Sun Sentinel: Lifestyle*, August 1994.

Melton, J. Gordon. *New Age Encyclopedia*. Detroit, MI: Gale Research, 1990.

Meyer, Clarence. *American Folk Medicine*. Glenwood, IL: Meyerbooks Publishing, 1973.

Meyer, Clarence. *Old Ways Rediscovered*. Glenwood, IL: Meyerbooks Publishing, 1988.

Mills, Simon, M.A., and Steven J. Finando, Ph.D. *Alternatives in Healing*. New York, NY: New American Library, 1988.

Ming, Ou, Xu Honghua, Li Yanwen, and Luo Hesheng. *An Illustrated Guide to Antineoplastic Chinese Herbal Medicine*. Hong Kong: The Commercial Press Ltd., 1990.

Mitton, F., and V. Mitton. *Mitton's Practical Modern Herbal*. New York, NY: Arco Publishing, 1984.

Mollen, Art. *Dr. Mollen's Anti-Aging Diet*. New York, NY: Penguin Books, 1992.

Moore, Michael. *Medicinal Plants of the Mountain West*. Santa Fe, NM: Museum of New Mexico Press, 1979.

Morgan, Dr. Brian, L.G. *Nutrition Prescription*. New York, NY: Crown, 1987.

Moser, P. W. "In Cod We Trust," *Hippocrates*, September 1993.

Mowrey, Daniel B. *Herbal Tonic Therapies*. New Canaan, CT: Keats Publishing Inc., 1993.

Mowrey, Daniel B. *The Scientific Validation of Herbal Medicine*. New Canaan, CT: Keats Publishing Inc., 1986.

Murray, Michael T., M.D. *Alternatives to Over-the-Counter and Prescription Drugs.* New York, NY: William Morrow & Co. Inc.,

Null, Gary. *Reverse the Aging Process Naturally.* New York, NY: Villard Books, 1993.

O'Brien, Jim. "Bible Food That Fights Ulcers, Cancer and More," *Your Health*, March 1994.

O'Brien, Jim. "Shiitake: The Healing Power of Mushrooms," *Your Health*, March 1995.

Ody, Penelope. *The Complete Medicinal Herbal.* New York, NY: Dorling Kindersley, 1993.

Olkin, Sylvia Klein. "Women's Health," *East West*, April 1990.

Ornish, Dean, M.D. *Dr. Dean Ornish's Program for Reversing Heart Disease.* New York, NY: Ballantine Books, 1990.

Ornish, Dean, M.D. *Stress, Diet and Your Heart.* New York, NY: Penguin Books, 1982.

Panati, Charles. *Browser's Book of Beginnings.* Boston, MA: Houghton Mifflin Company, 1984.

Panati, Charles. *Extraordinary Origins of Everyday Things.* New York, NY: Harper & Row Publishers,1987.

Pennisi, Elizabeth. "Pharming Frogs: Chemist Finds Precious Alkaloids in Poisonous Amphibians," *Science News*, July 18, 1992.

Peterson, Nicola. *Herbs and Health.* London, England: Webb & Bower, 1989.

Pitcairn, Dr. Richard H., D.V.M., Ph.D., and Susan Hubble Pitcairn. *Dr. Pitcairn's Complete Guide to Natural Health for Dogs and Cats.* Emmaus, PA: Rodale Press, 1982.

Pitchford, Paul. *Healing With Whole Foods.* Berkeley, CA: North Atlantic Books, 1993.

Pratt, Steven. "Love Starved? Pass the Asparagus," *Sun Sentinel: Lifestyle,* February 1995.

Prevention Magazine, Editors of the Health Books. *The Complete Book of Natural and Medicinal Cures.* Emmaus, PA: Rodale Press, 1994.

Rechelbacher, Horst. *Rejuvination: A Wellness Guide for Men and Women.* Rochester, NY: Thorsons Publishers, 1987.

Rinzler, Carol Ann. *The Dictionary of Medical Folklore.* New York, NY: Thomas Y. Crowel, 1979.

Rosenfeld, Isadore, M.D. *Doctor, What Should I Eat?* New York, NY: Random House, 1995.

Santillo, Humbart, M.D. *Natural Healing With Herbs.* Presscott, AZ: Hohm Press, 1984.

Scheer, J. F. "Propolis for Fighting Bacteria," *Better Nutrition for Today's Living,* September 1991.

Scheer, James F., and Maureen Soloman. *Foods That Heal.* Meno Park, CA: Stratford Publications, 1989.

Scher, Stephen K. "Botanicals - Myth and Reality," *Cosmetics and Toiletries,* June 1991.

"Scientists Report Garlic Can Contribute to Cancer Prevention and Treatment," *Cancer Weekly,* June 15, 1992

Sharon, Michael. *Complete Nutrition: How To Live In Total Health.* London, England: Prion Books, 1989.

Smith, Trevor. *A Doctor's Guide to Remedies for Common Ailments.* New York, NY: Thorsons Publishers, Inc., 1982.

Spaulding, C.E., D.V.M. *A Veterinary Guide for Animal Owners.* Emmaus, PA: Rodale Press, 1976.

Spoerke, David G. Jr. *Herbal Medications.* Woodbridge, NJ: Woodbridge Press Publishing, 1980.

Steiner, Richard P. *Folk Medicine: The Art and the Science.* Washington DC: American Chemical Society, 1986.

Stephenson, Joan, Ph.D. *Harvard Health Letter*, July 1993.

Stolzenburg, William. "Garlic Medicine: Cures in Cloves? (Report on First World Congress on the Health Significance of Garlic and Garlic Constituents)," *Science*, September 8, 1990.

Strehlow, Dr. Wighard, and Gottfried Hertzka, M.D. *Hildegard of Bingen's Medicine.* Santa Fe, NM: Bear & Company, 1988.

Subak-Sharpe, Genell J., ed., Morton Bogdonoff, M.D., and Rubin Bressler, M.D., medical eds. *The Physicians' Manual for Patients.* New York, NY: Times Books, 1984.

"Summer Harvest," *Weight Watchers Magazine*, August 1992.

"Sweet and Sour Shiitake Salad," *Shiitake News*, March 1993.

Tang, Stephen, and Martin Palmer. *Chinese Herbal Prescriptions.* London, England: Rider and Company, 1987.

Taub, Edward A. *The Wellness Rx.* Edgewood Cliffs, NJ: Prentice Hall, 1994.

Tenney, Louise. *Health Handbook*. Pleasant Grove, UT: Woodland Books.

Tenney, Louise. *Today's Herbal Health*, 3rd Edition. Provo, UT: Woodland Books, 1992.

Theiss, Barbara and Peter. *The Family Herbal*. Healing Arts Press, 1989.

Thompson, Robert. *The Grosset Encyclopedia of Natural Medicine*. New York, NY: Grosset & Dunlap Publishers, 1990.

Tierra, Lesley, L. A.C., Herbalist. *The Herbs of Life*. Freedom, CA: The Crossing Press, 1992.

Tierra, Michael C.A., N.D. *The Way of Herbs*. New York, NY: Pocket Books/ Simon & Schuster, 1990.

Trac, Debora, Editor. *The Doctor's Book of Home Remedies*. Emmaus, PA: Rodale Press, 1980.

Trubo, Richard. "Healthy Teeth for Life," *Woman's World*, April 1995.

Tyler, Varro. *The Honest Herbal*. New York: Pharmacal Press, 1993.

University of California, Berkeley, eds. *The Wellness Encyclopedia*. New York, NY: Houghton Mifflin Co.

Vogel, H.C.A. *The Nature Doctor: A Manual of Traditional and Complementary Medicine*. New Canaan, CT: Keats Publishing Inc., 1991.

Vukovic, Laurel. "Home Remedies," *Natural Health*, November/December 1994.

Wade, C. *Bee Pollen and Your Health*. New Canaan, CT: Keats Publishing Inc., 1978.

Watson, Cynthia, M.D. "Eat, Drink and Make Love," *Mademoiselle*, May 1993.

Weil, Andrew. *Natural Health, Natural Medicine*. Boston, MA: Houghton Mifflin, Co., 1990.

Weiner, Michael A. *Herbs That Heal: Rx For Herbal Healing*. Mill Valley, CA: Quantum Books, 1994.

Weiner, Michael, Ph.D. *Weiner's Herbal: The Guide to Herb Medicine*. Mill Valley, CA: Quantum Books, 1990.

Weiss, Gaea, and Shandor Weiss. *Growing and Using Healing Herbs*. Emmaus, PA: Rodale Press, 1985.

Wilen, Joan, and Lydia Wilen. *Live and Be Well*. New York, NY: Harper Collins, 1992.

Wilen, Joan, and Lydia Wilen. *More Chicken Soup and Other Folk Remedies*. New York, NY: Fawcett Columbine, 1986.

Willix, Robert D., M.D., FACM. *Health & Longevity*, Baltimore, MD: January 1994; February 1994; April 1994; June 1994; July 1994; September 1994; October 1994; November 1994; December 1994; March 1995; April 1995.

Wilson, Roberta. "Tips on Natural Deodorants," *Delicious!*, March 1993.

Wolff, Michael, with Peter Rutten, Albert F. Bayers III, and the World Bank Research Team. *Where We Stand*. New York, NY: Bantam Books, 1992.

Wood, Cedric Stephen, P.E., ed. *Cracker Cures*. Fort Ogden, FL: Peace River Historical Society, 1976.

Woodier, Olwen. "Quick! The Plant That Heals," *Woman's Day*, May 1988.

Zhao, Zhang Da. *Keeping in Good Health and Beauty*. Hong Kong: Hai Feng Publishing Co., 1992.

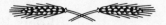

INDEX

B

Bach system 16, 475
Backache 127 - 132
    exercises 128 - 129
Bad breath 133 - 136
Baking soda 125, 142, 387, 413, 487
Baldness 137 - 138
Banana 34, 196, 276, 279, 301, 391,
    413, 448, 459, 463, 506
Barley 196, 296, 305, 345, 383, 495
Barrenwort 315
Basil 191, 435, 459
Bay 464
Bayberry 253, 451
Beans 31, 48, 160
Bedwetting 320
Bee propolis 367
Bergamot oil 489
Beta-carotene 440
Betel nuts 253
Betony 213
Bilberry 499
Bioflavonoids 99
Birch bark 127, 283, 451
Bitter gourd 499
Bitterroot 224
Black beans 127
Blackberry leaf 229, 253, 291, 363,
    455
Black cohosh 363, 418
Black currant 93, 203, 383, 431, 500
Black strap molasses 112, 296, 417,
    497
Black walnut shell 276

Blisters 139 - 140
Blueberry 20, 224, 230, 495
Body odor 141 - 142
Boils 143 - 144
Borage 173, 219, 239, 247, 254,
    415, 467
Boron 247
Bran 47, 196, 402, 447
Breast feeding 414 - 415
Brewer's yeast 38, 201, 401
Broccoli 31, 43, 160
Bromelain 363
Bronchitis 145 - 148
Broth 232
Bruises 149 - 152
Brussels sprouts 32, 44, 161
Bulgur 512
Burdock 137, 149, 154, 161, 207,
    239, 411
Burnet 167
Burns 153 - 156
Buttermilk 375, 445, 448, 449

C

Cabbage 43, 139, 196, 204, 243,
    349, 464
Caffeine 18, 110, 221, 247, 358, 422
Calcium 171, 296, 306, 321, 331,
    337, 356, 363, 368, 379, 421
Calendula 177, 213, 227, 243, 359,
    391, 418, 443, 477, 498
Calluses 201
Camphor 375

H

M

N

Vitamin E 53, 126, 155, 168, 179,
    267, 359, 365, 386, 417, 419,
    424, 436, 507
Vomiting 503 - 504

W

Walnuts 199, 346
Warts 505 - 508
Water 92, 10l, 172, 199, 234, 346,
    350, 359, 441, 443, 453, 479,
    517
Watercress 226, 241
Weight control 509 - 514
    exercises 510
Wheat bran 335
Wheat germ 359, 386
Wheat germ oil 268, 446
Wheat grass 166
Whey 490
Whipped cream 448
Wild yam 339, 357, 365
Willow bark 115
Wine concentrate 179
Wintergreen 115, 485
Witch hazel 141, 150, 246, 268,
    277, 302, 329, 381, 393,
    443, 465
Wood betony 475
Wormwood 465

Y

Yams 425
Yarrow 256, 277, 308, 393, 418,
    485, 498, 517
Yeast infections 515 - 520
Yerba mate 97, 252, 287, 335
Yoga 6 - 10, 26, 73, 115, 472
    breathing 73
    positions 8-10, 472
Yogurt 23, 35, 46, 97, 185, 218,
    231, 232, 294, 358, 400, 443,
    448, 479, 520
Yucca 218, 434

Z

Zinc 54, 92, 174, 179, 228, 335,
    354, 401, 416, 441, 520

ABOUT THE EDITORS

GLENN W. GEELHOED, M.D.

Glenn W. Geelhoed received his M.D. degree cum laude from the University of Michigan. Following his surgical internship at Harvard, he served at the National Cancer Institute. After completing his surgical residency, he joined the faculty at George Washington University in 1975. He was appointed clinical scholar of the Robert Wood Johnson Foundation. He is a member of the Society of University Surgeons and The American College of Surgeons, and is a past president of the Washington Academy of Surgeons. He was selected the James IV Traveling Scholar of 1986, and inducted into the Academie de Chirurgie de Paris in 1990.

Dr. Geelhoed has been a frequent visiting professor in most of the United States and on all continents. He is a widely published author accredited with several books and over 350 published journal articles. Because of his strong interest in global health, he completed a Doctorate in Tropical Medicine and Hygiene at the University of London School of Hygiene and Tropical Medicine in 1990, and a Master's degree in International Affairs from the Elliott School of International Affairs at George Washington University in 1991. Currently, as George Washington University Professor of International Medical Education, he is developing and directing an international health center.

In 1996, Dr. Geelhoed was appointed Senior Fulbright Scholar to Africa.

JEAN BARILLA, M.S.

Jean Barilla is a medical writer, biomedical researcher, lecturer, and health consultant. She received her Master's degree in Biology from New York University and completed two years of medical school as part of a graduate program in biochemistry at the University of South Alabama College of Medicine. Ms. Barilla has been a biologist for the U.S. Food and Drug Administration and a lecturer in Biology at the City University of New York.

Ms. Barilla's publications have appeared in medical journals, medical-legal textbooks, magazines, and newspapers. She is a member of the American Medical Writers Association. She currently lives in Connecticut and writes and edits educational materials for physicians, healthcare personnel, and the general public.